Perioperative Management

Editor

PAUL J. SCHENARTS

SURGICAL CLINICS OF NORTH AMERICA

www.surgical.theclinics.com

Consulting Editor
RONALD F. MARTIN

April 2015 • Volume 95 • Number 2

ELSEVIER

1600 John F. Kennedy Boulevard • Suite 1800 • Philadelphia, Pennsylvania, 19103-2899

http://www.surgical.theclinics.com

SURGICAL CLINICS OF NORTH AMERICA Volume 95, Number 2
April 2015 ISSN 0039–6109, ISBN-13: 978-0-323-35986-3

Editor: John Vassallo, j.vassallo@elsevier.com
Developmental Editor: Colleen Viola

Surgical Clinics of North America (ISSN 0039–6109) is published bimonthly by Elsevier Inc., 360 Park Avenue South, New York, NY 10010-1710. Months of publication are February, April, June, August, October, and December. Business and Editorial Offices: 1600 John F. Kennedy Blvd., Suite 1800, Philadelphia, PA 19103-2899. Periodicals postage paid at New York, NY and additional mailing offices. Subscription prices are $370.00 per year for US individuals, $627.00 per year for US institutions, $180.00 per year for US students and residents, $455.00 per year for Canadian individuals, $793.00 per year for Canadian institutions, $510.00 for international individuals, $793.00 per year for international institutions and $250.00 per year for Canadian and foreign students/residents. To receive student/resident rate, orders must be accompanied by name of affiliated institution, date of term, and the *signature* of program/residency coordinator on institution letterhead. Orders will be billed at individual rate until proof of status is received. Foreign air speed delivery is included in all *Clinics* subscription prices. All prices are subject to change without notice. POSTMASTER: Send address changes to *Surgical Clinics*, Elsevier Health Sciences Division, Subscription Customer Service, 3251 Riverport Lane, Maryland Heights, MO 63043. **Customer Service (orders, claims, online, change of address): Telephone: 1-800-654-2452 (U.S. and Canada); 314-447-8871 (outside U.S. and Canada). Fax: 314-447-8029. E-mail: journalscustomerservice-usa@elsevier.com (for print support); journalsonline support-usa@elsevier.com (for online support)**.

Reprints. For copies of 100 or more, of articles in this publication, please contact the Commercial Reprints Department, Elsevier Inc., 360 Park Avenue South, New York, New York 10010-1710. Tel. 212-633-3874, Fax: 212-633-3820, E-mail: reprints@elsevier.com.

The Surgical Clinics of North America is also published in Spanish by McGraw-Hill Interamericana Editores S.A., P.O. Box 5-237 06500 Mexico D.F. Mexico; and in Portuguese by Interlivros Edicoes Ltda., Rua Comandante Coelho 1085, CEP 21250, Rio de Janeiro, Brazil; and in Greek by Paschalidis Medical Publications, Athens Greece.

The Surgical Clinics of North America is covered in *MEDLINE/PubMed (Index Medicus), EMBASE/Excerpta Medica, Current Contents/Clinical Medicine, Current Contents/Life Sciences, Science Citation Index*, and *ISI/BIOMED*.

Contributors

CONSULTING EDITOR

RONALD F. MARTIN, MD
Staff Surgeon, Department of Surgery, Marshfield Clinic, Marshfield, Wisconsin; Clinical Associate Professor, University of Wisconsin School of Medicine and Public Health, Madison, Wisconsin; Colonel (ret.), Medical Corps, United States Army Reserve

EDITOR

PAUL J. SCHENARTS, MD, FACS
Professor and Vice Chairman for Academic Affairs, Chief of Trauma, Surgical Critical Care and Emergency Surgery, Department of Surgery, College of Medicine, University of Nebraska Medical Center, Omaha, Nebraska

AUTHORS

MARCUS BALTERS, MD
Assistant Professor, Department of Surgery, Creighton University, Omaha, Nebraska

CHRISTOPHER P. BRANDT, MD
Chair, Department of Surgery, MetroHealth Medical Center, Professor of Surgery, Case Western Reserve University, Cleveland, Ohio

KEELY L. BUESING, MD
Assistant Professor, Division of Trauma & Surgical Critical Care, Department of General Surgery, University of Nebraska Medical Center, Omaha, Nebraska

RAMON F. CESTERO, MD, FACS
Division of Trauma and Emergency Surgery, Assistant Professor, Department of Surgery, UT Health Science Center San Antonio, San Antonio, Texas

STEPHEN W. DAVIES, MD
Department of Surgery, University of Virginia, School of Medicine, Charlottesville, Virginia

ZACHARY DeBOARD, MD
Senior Resident, Surgical Education Department, Santa Barbara Cottage Hospital, Santa Barbara, California

DAVID DENNING, MD, FACS
Department of Surgery, Marshall University Joan C. Edwards School of Medicine, Huntington, West Virginia

DANIEL L. DENT, MD, FACS
Division of Trauma and Emergency Surgery, Department of Surgery, UT Health Science Center San Antonio, San Antonio, Texas

WADE G. DOUGLAS, MD, FACS
Department of Clinical Sciences, Florida State University College of Medicine, Tallahassee, Florida

CHARITY H. EVANS, MD, MHCM
Department of Surgery, University of Nebraska Medical Center, Omaha, Nebraska

KRISTIN A. FLOWERS, MD
Department of General Surgery, University of Nebraska Medical Center, Omaha, Nebraska

JEFFREY M. GAUVIN, MD, MS, FACS
Director of Surgical Education, Surgical Education Department, Santa Barbara Cottage Hospital, Santa Barbara, California

MATTHEW GOEDE, MD
Assistant Professor, Department of Surgery, College of Medicine, University of Nebraska, Omaha, Nebraska

JOHN M. GREEN, MD, FACS
Associate Professor and Program Director, Department of Surgery, Carolinas Medical Center, Charlotte, North Carolina

MEGHAN E. HALUB, MD
Department of Surgical Education, Iowa Methodist Medical Center, Des Moines, Iowa

JASON ISA, MD
The Queen's Medical Center, University of Hawaii, Honolulu, Hawaii

JASON M. JOHANNING, MD, FACS
Professor, Department of Surgery, University of Nebraska Medical Center, Omaha, Nebraska

JANE LEE, MD, PhD
Department of Surgery, University of Nebraska Medical Center, Omaha, Nebraska

KENJI L. LEONARD, MD
Department of Surgery, The Brody School of Medicine, East Carolina University, Greenville, North Carolina

JESSICA LOVICH-SAPOLA, MD, MBA
Associate Program Director, Anesthesia Residency, MetroHealth Medical Center, Assistant Professor, Case Western Reserve University, Cleveland, Ohio

ALYSON A. MELIN, DO
General Surgery Resident, Department of Surgery, University of Nebraska Medical Center, Omaha, Nebraska

SHARON MORAN, MD, FACS
The Queen's Medical Center, University of Hawaii, Honolulu, Hawaii

BARGHAVA MULLAPUDI, MD
Department of General Surgery, University of Nebraska Medical Center, Omaha, Nebraska

PETER A. NAJJAR, MD
Resident, Department of Surgery; Fellow, Patient Safety and Quality, Center for Clinical Excellence, Brigham and Women's Hospital, Harvard Medical School, Boston, Massachusetts

MELISSA K. RUHLMAN, MD
Department of Surgery, University of Nebraska Medical Center, Omaha, Nebraska

PAUL J. SCHENARTS, MD, FACS
Professor and Vice Chairman for Academic Affairs, Chief of Trauma, Surgical Critical Care and Emergency Surgery, Department of Surgery, College of Medicine, University of Nebraska Medical Center, Omaha, Nebraska

LISA L. SCHLITZKUS, MD
Assistant Professor, Department of Surgery, University of Nebraska Medical Center, Omaha, Nebraska

RICHARD A. SIDWELL, MD
Program Director, General Surgery Residency, Iowa Methodist Medical Center, Des Moines, Iowa; Adjunct Clinical Professor, Department of Surgery, University of Iowa Carver College of Medicine, Iowa City, Iowa

DOUGLAS S. SMINK, MD, MPH
Program Director, General Surgery Residency; Vice Chair for Education, Department of Surgery, Brigham and Women's Hospital, Harvard Medical School, Boston, Massachusetts

CHARLES E. SMITH, MD
Director, Cardiothoracic and Trauma Anesthesia, MetroHealth Medical Center, Professor of Anesthesia, Case Western Reserve University, Cleveland, Ohio

SUSAN STEINEMANN, MD, FACS
The Queen's Medical Center, University of Hawaii, Honolulu, Hawaii

MELISSA K. STEWART, MD
Resident, General Surgery; Fellow, Anesthesia Critical Care, Vanderbilt University Medical Center, Nashville, Tennessee

AMBER TAYLOR, MD
Chief Resident, Surgical Education Department, Santa Barbara Cottage Hospital, Santa Barbara, California

KYLA P. TERHUNE, MD
Associate Professor, Department of Surgery, Vanderbilt University Medical Center, Nashville, Tennessee

ZACHARY TORGERSEN, MD
Department of Surgery, Creighton University, Omaha, Nebraska

EKONG UFFORT, MD
Department of Surgery, Marshall University Joan C. Edwards School of Medicine, Huntington, West Virginia

BRETT H. WAIBEL, MD, FACS
Assistant Professor, Division of Trauma and Acute Care Surgery, Department of Surgery, The Brody School of Medicine, East Carolina University, Greenville, North Carolina

MATTHEW WHEELER, MD
Department of Surgery, College of Medicine, University of Nebraska, Omaha, Nebraska

Contents

Foreword: Perioperative Management xiii

Ronald F. Martin

Preface: Perioperative Management xv

Paul J. Schenarts

Cardiac Risk Stratification and Protection 217

Meghan E. Halub and Richard A. Sidwell

The goal of preoperative cardiac evaluation is to screen for undiagnosed cardiac disease or to find evidence of known conditions that are poorly controlled to allow management that reduces the risk of perioperative cardiac complications. A careful history and physical examination combined with the procedure-specific risk is the cornerstone of this assessment. This article reviews a brief history of prior cardiac risk stratification indexes, explores current practice guidelines by the American College of Cardiology and the American Heart Association Task Force, reviews current methods for preoperative evaluation, discusses revascularization options, and evaluates perioperative medication recommendations.

Prevention of Postoperative Pulmonary Complications 237

Amber Taylor, Zachary DeBoard, and Jeffrey M. Gauvin

Postoperative pulmonary complications (PPCs) occur frequently among general surgical patients. The spectrum of illness is broad and includes preventable causes of morbidity and death. Careful preoperative evaluation can identify undiagnosed and undertreated illness and allow for preoperative intervention. Optimization of patient, surgical, and anesthetic factors is crucial in the prevention of PPCs.

Perioperative Nutrition 255

Zachary Torgersen and Marcus Balters

Perioperative nutrition is a vitally important yet often overlooked aspect of surgical care. Significant disparity exists between evidence-based recommendations and practices encouraged by traditional surgical teaching. The metabolic response to surgical stress is complex. Poor nutrition has been demonstrated to correlate with adverse surgical outcomes. Perioperative nutrition encompasses preoperative, intraoperative, and postoperative care. Preoperative nutritional assessment identifies at-risk patients who benefit from supplementation before surgery. Prehabilitation seeks to prepare patients for the impending surgical stress. Immunonutrition seems to provide a benefit, although its precise mechanisms are unknown. This article provides a review of the current state of perioperative nutrition.

levels and metabolic acidosis. This review discusses the major endpoints of resuscitation in clinical use.

Optimal Glucose Management in the Perioperative Period 337

Charity H. Evans, Jane Lee, and Melissa K. Ruhlman

Hyperglycemia is a common finding in surgical patients during the perioperative period. Factors contributing to poor glycemic control include counterregulatory hormones, hepatic insulin resistance, decreased insulin-stimulated glucose uptake, use of dextrose-containing intravenous fluids, and enteral and parenteral nutrition. Hyperglycemia in the perioperative period is associated with increased morbidity, decreased survival, and increased resource utilization. Optimal glucose management in the perioperative period contributes to reduced morbidity and mortality. To readily identify hyperglycemia, blood glucose monitoring should be instituted for all hospitalized patients.

Essentials of Sepsis Management 355

John M. Green

Despite remarkable advances in the knowledge of infection and human response to it, sepsis continues to be one of the most common challenges surgeons and critical care providers face. Surgeons confront the problem of infection every day, in treating established infections or reacting to a consequence of surgical intervention. Infections after surgery continue to be a problem despite massive efforts to prevent them. Patients rely on the surgeon's ability to recognize infection and treat it. Also, preventing nosocomial infection and antibiotic resistance is a primary responsibility. This article describes diagnostic and therapeutic measures for sepsis in the perioperative surgical patient.

Transfusion and Management of Surgical Patients with Hematologic Disorders 367

Wade G. Douglas, Ekong Uffort, and David Denning

Clinical trials have provided guidance in developing triggers for transfusing in the hemodynamically stable patient. These studies have identified that improved outcomes can be obtained in the massively transfused patient when platelets and fresh frozen plasma are transfused with packed red blood cells. Studies that characterize the complications of transfusions, such as transfusion-related acute lung injury and poor cancer-related outcomes, are discussed. Emerging data that characterize the risk factors associated with transfusion-related acute lung injury and suggest metastasis and local recurrence occur at a higher rate in the transfused patient are discussed. Hematologic disorders commonly encountered by surgeons are discussed.

Perioperative Management of Obese Patients 379

Kenji L. Leonard, Stephen W. Davies, and Brett H. Waibel

Obesity prevalence has quadrupled since the 1980s in the United States. It is estimated that 30% of the population is obese or has a body mass index of greater than or equal to 30 as defined by the World Health Organization.

Surgeons are likely to engage in the care of obese patients and need to be adept in every aspect of the patients' care in order to have a successful hospital course. There is significant controversy in perioperative management of obese patients. This article discusses perioperative management of obese patients to provide guidelines, education, and discussion of current issues.

Perioperative Management of Elderly Patients **391**

Lisa L. Schlitzkus, Alyson A. Melin, Jason M. Johanning, and Paul J. Schenarts

The older population only represents 13.7% of the US population but has grown by 21% since 2002. The centenarian population is growing at a faster rate than the total US population. This unprecedented growth has significantly increased surgical demand. The establishment of quality and performance improvement data has allowed researchers to focus attention on the older patient population, resulting in an exponential increase in studies. Although there is still much work to be done in this field, overlying themes regarding the perioperative management of elderly patients are presented in this article based on a thorough literature review.

Perioperative Management in the Patient with Substance Abuse **417**

Sharon Moran, Jason Isa, and Susan Steinemann

Drug and alcohol use is a pervasive problem in the general population and in those requiring anesthesia for an operation. History and screening can help delineate those who may be acutely intoxicated or chronic drug and alcohol users. Both acute intoxication and chronic abuse of these substances present challenges for anesthetic management during and after an operation. The clinician should be aware of problems that may be encountered during any part of anesthesia or postoperative care.

Management of Pregnant Patients Undergoing General Surgical Procedures **429**

Melissa K. Stewart and Kyla P. Terhune

Pregnant patients have a 0.2% to 0.75% chance of developing a medical condition that requires a general surgical intervention during pregnancy. To safely and appropriately care for patients, surgeons must be cognizant of the maternal physiologic changes in pregnancy as well as of the unique risk to both mothers and fetuses of diagnostic modalities, anesthetic care, operative intervention, and postoperative management. Surgeons can be assured that, if these risks are understood and considered, operating during pregnancy, even in the abdomen, can be safely undertaken.

Advance Directives, Living Wills, and Futility in Perioperative Care **443**

Matthew Goede and Matthew Wheeler

Patient autonomy is preserved through the use of advance directives. A living will defines treatment by establishing parameters under which patients want to be treated. A durable power of attorney for health care establishes a surrogate for patients if they are unable to make decisions

for themselves. In the perioperative setting, advance directives are applied with significant variation between surgeons, likely due to surgeons implying from informed consent discussions that patients want to pursue aggressive treatment. Futility is a rare occurrence in patient care that is difficult to define; however, there are some classic surgical conditions in which futility is part of the decision process.

SURGICAL CLINICS OF NORTH AMERICA

FORTHCOMING ISSUES

June 2015
Surgical Approaches to Esophageal Disease
Dmitry Oleynikov, *Editor*

August 2015
Simulation in Surgical Training and Practice
Kimberly M. Brown and John T. Paige, *Editors*

October 2015
Cancer Screening and Genetics
Christopher L. Wolfgang, *Editor*

RECENT ISSUES

February 2015
Caring for the Geriatric Surgical Patient
Fred A. Luchette, *Editor*

December 2014
Surgical Infections
Robert G. Sawyer and Traci L. Hedrick, *Editors*

October 2014
Melanoma
Kimberly M. Brown and Celia Chao, *Editors*

August 2014
Management of Burns
Robert L. Sheridan, *Editor*

ISSUE OF RELATED INTEREST

Primary Care: Clinics in Office Practice
June 2014 (Vol. 41, Issue 2)
Screening and Prevention in Primary Care
Mack T. Ruffin and Cameron G. Shultz, *Editors*
Available at: www.primarycare.theclinics.com

Foreword
Perioperative Management

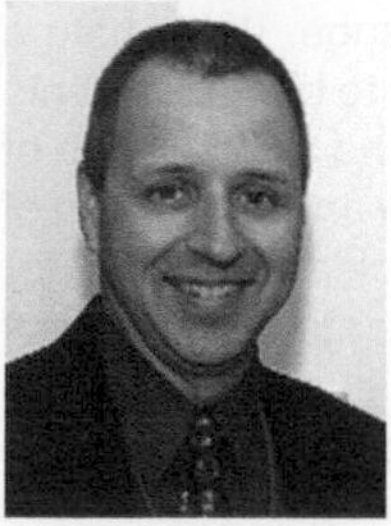

Ronald F. Martin, MD
Consulting Editor

Surgery is a way of life, a state of mind, a discipline, occasionally a passion—it is not specifically an operation. Operations are procedures that surgeons perform in operating rooms as part of their craft. I have written this before, and I will most likely write it again. Over the years, some people, not the least of whom include those who edit the *Oxford English Dictionary*, have stated that the word "surgery" can be used synonymously with "operation." I would submit that even if the master wordsmiths are okay with this, we as surgeons should not be. The term "Surgery" should be all encompassing. After all, your average dictionary editor will rarely, if ever, be asked to take someone to the operating room, but you will.

The distinction is important because it reaffirms the need to consider all the things that happen prior to going to the operating room and all the things that will happen after we leave the OR. For the majority of patients undergoing operations in the inpatient setting, a much larger fraction of time will be spent in the hospital outside of an operating room than in one. Conversely, since the era of same-day admission, nearly all clinical decision-making and patient preparation are not only done outside of the OR but also are done outside of the hospital, either in the office setting or at the patient's home.

At the institution for which I work, I have the responsibility of moderating the weekly morbidity and mortality conference. We try to keep the discussions organized to identify decision points and see where we might have made better decisions with the benefit of hindsight; occasionally we succeed. One clear trend that emerges, though, is that the majority of possibly preventable complications we see are the results of error chains that started well before the operation commenced. We have our share of complications that occur in the postoperative period as well, but even those postoperative complications frequently stem back to some nonaddressed, or incompletely addressed, problem that was or should have been known preoperatively. A distinct minority of the complications we see stem from the actual operation itself.

Surg Clin N Am 95 (2015) xiii–xiv
http://dx.doi.org/10.1016/j.suc.2015.02.002
0039-6109/15/$ – see front matter

How things get missed in either detection or action is a complex problem. In our organization, as well as many others, there is an increasing fractionation of responsibility for perioperative care. Patients get "cleared for surgery" by internists, cardiologists, and others. Postoperative patients are "medically managed" by hospitalists. Even within our own specialty, we see patients operated on by people who were not involved in the initial evaluation because there was a shift change. While I am a true believer that team care is here to stay and on the whole is likely to benefit patients if used properly, there is a huge difference in coordination of care and fractionation of care just as there is a difference between delegation of responsibility and abdication of responsibility. I still maintain that only the operating surgeon can "clear" a patient for an operation. Surgeons have long prided themselves on their breadth and depth of knowledge. At the level of our board certification, we expect that successful candidates for board certification will demonstrate sufficient knowledge of preoperative and postoperative care as well as operative and procedural knowledge.

When I was first in residency training, my chairman informed me that, "a surgeon is an internist who has completed his training." I don't recommend you share that particular line in today's world, especially at a medical staff gathering, for instance. However, political incorrectness aside, the sentiment that becoming a surgeon doesn't preclude one from being a doctor is still good advice. Keeping track of those aspects of care that our nonoperative colleagues may focus on is a good idea on many levels if for no other reason than it lets us communicate more efficiently and effectively with our colleagues when collaboration is required.

Dr Schenarts, who, parenthetically, trained in the same crucible as I, along with his colleagues, have done an excellent job of collecting current and useful information about the preoperative and postoperative care of patients. Perhaps most importantly, they provided us with easy to understand and useful information about best current practices to minimize preventable errors. Also, there is an excellent article about advanced directives, living wills, and futility that I highly commend to you as it addresses issues that always seem to confound people where I work.

Both internal and external pressures on our practices will necessitate the adoption of team-based care and shared responsibility. That will limit surgeon autonomy to some degree and that may not be a bad thing. This, however, will not limit the need for us surgeons to be leaders of these team efforts as it will most likely benefit our patients as well as ourselves. To lead effectively, we will need to be well versed in our understanding of all matters of patient care. This issue of the *Surgical Clinics of North America* should give you an excellent platform to update and increase your level of knowledge on perioperative care.

Ronald F. Martin, MD
Department of Surgery
Marshfield Clinic
1000 North Oak Avenue
Marshfield, WI 54449, USA

E-mail address:
Martin.ronald@marshfieldclinic.org

Preface
Perioperative Management

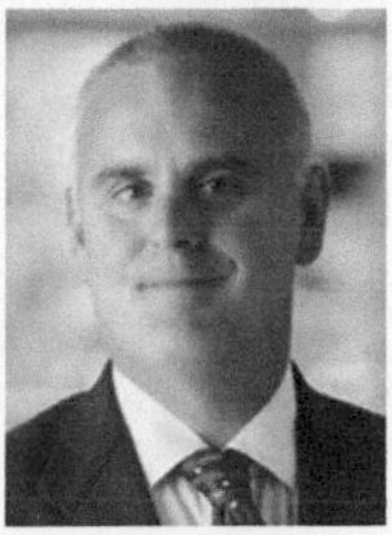

Paul J. Schenarts, MD, FACS
Editor

I recall a discussion as an intern about perioperative care with my then chief resident who said, "If you take care of the small things, the big things take care of themselves." That chief resident, Ronald Martin, MD, FACS, is now the Consulting Editor of *Surgical Clinics of North America.* I seriously doubt he knew he was quoting the poet Emily Elizabeth Dickinson, but, when faced with a complex clinical situation, I frequently reflect on the wisdom of Ron's statement and continue to apply this philosophy to every aspect of my practice. When asked to serve as editor for an issue on perioperative management, I knew immediately that this philosophy would guide the approach.

The modern surgical patient is often of advanced age, takes multiple medications, and has multiple associated medical problems which would have led to their demise in earlier years. At no point in history has the need for a detail-oriented and careful approach to perioperative care been more important.

In this issue of *Surgical Clinics of North America*, teams of authors from across the United States, from both university-based and non-university-based practices, have come together to produce an issue that provides both a comprehensive review and pragmatically useful guidance. It is hoped that the information contained within this issue will be of value to practicing surgeons and surgical trainees, but also to nonsurgeons, who frequently collaborate in the care of our patients. It has been a true honor to work with each of my fellow authors. I thank them for their time, efforts, and steadfast commitment to putting out an excellent issue. I would also like to thank the editorial staff at Elsevier for their assistance, and at times, great patience. Finally, I would like

Surg Clin N Am 95 (2015) xv–xvi
http://dx.doi.org/10.1016/j.suc.2015.02.001

to thank my former chief resident for his confidence in me by asking me to serve as an editor. This has truly been a highpoint in my academic career.

Paul J. Schenarts, MD, FACS
Surgical Critical Care & Emergency Surgery
Department of Surgery
University of Nebraska
College of Medicine
983280 Nebraska Medical Center
Omaha, NE 68198-3280, USA

E-mail address:
paul.schenarts@unmc.edu

Cardiac Risk Stratification and Protection

Meghan E. Halub, MD[a], Richard A. Sidwell, MD[b,c,*]

KEYWORDS

- Cardiac evaluation • Preoperative evaluation • Cardiac risk assessment

KEY POINTS

- Preoperative history and physical examination should be directed at assessment of known cardiac conditions (ischemic heart disease, heart failure), comorbidities that increase the chance of perioperative cardiac complications (diabetes requiring insulin, renal insufficiency, cerebrovascular disease), and patient functional status.
- Guidelines for perioperative cardiovascular evaluation are continuously updated by the American College of Cardiology and the American Heart Association and provide an algorithmic approach to this evaluation.
- Guidelines for the use of beta-blockers and statins in the perioperative period are in evolution.

INTRODUCTION

Cardiac risk assessment is important in the preoperative evaluation of surgical patients. The heart, although seemingly simple in its 4-chamber design, must be thoroughly evaluated before surgery because of the significant risks that can be incurred. It is estimated that cardiovascular complications cause half of all morbidity and mortality experienced in the perioperative period for patients undergoing noncardiac surgery, with even higher rates among vascular patients.[1]

Cardiovascular disease is the leading cause of death in the United States. Thus, it is no surprise that it is a significant contributing factor to perioperative morbidity and mortality.[2,3] The population of persons aged 65 years and older is estimated to increase 25% to 35% in the next 30 years, and this is the age group in which the largest number of operations is performed.[4] It is also estimated that the number of surgical

The authors have nothing to disclose.
[a] Department of Surgical Education, Iowa Methodist Medical Center, 1415 Woodland Avenue, Suite 140, Des Moines, IA 50309, USA; [b] General Surgery Residency, Iowa Methodist Medical Center, 1415 Woodland Avenue, Suite 140, Des Moines, IA 50309, USA; [c] Department of Surgery, University of Iowa Carver College of Medicine, Iowa City, IA, USA
* Corresponding author. General Surgery Residency, 1415 Woodland Avenue, Suite 140, Des Moines, IA 50309.
E-mail address: richard.sidwell@unitypoint.org

Surg Clin N Am 95 (2015) 217–235
http://dx.doi.org/10.1016/j.suc.2014.11.007
surgical.theclinics.com
0039-6109/15/$ – see front matter

procedures in this age group will increase from 6 million to 12 million over the next 30 years.[4]

Every year, approximately 27 million patients undergo a noncardiac operation in the United States; 8 million, or 30%, have significant underlying coronary artery disease (CAD) or other cardiac conditions at the time of their procedure.[1,3,5] Of people undergoing noncardiac surgery, 1 million, or 3%, of these patients will experience perioperative cardiac complications.[3,6] The mortality after perioperative myocardial infarction (MI) has been quoted to be as high has 40% to 50% and tends to occur on postoperative day 3.[5]

Because of the risk of a cardiac event, emphasis must be placed on the preoperative cardiac evaluation. The goal of the preoperative evaluation is to screen broadly for undiagnosed disease or to find evidence of known conditions that are poorly controlled. The preoperative evaluation also helps determine if an additional cardiac work-up is necessary for patients. It also helps define realistic risks and goals for the forthcoming procedure, involves additional care teams, and helps determine whether the procedure is a realistic option. There are some cases when canceling an operation is necessary so that an underlying cardiac problem can be evaluated and managed to improve the safety of patients.[7]

Operations with major extracellular shift causing hemodynamic stress, prolonged operative times, or extensive anatomic dissections or that are performed on an urgent or emergent basis place patients at the highest risk for a cardiac event (**Table 1**).[2,4,5] Patients can be placed into low-, intermediate-, or high-risk groups, with cardiac event rates being 1% or less, 1% to 5%, or 5% or more, respectively. Patients need to be medically optimized in the preoperative period, if possible.[8] Some patients may never

Table 1
Cardiac risk stratification for noncardiac surgical procedures

Risk[a,b]	Example
High (≥5% cardiac risk)	Emergent major operations, particularly elderly Aortic or major vascular surgery Peripheral vascular surgery Upper abdominal
Intermediate (1%–5% cardiac risk)	Intraperitoneal and intrathoracic surgery Carotid endarterectomy Head and neck surgery Gynecologic surgery Neurosurgery Orthopedic surgery Urologic surgery
Low (≤1% cardiac risk)	Endoscopic procedures Superficial procedures Cataract surgery Breast surgery Ambulatory surgery

[a] Cardiac events include fatal and nonfatal cardiac events.
[b] This table incorporates perioperative cardiovascular events within 30 days after surgery.[12]

Adapted from Fleisher LA, Beckman JA, Brown KA, et al. 2009 ACCF/AHA focused update on perioperative beta blockade incorporated into the ACC/AHA 2007 guidelines on perioperative cardiovascular evaluation and care for noncardiac surgery: a report of the American College of Cardiology Foundation/American Heart Association task force on practice guidelines. Circulation 2009;120:169–276; and Mukherjee D, Eagle KA. Perioperative cardiac assessment for noncardiac surgery: eight steps to the best possible outcome. Circulation 2003;107:2771–74.

be medically stable enough for such surgery, and the discussion of the benefits versus the risks of surgery must be explored.

Overall, the goal of any operation is to perform a procedure that will improve the patient's life. The objective of the perioperative evaluation is to find patients who are best suited for the procedure and will have the best outcome by minimizing morbidity and mortality. All patients require a history and physical examination, and this may be the only necessary evaluation for some patients. However, other patients may require further evaluation by a cardiologist or internist; some may even need an invasive cardiac procedure before a noncardiac surgery to optimize cardiac function to avoid perioperative events, such as MI, stroke, renal failure, and death. It is a delicate balance to determining which patients need this additional evaluation while avoiding unnecessary testing that delays surgical treatment and increases the cost of care.[9]

The objective of this article is to give a broad overview of the preoperative cardiac risk stratification and current recommendations for preoperative care. By far the most common cardiac issue confronted by the surgeon in the preoperative evaluation in noncardiac surgery is ischemic heart disease, so it is necessary to be familiar with how to perform an adequate preoperative cardiac evaluation to minimize this risk.[10] This article reviews a brief history of prior cardiac risk stratification indexes, explores the current practice guidelines by the American College of Cardiology (ACC) and the American Heart Association (AHA) Task Force, reviews current methods for preoperative evaluation, discusses revascularization options, and evaluates perioperative medication recommendations.

EVOLUTION OF RISK STRATIFICATION

Introduced in 1963, the American Society of Anesthesiologist's (ASA) Physical Classification System (**Table 2**)[3] was one of the first classifications systems used to assess the general risk for patients undergoing surgery. It is known from the National Surgical Quality Improvement Program that patients with an ASA score of 3 have increased odds for perioperative morbidity and mortality (3.4 odds ratio [OR], 95% confidence interval [CI] 2.7–4.7) and those with an ASA score of 4/5 have even higher odds of complications (8.1 OR, 95% CI 6.0–11.0).[3] Although this classification system is a significant independent predictor of perioperative complications, it is still recommended that patients undergoing a procedure more involved than a skin biopsy should have a thorough risk assessment.[3,8]

Table 2
ASA classification system

ASA Class	Description
I	Healthy patients
II	Mild/well-controlled diseases
III	Severe/multiple systemic diseases that limit activity but not incapacitating
IV	Life-threatening diseases that are incapacitating
V	Severely ill patients who may not survive without surgery in 24 h
VI	Brain dead patients for organ procurement
E	Emergency operation

From Saklad M. Grading of patients for surgical procedures. Anesthesiology 1941;2:281–4.

Over the past 50 years, the derivation of a standard cardiac risk index system has been evaluated and modified. Starting in 1977, the first set of multifactorial risk factors was evaluated by Goldman and colleagues,[11] and the original cardiac index (or the Goldman Cardiac Index) was created (**Table 3**).[12,13] This system was later updated in 1986 by Detsky and colleagues,[14] which also created a point system to identify patients with high cardiac risk, and incorporated patients with CAD, angina, recent MI, and heart failure (HF) (**Table 4**).[13] A few years later in 1989, Eagle and colleagues[15] evaluated patients who had undergone cardiac evaluation with nuclear medicine and found 5 predictive cardiac risk factors for patients undergoing vascular procedures, and they created the Eagle Cardiac Index (**Table 5**).[16]

Finally, in 1999 Lee and colleagues[17] derived and validated the Revised Cardiac Risk Index (RCRI) after evaluating 4315 patients aged 50 years and older and incorporated 6 criteria to estimate patients' overall risk in noncardiac operations (**Table 6**). This system was found to be relatively inexpensive and less time consuming compared with other indices and has been used in the most current recommendations created by the ACC/AHA Task Force, which is described next.[12,18]

PERIOPERATIVE CARDIAC EVALUATION FOR NONCARDIAC SURGERY

In 2009, the ACCF/AHA Task Force published their most recent guidelines for perioperative cardiovascular evaluation for patients undergoing noncardiac surgery. This set of guidelines has been evaluated and updated since 1996, and it has served as an excellent protocol for surgeons in determining the extent of preoperative evaluation necessary in order to optimize care.[4,5,10] These clinical recommendations were updated in 2002 and extensively revised in 2007.[10] It has been shown that as many as 40% of cardiology consultations offer no further intervention and recommend proceeding with surgery.[4] Therefore, the surgeon acts as an important filter in determining which patients would benefit from further cardiac evaluation rather than sending all patients to a cardiologist or internist preoperatively.

Patients with known CAD or new onset of signs or symptoms suggestive of CAD need a baseline cardiac assessment.[4] The surgeon is tasked with determining what additional work-up is necessary in conjunction with a detailed perioperative history and physical. Specifically, determining the additional work-up needed in those patients older than 50 years is emphasized because the RCRI (see **Table 6**) was derived from this patient population.[17]

Table 3
The Goldman Cardiac Index

Risk Factor	Points	Cardiac Complication Rate
1. Third heart sound or jugular venous distention	11	0–5 points: 1%
2. Recent MI within 6 mo	10	6–12 points: 7%
3. Nonsinus rhythm or premature atrial contraction on electrocardiogram	7	13–15 points: 14% >26 points: 78%
4. >5 premature ventricular contractions	7	
5. Age >70 y	5	
6. Emergency operations	4	
7. Poor general medical conditions	3	
8. Intrathoracic, intraperitoneal, or aortic surgery	3	
9. Important valvular aortic stenosis	3	

From Goldman L, Caldera DL, Nussbaum SR, et al. Multifactorial index of cardiac risk in noncardiac surgical procedures. N Engl J Med 1977;297:845–50.

Table 4
Detsky modified multifactorial index

Risk Factor[a]	Points
1. Class 4 angina	20
2. Suspected critical aortic stenosis	20
3. MI within 6 mo	10
4. Alveolar pulmonary edema within 1 wk	10
5. Unstable angina within 3 mo	10
6. Class 3 angina	10
7. Emergency situation	10
8. MI >6 mo	5
9. Alveolar pulmonary edema resolved >1 wk	5
10. Rhythm or other than sinus or PACs on ECG	5
11. >5 PVCs any time before surgery	5
12. Poor general medical status	5
13. Age >70 y	5

Abbreviations: ECG, electrocardiogram; PACs, premature atrial contractions; PVCs, premature ventricular contractions.
[a] Greater than or equal to 15 points equals a high risk of cardiac complications.
From Detsky AS, Abrams HB, Forbath N, et al. Cardiac assessment for patients undergoing noncardiac surgery: a multifactorial clinical risk index. Arch Intern Med 1986;146:2131–4.

The initial history and physical examination of patients is key in determining what diseases patients may have been treated for or discovering a new underlying disease, and it is required in all nonemergent patient populations. When determining a cardiac history, patients should be questioned about any history of unstable coronary syndromes, angina, MI, HF, valvular disease, or arrhythmia (**Table 7**).[4,9,19] If patients have a known cardiac history, it should also be determined what prior interventions have been undertaken, including pacemaker placement, percutaneous coronary intervention, or cardiac surgery.[20] Many times, patients have associated diseases like diabetes, hypertension, or renal disease; these should also be documented.[8]

During the history and physical examination, the patients' baseline functional capacity should be determined.[21] Functional capacity correlates positively with

Table 5
Eagle's criteria for cardiac risk assessment

Risk Factor (Each 1 Point)	Score	Risk of Cardiac Complications (95% CI)
1. Age >70 y		
2. Diabetes	0	3.1% (0%–8%)
3. Angina	1–2	29.6% (16%–44%)
4. Q waves on electrocardiogram	≥3	50.0% (29%–71%)
5. Ventricular arrhythmia		

From Eagle KA, Brundage BH, Chaitman BR, et al. Guidelines for perioperative cardiovascular evaluation for noncardiac surgery. Report of the American College of Cardiology/American Heart Association task force on practice guidelines. Committee on Perioperative Cardiovascular Evaluation for Noncardiac Surgery. Circulation 1996;93(6):1278–317; with permission.

Table 6
RCRI

Risk Factors (1 Point Each)	Score	Risk of Cardiac Complications (95% CI)
1. HF		
2. Cerebrovascular disease	0	0.4% (0.05–1.5)
3. Ischemic heart disease	1	0.9% (0.4–2.1)
4. Diabetes requiring insulin	2	7% (3.9–10.3)
5. Creatinine >2.0 mg/dL	≥3	≥11% (5.8–18.4)
6. Undergoing suprainguinal vascular, intraperitoneal, or intrathoracic surgery		

All risk factors are based on history of these diseases or active diseases found on physical examination or study.[4]

From Lee TH, Marcantonio ER, Mangione CM, et al. Derivation and prospective validation of a simple index for prediction of cardiac risk of major noncardiac surgery. Circulation 1999;100:1043–90; with permission.

oxygen uptake found on treadmill testing.[20] The functional capacity is expressed as metabolic equivalents (METs), whereby resting (also called basal) oxygen consumption is roughly 1 MET.[5,21,22] Functional capacity is generally classified as excellent (>10 METs), good (7–9 METs), moderate (4–6 METs), or poor (≤4 METs).[21] Perioperative cardiac risks are increased in patients unable to reach 4 METs.[1,2,5,22] Patients who cannot walk 4 blocks or climb 2 flights of stairs, for example, are considered to have poor functional capacity.[18,21,23]

Table 7
Active cardiac conditions requiring further evaluation and treatment before noncardiac surgery

Condition	Examples
Unstable coronary symptoms	Stable or severe angina Recent or acute MI
Decompensated HF	
Significant arrhythmias	High-grade atrioventricular block Mobitz II atrioventricular block Third-degree heart block Symptomatic ventricular arrhythmias Supraventricular arrhythmias with uncontrolled rate (>100 beats per min) Symptomatic bradycardia Newly recognized ventricular tachycardia
Severe valvular disease	Severe aortic stenosis (mean pressure gradient >40 mm Hg, valve area <1 cm^2, symptomatic) Symptomatic mitral stenosis (dyspnea, exertional syncope, HF)

Adapted from Fleisher LA, Beckman JA, Brown KA, et al. 2009 ACCF/AHA focused update on perioperative beta blockade incorporated into the ACC/AHA 2007 guidelines on perioperative cardiovascular evaluation and care for noncardiac surgery: a report of the American College of Cardiology Foundation/American Heart Association task force on practice guidelines. Circulation 2009;120:169–276; and Fleisher LA. Cardiac risk stratification for noncardiac surgery: update on the American College of Cardiology/American Heart Association 2007 guidelines. Cleve Clin J Med 2009;76(4):9–15.

When evaluating patients by physical examination, vital signs, carotid pulse and bruits, auscultation of the lungs, auscultation of heart for S3 and S4 sounds or arrhythmias, abdominal palpation, and extremity evaluation are all crucial in determining the cardiac status of patients and can also be key to discovering underlying disease.[4,20] If patients have known comorbidities, such as diabetes or hypertension, evaluation of medical control of these conditions also needs to be performed.[9] Diabetes is the most common comorbidity associated with cardiac disease; if present, suspicion should be heightened for CAD.[13] Also, preoperative hemoglobin A_{1c} is of value because it may alter perioperative diabetic management.[9,13] If laboratory or radiographic data are available, it should be reviewed. The decision to perform additional preoperative testing should be based on the findings of the history, physical examination, and clinical judgment of the surgeon.[8,9,20]

Fig. 1 represents the preoperative cardiac evaluation algorithm for noncardiac surgery as proposed in the "2009 Updated ACCF/AHA Guidelines on Perioperative Cardiovascular Evaluation and Care for Noncardiac Surgery."[4] As can be seen, there are 5 steps in the algorithm that can help the surgeon tailor the cardiac evaluation for preoperative patients.

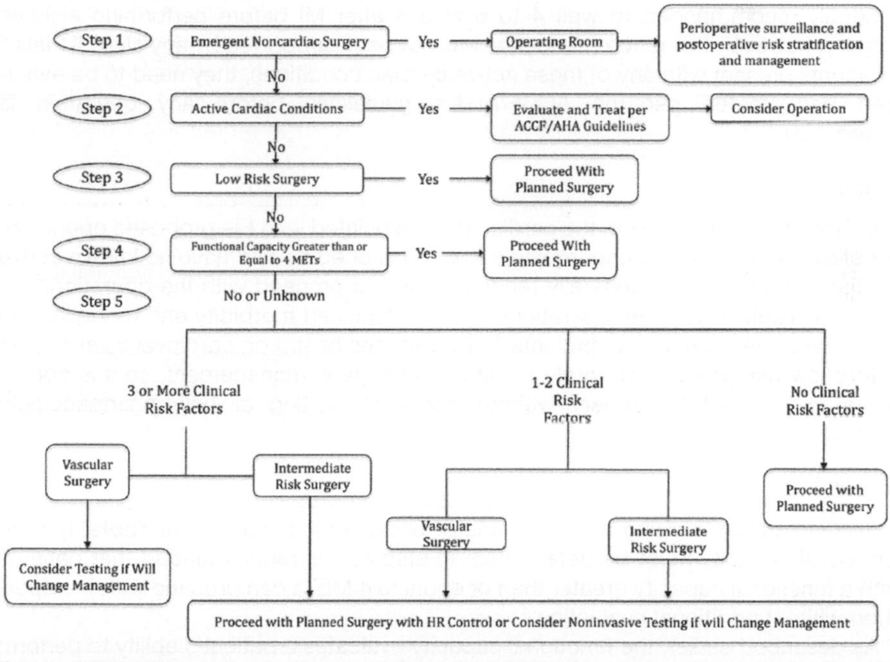

Fig. 1. ACCF/AHA's perioperative guidelines algorithm for noncardiac surgery. Encompasses active clinical conditions, known cardiovascular disease, or cardiac risk for patients aged 50 years and older. HR, heart rate. [a] Active cardiac conditions as described in **Table 7**. [b] Low-, intermediate-, and high-risk surgeries as described in **Table 1**. [c] Risk factors as described in **Table 6**. (*Adapted from* Fleisher LA, Beckman JA, Brown KA, et al. 2009 ACCF/AHA focused update on perioperative beta blockade incorporated into the ACC/AHA 2007 guidelines on perioperative cardiovascular evaluation and care for noncardiac surgery: a report of the American College of Cardiology Foundation/American Heart Association task force on practice guidelines. Circulation 2009;120:169–276; with permission.)

Step 1

Determining if the surgery is emergent is step 1 of the algorithm. If so, it is recommended that patients immediately proceed to the emergent operation; only the most necessary tests and interventions are performed.[4] These tests and interventions may be limited to simple evaluations, such as vitals, essential laboratory values, electrocardiogram (ECG), and urine analysis, so the procedure will not be delayed. Cardiac complications are 2 to 5 times more likely to occur with emergent surgical procedures.[4,24] Because these surgical emergencies eliminate the ability for a preoperative cardiac optimization, a more thorough investigation and monitoring must be performed once patients are stable postoperatively.[4] If there is concern for a cardiac abnormality, it is suggested that transesophageal echocardiography be used intraoperatively to evaluate for a potential cardiac event in emergent patients.[8]

Step 2

Step 2 is determining if patients have an active cardiac condition, which is a substantial perioperative risk.[10,13] Active cardiac conditions are defined in these guidelines as unstable coronary syndromes, decompensated HF, significant arrhythmias, and severe valvular disease, with examples given in **Table 7**.[4] An acute MI is defined as within 7 days, and recent MI is between 7 days to 1 month before evaluation.[3] It is generally recommended to wait 4 to 6 weeks after MI before performing elective surgery; however, this recommendation has not been supported by any clinical trials.[3] If patients present with any of these active cardiac conditions, they need to be evaluated and treated per the ACCF/AHA's guidelines before any operation is undertaken.[4,13]

Step 3

The third step is determining the cardiac risk associated with the proposed operation. For step 3, if patients are undergoing a low-risk procedure and have no known active cardiac conditions, it is generally recommended to proceed with the operation.[4] As shown in **Table 1**, low-risk operations have a combined morbidity and mortality rate 1% or less even in high-risk patients.[4] Interventions based on cardiovascular testing before low-risk procedures rarely result in a change in management, so it is appropriate to proceed to surgery without additional testing or new pharmacologic therapy.[8,10]

Step 4

If patients are undergoing an intermediate- or high-risk surgery (see **Table 1**), their functional capacity must be determined. In step 4, it is recommended that patients with a functional capacity greater than or equal to 4 METs can proceed with the operation without additional evaluation.[4]

As described earlier, the functional capacity evaluates a patient's ability to perform daily activities and is a reliable predictor of cardiac events.[3,4] One of the benefits of this algorithm is that it takes into account that the perioperative and long-term cardiac risks are increased in patients unable to meet a 4-MET minimum.[3,23] In a series evaluating 600 patients undergoing noncardiac surgery, Reilly and colleagues[23] showed that self-reported poor exercise tolerance ($\leq$4 METs) was associated with increased perioperative cardiac risk and the likelihood of a serious complication occurring was inversely related to the number of blocks that could be walked or flights of stairs that could be climbed. In their study, patients reporting poor exercise tolerance had more perioperative complications compared with patients with good functional capacity (20.4% vs 10.4%; *P*<.001), including myocardial ischemia and cardiovascular and neurologic events.[23]

Step 5

If the patients' functional capacity is unknown or less than 4 METs, the number of clinical risk factors as described by the RCRI (see **Table 6**) helps determine if the patients require further cardiac evaluation. For step 5 of the algorithm, if patients have no clinical risk factors, then they are able to proceed with the planned operation.[4]

If patients have 1 to 2 clinical risk factors, the ACCF/AHA's guidelines recommend 2 possible options. The first is to proceed with surgery with heart rate control with beta-blockade. Alternatively, the physician can consider preoperative cardiac testing if it is thought that it will result in a change in patient management.[4,10]

In patients with 3 or more clinical risk factors, the surgery associated cardiac risk (see **Table 1**) is important in determining the care. For the patient population undergoing intermediate-risk surgery, there are insufficient data to determine the best strategy.[4] However, there are 2 suggestions: proceed with surgery with beta-blockade or undergo further cardiac testing if it is expected to result in a change in patient management.[4,10] In the same population undergoing vascular or other high-risk surgery, there is a higher incidence of underlying CAD; therefore, additional cardiac testing is recommended if it will change management.[4] Faggiano and colleagues[6] found that intensive cardiac preoperative evaluation with noninvasive diagnostic tests in patients undergoing high-risk surgery had reductions in cardiac morbidity and mortality and recommended noninvasive preoperative testing for patients in this population.

Overview of Recommendations

Although this algorithm is useful for directing the surgeon in the preoperative cardiac evaluation for patients, it must be remembered that morbidity and mortality vary significantly between procedures and institutions.[4,19] A study performed at the University of Michigan demonstrated that the implementation of these guidelines in an internal medicine preoperative assessment clinic led to a more appropriate use of preoperative stress testing and beta-blocker therapy, while keeping the rate of cardiac complications low.[16]

The ACCF/AHA's guidelines give a framework for the perioperative intervention strategy, but patient risks and preoperative care must be individualized. In the end, it is up to the surgeon to determine the risk incurred by the patients and when there is a need for further evaluation.

SUPPLEMENTAL CARDIAC EVALUATION

After working through the aforementioned algorithm, the surgeon must determine if supplemental testing is necessary. This section explores the ACCF/AHA Task Force's recommendations for supplemental cardiac evaluation.

Electrocardiogram

The standard 12-lead ECG is a frequent starting point for perioperative testing. According to the ACCF/AHA, preoperative resting ECG testing guidelines are as follows:

- ECG is recommended for patients with at least 1 clinical risk factor who are undergoing vascular or intermediate-risk surgery.
- ECG is recommended for patients with known congestive HF, peripheral artery disease, or cerebrovascular disease who are undergoing an intermediate or high-risk procedure.

- ECG is reasonable to perform in patients with no risk factors undergoing vascular surgery.
- ECG is not indicated in asymptomatic patients undergoing low-risk procedures.[4,9,18]

The general consensus is that an ECG, if necessary, be performed within 30 days of the procedure.[20] In the aforementioned recommendations, clinical risk factors are defined as those from the RCRI (see **Table 6**). When Lee and colleagues[17] developed the RCRI, the presence of a pathologic Q wave on the preoperative ECG was associated with a 2.4-fold increased risk of fatal and nonfatal events.[12] One single-center study showed that patients with abnormal preoperative ECGs had higher rates of perioperative cardiovascular events compared with those with normal ECGs (16.0% vs 6.4%; *P*<.001), and prolonged QTc interval was associated with a 13% increased risk of perioperative cardiac event.[12]

Exercise Stress Testing: Evaluation of Myocardial Ischemia and Functional Capacity

If patients are found to have an abnormal ECG or the functional capacity has not yet been evaluated, exercise stress testing can be used to identify the presence of myocardial ischemia, to determine a patient's functional capacity, and to evaluate hemodynamic response.[10,13,22] The exercise stress test is preferred over the pharmacologic stress test because of its ability to determine all of these factors.[3,10,22] Of the patients who undergo exercise stress testing who have a normal ECG and do not have a cardiac history, 20% to 50% will have an abnormal exercise ECG. A total of 35% to 50% of patients with a prior history of MI or who have an abnormal resting ECG will have abnormalities on exercise stress testing.[4] When performing the exercise stress test, the onset of myocardial ischemia at low exercise workloads is associated with a significantly increased risk of perioperative cardiac events.[20]

According to the ACCF/AHA Task Force, the following are recommendations regarding noninvasive stress testing before noncardiac surgery:

- It is reasonable to perform noninvasive stress testing in patients with 3 or more clinical risk factors and a functional capacity 4 METs or less who require vascular surgery if it will alter preoperative management.
- It may be considered for patients with 1 to 2 clinical risk factors and a functional capacity of 4 METs or less who require intermediate-risk or vascular surgery.
- Noninvasive stress testing is not useful for patients with no clinical risk factors undergoing intermediate-risk surgery or patients undergoing low-risk surgery.[4]

Some patients are unable to exercise to increase myocardial oxygen demand to a level needed for optimal cardiac stress evaluation, and attempts to determine myocardial ischemia must be done with pharmacologic stress testing.[13] The most commonly used methods are the dobutamine stress echocardiography (DSE) and intravenous dipyridamole myocardial perfusion imaging with thallium-201 and technetium-99m.[1,4,13] DSE and dipyridamole nuclear imaging have high negative predictive values, 90% to 100% and 97% to 100%, respectively, in evaluating for ischemia.[1,5] Studies have shown that reversible perfusion defects (demonstrating jeopardized myocardium) indicate the greatest risk of a cardiac event, and the risk of events increases with extent of the reversible defect.[4] Conversely, studies show that a fixed perfusion defect does not serve as a predictor of perioperative cardiac events.[4]

If perfusion defects are found via exercise, dobutamine, or dipyridamole testing then it may be necessary for patients to undergo additional evaluation by angiography.[25] Angiography is used to define anatomic abnormalities requiring intervention but should only be performed if it will alter perioperative management.[3,13] Overall, stress testing should no longer be considered a routine step in the preoperative evaluation unless it will significantly affect patient management.[10]

PERIOPERATIVE THERAPY: REVASCULARIZATION WITH CORONARY ARTERY BYPASS GRAFT AND PERCUTANEOUS CORONARY INTERVENTION

If patients are found to have significant CAD in the preoperative evaluation, the next determination to be made is if they require revascularization. Some patients may undergo coronary artery bypass grafting (CABG), whereas others may receive percutaneous coronary intervention (PCI). The ACCF/AHA Task Force has class I, level A recommendations that show coronary revascularization before noncardiac surgery is useful in

- Patients with stable angina who have significant left main coronary artery stenosis
- Patients with stable angina who have 3-vessel disease
- Patients with stable angina who have 2-vessel disease with significant proximal left anterior descending stenosis and either ejection fraction of 50% or less or demonstrable ischemia on noninvasive testing
- Patients with high-risk unstable angina or non-ST segment elevation MI or with acute ST-elevation MI[4]

Determining which intervention is necessary is often at the discretion of the cardiology consultant, and risks and benefits must be weighed. Generally, patients who need CABG before noncardiac procedures are found to have high-risk coronary anatomy.[4] Studies have shown that patients with previous successful coronary bypass have a low perioperative mortality rate with noncardiac procedures and that their mortality rate is comparable to the surgical risk for other patients who have no clinical CAD.[4,5] These patients also have lower rates of perioperative MI compared with those patients undergoing PCI, which is attributable to more thorough revascularization with the CABG.[18]

After a CABG procedure, it is recommended that patients wait 4 to 8 weeks before proceeding with noncardiac surgery.[10] For patients recommended for a CABG, it must be remembered that the benefit of the noncardiac operation should outweigh the morbidity and mortality of both the cardiac revascularization and the planned noncardiac procedure.[5,8]

PCI is another method of coronary artery revascularization in the preoperative period. There are currently 3 methods of percutaneous revascularization: balloon angioplasty, bare metal stents, and drug-eluting stents (DES). Coronary stents are now used in more than 80% of PCIs.[2] Each of these comes with different risks and benefits; but studies have found PCI before noncardiac surgery is of no value in preventing perioperative events, except in those patients who have an acute coronary syndrome, such as ST-elevation MI, unstable angina, and non-ST-elevation MI. In these situations, PCI would independently be recommended per the ACC/AHA's guidelines.[1,2,4] This intervention usually includes patients with significant left main CAD and those with 3-vessel CAD.[10] Once again, the cardiology consultant exercises the discretion in determining the type of intervention. Selection of patients for a CABG procedure versus PCI is beyond the scope of this article, but the topic is addressed in the ACCF/AHA's practice guidelines for PCI and CABG.[26–28]

If patients undergo balloon angioplasty for an acute coronary condition, it is recommended that the elective noncardiac procedure be delayed at least 2 to 4 weeks so sufficient time is allowed for the healing of the vessel injury at the balloon treatment site.[4] This type of intervention can be used for patients requiring urgent operations.[2] Patients that undergo this treatment should be kept on aspirin from the time of intervention through the perioperative period, if possible.[4] It is recommended that if patients require an elective noncardiac operation, that it be performed within 8 weeks of the balloon angioplasty because of the risk of restenosis at the angioplasty site and subsequent increased risk of perioperative cardiac events.[4]

The bare-metal stent is the next PCI option, and it can be used for mitigation of cardiac symptoms in patients requiring an elective noncardiac operation within 12 months.[4] Following bare-metal stent placement, it is recommended that dual antiplatelet therapy with a thienopyridine (ticlopidine or clopidogrel) and aspirin be administered for at least 4 to 6 weeks.[25,29] The risk of thrombosis of the bare-metal stent is highest at 2 weeks after placement and rare beyond 4 weeks of placement.[8,29] Following 4 weeks of dual antiplatelet therapy, aspirin should be continued lifelong, and thienopyridine therapy can be stopped.[18,30] Elective noncardiac operations should be delayed 4 to 6 weeks after the placement of bare-metal stents to allow for partial endothelialization of the stent, but these operations should be undertaken before 12 weeks when restenosis begins to occur.[4,5,30] It is recommended to allow 1 week after stopping thienopyridine therapy before surgery because of the increased risk of bleeding, although aspirin should be continued if possible.[4] Aspirin increases surgical bleeding by about 20%; however, if such bleeding can be tolerated during the procedure, then aspirin should be continued because the cardioprotective risks usually outweigh the risk of bleeding.[10,18]

The final PCI option is the DES, which is designed to reduce neointimal hyperplasia and lower restenosis rates.[4] These stents can be coated with sirolimus or paclitaxel, which actually can increase the risk of thrombosis and delay endothelialization and healing of the vessel.[4,31–33] For this reason, the US Food and Drug Administration's current recommendation is that dual antiplatelet therapy with a thienopyridine and aspirin be continued for 12 months after DES placement as long as patients are not at significant risk for bleeding.[4,33]

It has been shown that premature discontinuation of dual antiplatelet therapy with DES is associated with a markedly increased risk of stent thrombosis and subsequent MI or death.[8,18,31,32] After 12 months, it is recommended to continue with lifelong aspirin therapy. This therapy should be continued through the perioperative period of an elective noncardiac procedure.[18,29,33] Overall, elective noncardiac surgery should not be performed within 12 months of DES placement because of the increased risk of thrombosis with discontinuation of dual antiplatelet therapy.[33]

The type of intervention, the time frame before surgery, and the medical interventions required for each PCI are listed in **Table 8**. If thienopyridines must be discontinued prematurely before major surgery, then aspirin should be continued and thienopyridine therapy resumed as soon as possible.[4,10,19] It has been shown that a hypercoagulable condition develops 7 to 10 days after discontinuation of antiplatelet therapy and places patients at risk for a thrombotic cardiac event.[4,10,19]

As mentioned earlier, there is no current evidence that PCI before an elective noncardiac surgery is beneficial; patients that have indications for PCI in the preoperative setting are the same as those developed by the ACCF/AHA Task Force, regardless of an impending surgical procedure.[4] It is also not recommended that routine prophylactic coronary revascularization be performed in patients with stable CAD before noncardiac surgery.[4]

Two trials form the basis of these recommendations, with the first being the Coronary Artery Revascularization Prophylaxis (CARP) trial.[4] The purpose of the CARP trial

Table 8
PCI and time to noncardiac surgery

Intervention	Time Since PCI	Recommendation
Balloon angioplasty	<14 d	Delay for elective or nonemergent surgery
	>14 d	Proceed to operating room with aspirin
Bare-metal stent	<30–45 d	Delay for elective or nonemergent surgery Continue on dual antiplatelet therapy
	>30–45 d	Proceed to operating room with aspirin
DES	<1 y	Delay for elective or nonemergent surgery Continue on dual antiplatelet therapy
	>1 y	Proceed to operating room with aspirin

Adapted from Fleisher LA, Beckman JA, Brown KA, et al. 2009 ACC/AHA focused update on perioperative beta blockade incorporated into the ACC/AHA 2007 guidelines on perioperative cardiovascular evaluation and care for noncardiac surgery: a report of the American College of Cardiology Foundation/American Heart Association task force on practice guidelines. Circulation 2009;120:169–276; with permission.

was to determine if the use of prophylactic coronary revascularization before a high-risk operation reduced perioperative cardiac events when compared with optimized medical management.[13,18,34] After a mean follow-up of 30 days and 2.7 years, no difference in all-cause mortality or postoperative MI was found in either group, leaving the investigators to conclude that coronary-artery revascularization before elective vascular surgery among patients with stable cardiac symptoms was not recommended.[10,13,18,34] This study is criticized, however, because of the exclusion of some patients with 3-vessel disease and significant ischemia, and it lacked sufficient statistical power.[13]

To further address the situation, the second trial known as the Dutch Echocardiographic Cardiac Risk Evaluation Applying Stress Echocardiography (DECREASE-V) trial included these high-risk patients with evidence of significant ischemia undergoing vascular surgery.[18,35,36] This study confirmed that preoperative revascularization conferred no benefit when performed prophylactically to prevent cardiac events, and mortality was the same in medically optimized groups at 30 days and 1 year.[7,35,36] These studies highlight why the ACCF/AHA's guidelines indicate that routine prophylactic coronary revascularization is not recommended for patients with stable CAD before noncardiac surgery.[4,10,13]

PERIOPERATIVE MEDICAL THERAPY

Recommended guidelines on preoperative medical therapy were most recently updated in the "2009 ACCF/AHA Focused Update on Perioperative Beta Blockade Incorporated Into the ACC/AHA 2007 Guidelines on Perioperative Cardiovascular Evaluation and Care for Noncardiac Surgery" after the presentation of new clinical trials at scientific meetings of the ACCF, AHA, and European Society of Cardiology in 2008.[4,37] The following sections discuss beta-blocker and statin usage in accordance with current guidelines.

Beta-blockers

Perioperative beta-blocker use has been a significantly investigated and discussed topic. Beta-blockers have been shown to prevent cardiac ischemia by decreasing the heart rate and force of contraction, thereby decreasing myocyte oxygen demand.[7] The 2009 ACCF/AHA's focused update recommends the following:

- Beta-blockers should be continued in patients undergoing surgery who are receiving beta-blocker treatment of conditions with indications for the usage.
- Beta-blockers titrated to heart rate and blood pressure are probably recommended before vascular surgery for patients who are at a high cardiac risk because of CAD or ischemia on preoperative testing.
- Beta-blockers titrated to heart rate and blood pressure are reasonable for patients that have more than one clinical cardiac risk factor (see **Table 6**) on preoperative assessment for vascular surgery.
- Beta-blockers titrated to heart rate and blood pressure are reasonable for patients who are discovered to have CAD on the preoperative assessment or have more than one clinical cardiac risk factor (see **Table 6**) who are undergoing intermediate-risk surgery (see **Table 1**).[4]

The usefulness of beta-blockers is currently uncertain in 2 patient populations. The first are patients undergoing intermediate-risk or vascular surgery who only have a single clinical cardiac risk factor (see **Table 6**).[4] The second are patients undergoing vascular surgery with no clinical cardiac risk factors (see **Table 6**).[4] In a 2005 study by Lindenauer and colleagues,[38] more than 780,000 patients were evaluated retrospectively; it was determined that beta-blocker therapy was not associated with reducing cardiac risk in low-risk patients undergoing major noncardiac surgery.

Mangano and colleagues[24] performed the first randomized controlled trial to show a benefit of preoperative beta-blockade in 1996. They showed that atenolol decreased the mortality in patients from 21% to 10% at 2 years postoperatively. This study, however, did not show that atenolol significantly reduced the incidence of perioperative cardiac mortality.[24] In 1999, Poldermans and colleagues[39] showed in another randomized controlled trial that bisoprolol reduced the perioperative incidence of death from cardiac causes and nonfatal MI from 34.0% to 3.4% ($P<.001$) in more than 840 high-risk patients undergoing major vascular surgery. This study emphasized the importance of the preoperative evaluation in screening for high-risk patients who could benefit from medical therapy.[39] The study recommended that patients identified as high-risk receive beta-blockers 1 or 2 weeks before surgery with a heart rate goal of less than 70 beats per minute preoperatively and less than 80 beats per minute postoperatively.[39]

In 2008, Dunkelgrun and colleagues[40] further supported these 2 trials with the results of the DECREASE IV trial, which was a randomized controlled trial of bisoprolol and fluvastatin used in intermediate-risk patients undergoing noncardiac surgery.[41] More than 1060 enrolled patients were at least 40 years of age, scheduled for elective noncardiac surgery, naïve to statin and beta-blocker use, and had an estimated risk of perioperative death and MI of 1% to 6%.[40] Patients were randomized to use of beta-blocker therapy, statin therapy, a combination of both statin and beta-blocker, or no medications. Patients were started on medications at a median of 34 days before surgery and continued until postoperative day 30.[40] The end points of the study were 30-day cardiac death and MI, and it was shown that low-dose beta-blockers were cardioprotective in the intermediate-risk group without any increased incidence of stroke or mortality.[4,40] The DECREASE IV was stopped early secondary to slow enrollment, so the power of this study is limited.[37,41] This study did demonstrate that beta-blockers need to be started well in advance of surgery to allow appropriate titration. Further, although not adequately powered to achieve statistical significance, the study suggested patients treated with fluvastatin trended toward improved outcome.[40]

In 2008, the Perioperative Ischemic Evaluation (POISE) trial results were published showing that routine administration of high-dose beta-blockers in the absence of dose titration is not useful and may actually be harmful to patients undergoing noncardiac surgery.[42] The POISE trial was a randomized controlled trial that incorporated more than 8000 beta-blocker–naïve patients undergoing noncardiac surgery. In this trial, patients were randomized to start high-dose extended-release metoprolol 2 to 4 hours before surgery and continue for 30 days.[10,42] Patients were kept on metoprolol as long as their heart rate was greater than 50 beats per minute and their systolic blood pressure was greater than 100 mm Hg.[10] The end points evaluated were cardiovascular death, nonfatal MI, and nonfatal cardiac arrest.[42] This study found that although there was a reduction in cardiovascular death, MI, and cardiac arrest, this was offset by an increase in the risk of stroke, hypotension, bradycardia, and total mortality.[10,42] Overall, this study suggested that although beta-blocker therapy reduces the risk of perioperative cardiac events in high-risk patients, routine administration of high-dose, long-acting beta-blockers in beta-blocker–naïve patients without titration can actually increase mortality.[10,37]

The POISE study did not address patients who were already on beta-blocker therapy in accordance with the ACCF/AHA's current guidelines, and it is currently recommended that patients already on beta-blockers continue throughout the perioperative period.[10,37] Patients undergoing elective surgery for whom beta-blockers are recommended or reasonable (see earlier bullet points) should have the therapy initiated days to weeks before an elective operation, and this should be titrated to lowered heart rate without causing frank hypotension.[37] Beta-blockers should not be given to patients undergoing surgery who have absolute contraindications to beta-blockade.[4]

In titrating beta-blocker medications in any patient population, the ACCF/AHA's 2009 update recommends that patients be started on beta-blockers before surgery with titration to a goal heart rate between 60 and 65 beats per minute and with avoidance of frank hypotension.[4,10,40] A meta-analysis by Cucherat[43] found that each slowing of 10 beats per minute, while maintaining blood pressure, reduced the risk of cardiac death by 30%.

Interruption of beta-blocker therapy may lead to recurrent angina, arrhythmias, rebound hypertension, rapid atrial fibrillation, and MI in the perioperative period.[10,37] It has been shown that selective beta-blocker discontinuation increases the risk of MI in the first 30 days after cessation (relative risk [RR] 2.7, 95% CI 1.06–6.89) and 30 to 180 days after cessation (RR 2.44, 95% CI 1.07–5.59).[44] In more than 700 patients undergoing endovascular and open vascular surgery, it was shown that continuous beta-blocker use was significantly associated with decreased 1-year mortality compared with those who were not on beta-blockers (hazard ratio 0.4, 95% CI 0.2–0.7).[45] Overall, evidence shows that if beta-blockers are used, they should be appropriately titrated throughout the preoperative, intraoperative, and postoperative period to achieve heart rate control while avoiding hypotension. Patients already on beta-blockers should have this therapy continued through the perioperative period.[4]

Statins

Statin therapy has been shown to be effective in secondary prevention of cardiac events.[4] These medications work by inhibiting hydroxymethylglutaryl coenzyme A and have been shown to improve endothelial function, reduce vascular inflammation, stabilize atherosclerotic plaque, lower low-density lipoprotein cholesterol, and decrease matrix metalloproteinase and cell death.[4,40,46] The risks of statin therapy include myopathy and rhabdomyolysis.[40] The ACCF/AHA's current 2009 guidelines for statin medications are as follows:

- Patients who take a statin and are undergoing noncardiac surgery should have this therapy continued.
- Statin therapy is reasonable for patients undergoing vascular surgery with or without a risk factor.
- Statin therapy may be considered for patients with at least 1 clinical risk (see **Table 6**) factor undergoing intermediate risk procedures.[4]

Although much of the data that currently supports statin use are primarily from retrospective studies, case control studies, and small randomized controlled studies, the evidence suggests that statins are cardioprotective when used or continued during noncardiac surgery.[4,46] In 2005, The Statins for Risk Reduction In Surgery study retrospectively evaluated more than 1160 patients undergoing vascular surgery; it was found that patients receiving statins had significantly fewer cardiovascular complications (9.9%) than those patients who were not receiving statins (16.5%, $P = .001$).[47] Another retrospective study performed at the University of Rochester Medical Center showed through multivariate analysis that the use of statins was associated with decreased major cardiac complications, noncardiac complications, respiratory complications, and infectious complications.[48]

The exact mechanism through which statins confer possible benefits is still unknown, and it is currently recommended that more randomized controlled trials with prospective data would be beneficial to support perioperative statin usage.[46–48]

SUMMARY

Advances in the preoperative risk assessment have helped to decrease the frequency of cardiovascular complications associated with noncardiac surgery.[16,19] The major parameters that determine the risk of cardiac morbidity and mortality for patients undergoing noncardiac surgery are the risk of surgery, patient clinical characteristics, and patient functional capacity.[10] Nonfatal and fatal cardiac events are one of the biggest sources of perioperative morbidity and mortality; therefore, optimizing patients in the preoperative period is essential for surgeons who perform noncardiac operations.[24] Ultimately, everything comes down to the patients, and care must be individualized. All patients require some form of preoperative screening, ranging from a simple history and physical examination to invasive procedures. Therapy with beta-blockers and statins should be reviewed and considered. Surgeons must remain current on the recommendations for preoperative evaluation in order to optimize postoperative outcomes.

REFERENCES

1. Pannell LM, Reyes EM, Underwood SR. Cardiac risk assessment before non-cardiac surgery. Eur Heart J 2013;14:316–22.
2. Mukherjee D, Eagle KA. Perioperative cardiac assessment for noncardiac surgery: eight steps to the best possible outcome. Circulation 2003;107:2771–4.
3. Neumayer L, Vargo D. Principles of preoperative and operative surgery. Chapter 11. In: Sabiston text book of surgery: the biological basis of modern surgical practice, vol. 19, 19th edition. Philadelphia: Elsevier-Saunders; 2012. p. 211–39.
4. Fleisher LA, Beckman JA, Brown KA, et al. 2009 ACCF/AHA focused update on perioperative beta blockade incorporated into the ACC/AHA 2007 guidelines on

perioperative cardiovascular evaluation and care for noncardiac surgery: a report of the American College of Cardiology Foundation/American Heart Association task force on practice guidelines. Circulation 2009;120:169–276.
5. Akhtar S, Silverman DG. Assessment and management of patients with ischemic heart disease. Crit Care Med 2004;32(4):126–36.
6. Faggiano P, Bonardelli S, De Feo S, et al. Preoperative cardiac evaluation and perioperative cardiac therapy in patients undergoing open surgery for abdominal aortic aneurysms: effects on cardiovascular outcome. Ann Vasc Surg 2012;26:156–65.
7. Williams FM, Bergin JD. Cardiac screening before noncardiac surgery. Surg Clin North Am 2009;89:747–62 Elsevier Inc.
8. Cameron JL, Cameron AM. Preoperative preparation of the surgical patient. Current surgical therapy. 11th edition. Philadelphia: Elsevier-Saunders; 2014. p. 1163–8.
9. Feely MA, Collins CS, Daniels PR, et al. Preoperative testing before noncardiac surgery: guidelines and recommendations. Am Fam Physician 2013;87(6):414–8.
10. Freeman WK, Gibbons RJ. Perioperative cardiovascular assessment in patients undergoing noncardiac surgery. Mayo Clin Proc 2009;84(1):79–90.
11. Goldman L, Caldera DL, Southwick FS, et al. Cardiac risk factors and complications in noncardiac surgery. N Engl J Med 1977;297:845–50.
12. Biteker M, Duman D, Tekkesin AI. Predictive value of preoperative electrocardiography for perioperative cardiovascular outcomes in patients undergoing noncardiac, nonvascular surgery. Clin Cardiol 2012;35(8):494–9.
13. Hoeks SE, Willem-Jan F, van Kuijk JP, et al. Cardiovascular risk assessment of the diabetic patient undergoing noncardiac surgery. Best Pract Res Clin Endocrinol Metab 2009;23:361–73.
14. Detsky AS, Abrams HB, Forbath N, et al. Cardiac assessment for patients under going noncardiac surgery. A multifactorial clinical risk index. Arch Intern Med 1986;146(11):2131–40.
15. Eagle KA, Coley CM, Newell JB, et al. Combining clinical and thallium data optimizes preoperative assessment of cardiac risk before major vascular surgery. Ann Intern Med 1989;10:859–66.
16. Almanaseer Y, Mukherjee D, Kline-Rogers EM, et al. Implementation of the ACC/AHA guidelines for preoperative cardiac risk assessment in a general medicine preoperative clinic: improving efficiency and preserving outcomes. Cardiology 2005;103:24–9.
17. Lee TH, Marcantonio ER, Mangione CM, et al. Derivation and prospective validation of a simple index for prediction of cardiac risk of major noncardiac surgery. Circulation 1999;100:1043–90.
18. Holt NF. Perioperative cardiac risk reduction. Am Fam Physician 2012;85(3):239–46.
19. Fleisher LA. Cardiac risk stratification for noncardiac surgery: update on the American College of Cardiology/American Heart Association 2007 guidelines. Cleve Clin J Med 2009;76(4):9–15.
20. Graham L. ACC/AHA release guidelines on perioperative cardiovascular evaluation for noncardiac surgery. Am Fam Physician 2008;22(77):1748–51.
21. Sherwood ER, Williams CG, Prough DS. Anesthesiology principles, pain management, and conscious sedations. Chapter 16. In: Sabiston text book of surgery: the biological basis of modern surgical practice, vol. 19, 19th edition. Philadelphia: Elsevier-Saunders; 2012. p. 389–417.
22. Biccard BM. Relationship between the inability to climb two flights of stairs and outcomes after major non-cardiac surgery: implications for the preoperative assessment of functional capacity. Anaesthesia 2005;60:588–93.

23. Reilly DF, McNeely MJ, Doerner D, et al. Self reported exercise tolerance and the risk of serious perioperative complication. Arch Intern Med 1999;159:2185–92.
24. Mangano DT, Layug EL, Wallace A, et al. Effect of atenolol on mortality and cardiovascular morbidity after noncardiac surgery. N Engl J Med 1996;335: 1713–20.
25. Joehl RJ. Preoperative evaluation: pulmonary, cardiac, renal dysfunction and comorbidities. Surg Clin North Am 2008;85:1061–73 Elsevier-Saunders.
26. Eagle KA, Guyton RA, Davidoff R, et al. ACC/AHA 2004 guideline update for coronary artery bypass graft surgery: a report of the American College of Cardiology/American Heart Association task force on practice guidelines (committee to update the 1999 guidelines for coronary artery bypass graft surgery). Circulation 2004;110:340–437.
27. Hillis LD, Smith PK, Anderson JL, et al. 2011 ACCF/AHA guideline for coronary artery bypass graft surgery: a report of the American College of Cardiology Foundation/American Heart Association task force on practice guidelines. Circulation 2011;124:652–735.
28. Levine GN, Bates ER, Blankenship, et al. 2011 ACCF/AHA/SCAI guideline for percutaneous coronary intervention. A report of the American College of Cardiology Foundation/American Heart Association task force on practice guidelines and the society for cardiovascular angiography and interventions. Circulation 2011;124:574–651.
29. Grines CL, Bonow RO, Casey DE, et al. Prevention of premature discontinuation of dual antiplatelet therapy in patient with coronary artery stents. Circulation 2007; 115:813–8.
30. Nuttall GA, Brown MJ, Stombaugh JW, et al. Time and cardiac risk of surgery after bare-metal stent percutaneous coronary intervention. Anesthesiology 2008;109:588–95.
31. McFadden EP, Stabile E, Regar E, et al. Late thrombosis in drug-eluting coronary stents after discontinuation of antiplatelet therapy. Lancet 2004;364:1519–21.
32. Nasser M, Kapeliovich M, Markiewicz W. Late thrombosis of sirolimus eluting stents following noncardiac surgery. Catheter Cardiovasc Interv 2005;65:516–9.
33. Rabbitts JA, Buttal GA, Brown MJ, et al. Cardiac risk of noncardiac surgery after percutaneous coronary intervention with drug eluting stents. Anesthesiology 2008;109:596–604.
34. McFalls EO, Ward HB, Moritz TE, et al. Coronary-artery revascularization before elective major vascular surgery. N Engl J Med 2004;351:2795–804.
35. Boersma E, Poldermans D, Bax JJ, et al. Predictors of cardiac events after major vascular surgery. Role of clinical characteristics, dobutamine echocardiography, and B-blocker therapy. JAMA 2001;285:1865–73.
36. Poldermans D, Schouten O, Vidakovic R, et al. A clinical randomized trial to evaluate the safety of a noninvasive approach in high risk patients undergoing major vascular surgery: the DECREASE-V pilot study. J Am Coll Cardiol 2007; 49(17):1763–9.
37. Fleischmann KE, Beckman JA, Buller CE, et al. 2009 ACCF/AHA focused update on perioperative beta blockade: a report of the American College of Cardiology Foundation/American Heart Association task force on practice guidelines. Circulation 2009;120:2123–51.
38. Lindenauer PK, Pekow P, Wang K, et al. Perioperative beta-blocker therapy and mortality after major noncardiac surgery. N Engl J Med 2005;353:349–61.
39. Poldermans D, Boersma E, Bax JJ, et al. The effect of bisoprolol on perioperative mortality and myocardial infarction in high-risk patients undergoing vascular

surgery: Dutch echocardiographic cardiac risk evaluation applying stress echocardiography study group. N Engl J Med 1999;341:1789–94.
40. Dunkelgrun M, Boersma E, Schouten O, et al. Bisoprolol and fluvastatin for the reduction of perioperative cardiac mortality and myocardial infarction in intermediate risk patients undergoing noncardiovascular surgery: a randomized control trial (DECREASE- IV). Ann Surg 2009;249:921–6.
41. Schouten O, Poldermans D, Visser L, et al. Fluvastatin and bisoprolol for the reduction of perioperative cardiac mortality and morbidity in high risk patients undergoing noncardiac surgery: rationale and design of the DECREASE-IV study. Am Heart J 2004;148:1047–52.
42. Devereaux PJ, Yang H, Yusuf S, et al. Effects of extended release metoprolol succinate in patients undergoing noncardiac surgery (POISE Trial): a randomized controlled trial. Lancet 2008;371:1839–47.
43. Cucherat M. Qualitative relationship between resting heart rate reduction and magnitude of clinical benefits in post-myocardial infarction: a meta-regression of randomized clinical trials. Eur Heart J 2007;28:3012–9.
44. Teichert M, deSmet PA, Hofman A, et al. Discontinuation of beta-blockers and the risk of myocardial infarction in the elderly. Drug Saf 2007;30:541–9.
45. Hoeks SE, Scholte OP, Reimer WJ, et al. Increase of 1 year mortality after perioperative beta-blocker withdrawal in endovascular and vascular surgery patients. Eur J Vasc Endovasc Surg 2007;33:13–9.
46. Feldman LS, Brotman DJ. Perioperative statins: more than lipid lowering? Cleve Clin J Med 2004;116:96–103.
47. O'Neil-Callahan K, Katsimaglis G, Tepper MR, et al. Statins decrease perioperative cardiac complications in patient undergoing noncardiac vascular surgery: the Statins for Risk Reduction Surgery (StaRRS) study. J Am Coll Cardiol 2005; 45:336–42.
48. Iannuzzi JC, Rickles AS, Kelly KN, et al. Perioperative pleiotropic statin effects in general surgery. Surgery 2014;155:398–407.

Prevention of Postoperative Pulmonary Complications

Amber Taylor, MD, Zachary DeBoard, MD,
Jeffrey M. Gauvin, MD, MS*

KEYWORDS

• Postoperative • Pulmonary complications • COPD • Respiratory failure

KEY POINTS

- Postoperative pulmonary complications (PPCs) are common and infer greater risk of morbidity and mortality to surgical patients.
- Careful preoperative evaluation can identify undiagnosed and undertreated illness and allow for preoperative intervention.
- Surgical, anesthetic, and patient factors contribute to developing PPCs.
- Certain high-risk groups may benefit from presurgical optimization of known disease as well as specific postoperative maneuvers.
- Comorbidities that greatly increase risk include chronic obstructive pulmonary disease (COPD), obesity, obstructive sleep apnea (OSA), obesity hypoventilation syndrome (OHS), pulmonary hypertension (PH), and smoking.

INTRODUCTION

PPCs represent a significant burden of illness in surgical patients. The reported incidence is 5% for general surgical patients but as high as 20% in select groups undergoing high-risk procedures.[1–3] PPCs are as common as cardiac complications in general surgical patients.[4]

PPCs represent an important cause of mortality with rates as high as 25% depending on the operation and complication.[1] Abdominal surgical patients who develop postoperative pneumonia experience a 10-fold increase in mortality over those who do not, as well as longer length of stay.[5,6] In addition, PPCs increase 30-day readmission rates and may be a marker for decreased long-term survival in elderly hospitalized patients.[7] PPCs are more of a financial burden than cardiovascular or infectious complications after surgery, costing the United States $3.4 billion annually.[5,8]

The authors have nothing to disclose.
Surgical Education Department, Santa Barbara Cottage Hospital, 400 West Pueblo Street, Santa Barbara, CA 93105, USA
* Corresponding author.
E-mail address: jgauvin@sbch.org

Surg Clin N Am 95 (2015) 237–254
http://dx.doi.org/10.1016/j.suc.2014.11.002 surgical.theclinics.com

The spectrum of PPCs ranges from bronchospasm and atelectasis to pneumonia and respiratory failure. Atelectasis occurs in up to 90% of patients during an operation but is usually self-limited.[9] Pneumonia occurs in up to 15% of patients after surgery and has a high associated mortality rate.[5,10] Acute lung injury (ALI) is the most common cause of postoperative respiratory failure and is also associated with increased mortality.[11] The overall risk of acute respiratory distress syndrome (ARDS) among general surgical patients is approximately 0.2%; however, the risk is higher in subgroups with COPD and preexisting renal failure and those undergoing emergency surgery.[12]

A complex interplay of anesthetic factors, surgical factors, and patient factors contribute to the development PPCs. This review discusses the cause and prevention of PPCs in noncardiac surgical patients.

RISK ASSESSMENT

Smetana and colleagues[4] conducted a systematic review of preoperative pulmonary risk stratification for the American College of Physicians, which remains the most widely cited clinical guideline (**Table 1**). Based on these findings, there is good evidence that patients with congestive heart failure, American Society of Anesthesiologists (ASA)

Table 1
Risk factors for postoperative pulmonary complications

Patient-Related Factors[a]	Procedure-Related Factors[a]
Supported by good evidence	
Advanced age	Aortic aneurysm repair
ASA class ≥2	Thoracic surgery
Congestive heart failure	Abdominal surgery
Functional dependency	Upper abdominal surgery
Chronic obstructive pulmonary disease	Neurosurgery Prolonged surgery Head and neck surgery Emergency surgery Vascular surgery Use of general anesthesia
Supported by fair evidence	
Weight loss Impaired sensorium Cigarette use Alcohol use Abnormal results in chest examination	Perioperative transfusion
Good evidence *against* being a risk factor	
Well-controlled asthma	Hip surgery
Obesity	Genitourinary/gynecologic surgery
Insufficient data	
Obstructive sleep apnea[b] Poor exercise capacity	Esophageal surgery

Abbreviation: ASA, American Society of Anesthesiologists.

[a] Within each evidence category, risk factors are listed according to strength of evidence, with the first factor listed having the strongest evidence.

[b] Subsequent evidence indicates that this is a probable risk factor.

Adapted from Smetana GW. Postoperative pulmonary complications: an update on risk assessment and reduction. Cleve Clin J Med 2009;76(Suppl 4):S60–5.

class of 2 or greater, advanced age, COPD, and functional dependence have a higher risk of PPCs.[2,4,13,14]

A large, prospective multicenter trial by the ARISCAT (The Assess Respiratory Risk in Surgical Patients in Catalonia Group) group examined postoperative complications of general surgical patients in 59 hospitals in Spain. They identified 7 factors predictive of PCCs[3]:

1. Advanced age
2. Reduced preoperative peripheral capillary oxygen saturation (Spo_2)
3. Previous respiratory infection in the last month
4. Preoperative anemia (hemoglobin $\leq$10 g/dL)
5. Surgical incision close to the diaphragm
6. Longer duration of surgery
7. Emergency surgery

Other risk factors that have been linked to PPCs include decreased functional status, altered mental status, weight loss greater than 10% within the last 6 months, chronic kidney disease, diabetes mellitus, congestive heart failure, and significant alcohol use.[1,3,13,15–17]

Elderly patients have increased risk of PPCs even after adjusting for comorbidities.[4,18] Advanced age is accompanied by decreased elastic recoil of lung parenchyma, decreased chest wall compliance, decreased alveolar surface area, and decreased respiratory muscle strength.[18] Patients older than 70 years are at 3 times greater risk of experiencing a PPC.[19] Another article by Schlitzkus et al. in this issue addresses perioperative management of the elderly.

Gupta and colleagues[20] created a postoperative respiratory failure risk calculator based on National Surgical Quality Improvement Program (NSQIP) data, which considers ASA class, preoperative function, type of procedure, nature of surgery (emergent or elective), and presence of preoperative sepsis. This free calculator can be accessed at www.surgicalriskcalculator.com/.

PREOPERATIVE EVALUATION

History and Physical Examination

Prevention of PPCs begins with a thorough medical history. Special attention should be given to complaints related to underlying lung disease and smoking history. Exercise tolerance has been independently associated with improved survival after major abdominal operations.[21] Respiratory infection within 4 weeks and sputum production increase the risk of PPCs, as does alcohol use.[3,13,22,23]

Physical examination should pay careful attention to body habitus as well as cardiorespiratory signs. Severe obesity (body mass index >40 kg/m^2) increases the risk of unplanned tracheal intubation and complications in general.[24,25] A positive result in a cough test, whereby a patient attempts deep breathing and coughs involuntarily, is a predictor of PPCs.[3,26]

Laboratory Testing

Routine preoperative laboratory testing may help identify patients at increased risk. Preoperative anemia was established as an independent risk factor for PPCs by the ARISCAT study, and elevated blood urea nitrogen levels (>30 mg/dL) may also confer increased risk.[3,15]

Several studies have demonstrated the association between low serum albumin levels and PPCs, and a large systematic review by Smetana and colleagues[13,27] found good evidence to support serum albumin levels less than 30 g/L as a predictor for PPCs.[28] Patients with low serum albumin levels have significantly increased rates of reintubation, pneumonia, and failure to wean from mechanical ventilation.[28]

Routine arterial blood gas measurement is not indicated but may be useful to screen for OHS in at-risk patients to initiate positive airway pressure (PAP) therapy preoperatively, which can reduce morbidity and mortality (see later discussion).[29–31]

Other Investigations

There is some evidence that an abnormal finding on chest radiograph (CXR) may correlate with an overall increased risk of PPCs.[32,33] Findings that indicate subclinical heart failure or infection should delay elective surgery.[29] The American College of Physicians guidelines currently recommend preoperative CXRs in patients 50 years or older with known cardiopulmonary disease who are undergoing high-risk surgery.[13]

Routine preoperative pulmonary function tests (PFTs) are useful in thoracic surgical patients, but their role in nonthoracic surgery is limited to at-risk groups.[34] A forced expiratory volume at one second (FEV_1) less than 60% of predicted has been identified as a risk factor for PPCs.[35] PFTs should be ordered selectively in at-risk populations.[19]

Other interventions can be considered in patients with known risk factors such as PH, which usually mandates a preoperative electrocardiogram and right heart catheterization if the diagnosis is suspected.[36]

SURGICAL FACTORS

Postoperatively, inhibition of respiratory muscles contribute to pulmonary complications and are thought to be caused by the following[37,38]:

- Incisional pain
- Functional disruption from incisions
- Reflex inhibition of phrenic motor neuron output from traction of abdominal viscera

Surgical Site

Surgical site is perhaps the most important risk factor in the development of PPCs.[4] In particular, aortic surgery, thoracic surgery, and upper abdominal surgery carry the highest risk of PPCs, although neck operations also carry increased risk.[13,39] Patients undergoing open abdominal aortic aneurysm have a risk of developing PPCs that approaches 25%.[13] In general, the risk of PPCs increases with increasing proximity to the diaphragm.[18] Transverse or oblique incisions may have a mildly decreased risk of associated PPCs compared with vertical midline incisions.[40]

The benefits of laparoscopy include smaller incisions, decreased systemic inflammatory response, reduced postoperative pain, and improved pulmonary function. When compared with open surgery, patients undergoing laparoscopy have a lower incidence of PPCs.[41,42]

Regardless of surgical site, emergency surgery confers a greater risk of PPCs than elective cases.[13,15,16]

Analgesia

PPCs may occur less frequently in patients with either epidural or intravenous patient-controlled analgesia.[27,43] Segmental epidural blockade with local anesthetics can increase tidal volume and vital capacity and improve indices that reflect diaphragm activity after thoracic and upper abdominal surgery.[18,38,44] Several retrospective studies have demonstrated a decrease in PPCs among patients with epidural analgesia, and a large meta-analysis found the rate of pneumonia decreased from 12.8% to 7.5% in patients who received a postoperative epidural versus systemic analgesia.[45–47] However, randomized trials have failed to reproduce this benefit.[48–50]

Although the evidence is not strong, epidurals may infer protection from PPCs, especially in high-risk patients.[51] Pain control has special importance in select patient groups with underlying cardiorespiratory comorbidity, such as PH, whereby increases in vascular resistance due to catecholamine release can have deleterious effects on cardiac function. Multimodal analgesia that minimizes narcotic use may also reduce PPCs.[52]

Anesthesia

Several factors contribute to the harmful effects of general anesthesia on the lungs[38,53]:

- Instrumentation alters mucociliary function, promoting retention of secretions.
- Administered drugs release circulating mediators causing bronchoconstriction.
- There is decreased surfactant production.
- There is inhibition of alveolar macrophage activity.

General anesthesia causes an immediate and prolonged decrease in functional residual capacity (FRC) of up to 20% and is almost always associated with atelectasis.[54,55] Anesthesia causes immediate atelectasis in almost all patients as a result of chest wall deformation, decreased inspiratory muscle tone, and reduced FRC of the lung and may significantly impact gas exchange.[56–58] The physiologic response of the lungs and chest wall may be dose related, with higher doses causing uncoordinated respiratory function.[38,59] These effects can last into the postoperative period and contribute to overall complications.

Neuromuscular Blockade

Neuromuscular blocking agents are necessary for procedures that require muscle relaxation. Their use increases the risk for postoperative desaturation, unplanned reintubation, and postoperative residual curarization (PORC).[60,61] PORC is an incomplete recovery from nondepolarizing neuromuscular blocking agents and is a known risk factor for PPCs.[62]

Long-acting blockade agents can have residual effects up to 7 days postoperatively and are associated with an increased rate of PPCs, particularly pneumonia.[63,64] These drugs should be avoided in any patient at increased risk of PPCs, whereas medium-acting compounds are the preferred agents for most general surgical patients.[27,61,64]

Ventilator Strategies

There is strong evidence for the beneficial use of lower tidal volumes among patients with ALI, and all patients requiring mechanical ventilation may benefit from this strategy.[65,66] General surgical patients who undergo intraoperative mechanical ventilation with lower tidal volumes have lower levels of circulating inflammatory cytokines postoperatively[67] and may have a lower instance of pneumonia.[68] However, randomized studies to date fail to show major benefits of low intraoperative tidal volume strategies and a consensus is lacking.[11,66,69]

The use of positive end-expiratory pressure (PEEP) is generally a safe strategy that reduces the incidence and severity of atelectasis.[70–72] A Cochrane review of the use of intraoperative PEEP showed significant improvement in postoperative P/F ratios (PaO_2/FiO_2, the ratio of arterial oxygen concentration to the fraction of inspired oxygen) and reduced atelectasis.[58] Intraoperative recruitment maneuvers, such as the vital capacity maneuver whereby lungs are inflated to 40 cm H_2O for 15 seconds, can also reduce atelectasis.[73–75]

Fluids and Transfusion

There is good evidence that patients with ARDS benefit from restrictive fluid management, and patients undergoing major abdominal surgery may also benefit from a similar strategy.[76,77] However, the role of restrictive fluid strategies in preventing PPCs is not well studied. In a recent, large retrospective database analysis, higher amounts of intraoperative crystalloid infusion were a risk factor for developing ARDS.[12] A volume of 1.5 L has been proposed as the threshold above which postoperative ALI is significantly increased.[78]

Emergency surgery is a known risk for PPCs, and although blood transfusions are frequently unavoidable in emergencies, they are also associated with adverse outcomes including increased PPCs.[79,80] Specifically, patients who receive more than 4 units before surgery are at increased risk of PCCs.[81]

Nutrition

Low serum albumin level is an established risk factor for PPCs.[12,19,25,28] Preoperative protein depletion is associated with altered pulmonary dynamics and respiratory muscle function, which leads to a higher rate of pneumonia.[82] Weight loss of greater than 10% in the past 6 months is also an independent risk factor for PPCs.[81]

Despite the strong correlation between poor nutrition and an increased risk of PPCs, there is minimal evidence that routine total parenteral nutrition (TPN) modifies this risk; in fact, the use of TPN may increase complications.[27]

Deep Venous Thrombosis Prophylaxis

Pulmonary embolism (PE) is a rare but potentially fatal complication of surgery. More than 95% of PEs arise from deep venous thrombosis (DVT) of leg veins[83]; thus, prevention of PE is primarily aimed at prevention of DVT. Another article in this issue focuses entirely on this topic; however, given the high morbidity associated with pulmonary emboli, a brief discussion of venous thromboembolism and preventative measures are included here.

Surgery predisposes patients to DVT by several mechanisms, including immobilization, proinflammatory states, and preexisting disease. Cancer increases the risk of venous thromboembolism 7-fold.[84]

The American College of Chest Physicians guidelines recommend the following[85,86]:

- Patients undergoing moderate- or high-risk surgery should receive low-molecular-weight heparin or low-dose unfractionated heparin.
- Patients at high risk for bleeding should receive mechanical prophylaxis with intermittent pneumatic compression.
- Aspirin alone is inadequate to prevent DVT.

Warfarin is effective for DVT prophylaxis; however, it is often contraindicated in surgical patients because of its long half-life and increased risk of bleeding.[87] Not enough data exist to comment on the use of newer anticoagulant agents. Inferior vena cava filters reduce the incidence of pulmonary emboli but do not necessarily reduce mortality and are not routinely recommended for primary prevention.[85,88]

Nursing Interventions, Physiotherapy, and Pulmonary Rehabilitation

Deep breathing exercise, postural drainage, and pulmonary physiotherapy are simple exercises that pose minimal risk. However, there are limited data to suggest these measures significantly prevent PPCs. Some studies suggest that preoperative physiotherapy and pulmonary rehabilitation may preserve pulmonary function postoperatively, particularly in patients with COPD.[89] Chest physiotherapy might reduce PPCs in obese patients undergoing abdominal surgery.[90]

Spirometry is a simple and inexpensive intervention; however, it has not been proven to effectively prevent PPCs. A 2014 Cochrane review found no significant benefit of spirometry in the prevention of PPCs.[91,92] There is a lack of randomized control trials addressing this topic.

Noninvasive Ventilation

Minor reductions in PPCs have been observed with routine use of postoperative PAP. Several studies have demonstrated the role of continuous positive airway pressure (CPAP) in reducing atelectasis.[72,77] A recent meta-analysis of randomized control trials demonstrated that noninvasive ventilation reduces postoperative pneumonia and reintubation rates and may influence survival.[93]

Certain subgroups of patients benefit from PAP more than others. The severely obese and those with OSA have reduced rates of PPCs with the use of PAP therapy.[94,95] PAP should be continued postoperatively in anyone who used it before surgery and should be used as a rescue tactic in patients who experience postoperative respiratory distress.[29]

HIGH-RISK POPULATIONS

Patient-related factors pose additional risks for development of PPCs. Certain groups should be given careful consideration before any operation. The following is a discussion of these groups and management strategies that may reduce risk.

Obesity

Obesity is a disease of increasing prevalence worldwide and is associated with a spectrum of multisystem cormorbidities.[96,97] Particular to pulmonary physiology, obese patients have preexisting ventilation-perfusion mismatch due to underventilated and overperfused dependent lung tissue.[98] Increased lung blood volume and reduced chest wall compliance secondary to fat accumulation around the muscles of respiration reduces overall lung compliance.[98] On pulmonary function testing, obese patients have reduced FRC, forced vital capacity (FVC), and FEV_1 and are thus more prone to develop hypoxia in periods of apnea.[96,98]

Postoperatively, obese patients are more difficult to mobilize[98] and are at higher risk of venous thromboembolism.[96,99] Up to 30% of deaths in bariatric patients result from PE.[100] Although prevention of venous thromboembolism postoperatively is crucial, currently there is not enough evidence to recommend routine preoperative chemoprophylaxis.[101]

The mainstay of preoperative intervention for obesity is weight loss. Obese patients who decrease their weight by as little as 10% to 15% preoperatively can reduce the severity of sleep apnea by up to 50% and therefore reduce the risk of other PPCs.[102,103]

Obstructive Sleep Apnea

Although OSA is often related to obesity, it is also an independent risk factor for PPCs and is associated with other conditions that may affect overall perioperative performance.[1,104,105] Specifically, OSA is associated with hypoxemia and ARDS.[104,106–108] In a large national inpatient analysis by Memtsoudis and colleagues,[104] general surgical patients with OSA experienced significantly higher rates of ARDS as well as aspiration pneumonia, reintubation, and mechanical ventilation than matched controls. Preoperative optimization of OSA patients centers around 2 main components: disease identification and maximization of PAP therapy.

The true incidence of OSA is unknown; 3.2% of patients are diagnosed with the disease, but as many as 24% may be undiagnosed, and even those with known disease are often undertreated.[18,109,110] Patients who use CPAP preoperatively should be encouraged to continue it before surgery.[52]

Polysomnography remains the gold standard for diagnosis but may be difficult to obtain preoperatively. A thorough history can identify symptoms of daytime sleepiness, snoring, and partner-witnessed apnea episodes, all of which are associated with OSA. Physical examination findings might include a short, thick neck and obesity. In addition, questionnaires such as the Berlin, STOP (Snore-Tired-Obstruction-Pressure), and STOP-BANG (Snore-Tired-Obstruction-Pressure-BMI-Age-Neck-Gender) surveys can be useful for screening and diagnosis.[111,112]

Intraoperatively, several techniques have been shown to improve outcomes in patients with OSA. The pharyngeal dysfunction of OSA predisposes to higher rates of aspiration pneumonia; this can be partially countered by the use of short-acting neuromuscular blockers and acid-reducing medications.[104,113,114] General anesthesia should be avoided when possible, and shorter operative times lead to better outcomes.[115] In the setting of a general anesthetic, patients with OSA should be extubated fully awake and sitting upright to prevent airway obstruction.[115]

Postoperatively, OSA carries significant risk of hypoxemia and overall complications; this underscores the importance of immediate PAP therapy.[116,117] Opioids should be avoided when possible given the increased risk of respiratory depression. OSA patients may benefit from multimodal analgesia.[52]

Obesity Hypoventilation Syndrome (Pickwickian Syndrome)

OHS is characterized by a triad of obesity, daytime hypoventilation ($Paco_2 \geq 45$ and $Pao_2 \leq 70$), and sleep-disordered breathing without alternate cause.[29,118] OHS is distinct from obesity and OSA. The estimated prevalence is 0.15% to 0.3% of the general adult population and 10% to 20% of obese patients with OSA; however, it is likely underdiagnosed.[29,119,120] The vast majority of patients with OHS also suffer from OSA.[29]

OHS poses a greater risk for several disease states including PH.[29] When compared with obese patients without hypercapnia, patients with OHS have greater morbidity from cardiac causes as well as a higher overall mortality.[29,121,122]

Although the evidence is not strong, there may be benefits of postoperative PAP therapy for OHS.[94,95] Treatment with PAP for a period as short as 5 days can improve hypoventilation and sleep-disordered breathing in patients with OHS and should be considered preoperatively.[123] PAP therapy may even lower mortality in OHS.[29]

Asthma

Patients with well-controlled asthma tend to have normal levels in PFTs and arterial blood gas measurements and are not at risk for major PPCs.[19] However, patients with asthma with poor preoperative symptom control are at increased risk of minor complications, such as bronchospasm.[13,38,124]

Preoperative history should include medication review as well as the frequency and stimuli of attacks. An adjunct to preoperative examination is the forced expiratory time (FET), which is assessed by auscultation during expiration. FET values greater than 6 seconds correlate with abnormal FEV_1/FVC ratios and should prompt further investigations.[125] A patient's primary care physician can help optimize medications, and their involvement preoperatively is recommended. Patients should be advised to cease smoking at least 8 weeks before surgery, and certain patients may benefit from a brief course of corticosteroids.[126,127] Patients with asthma may also benefit from an increase in bronchodilator dosage preoperatively.[124]

Intraoperative measures to maximize management of patients with asthma include the following[125]:

- Careful intubation technique to prevent laryngeal spasm and edema
- Intubation and extubation in deep anesthesia
- Avoidance of drugs that may induce mast cell histamine release
- Use of volatile intravenous anesthetic drugs that promote bronchodilation
- Avoidance of anticholinesterase drugs

Postoperatively, adequate analgesia, bronchodilator administration, early mobilization, acid reflux prevention, and incentive spirometry are recommended.[19,27,128]

Chronic Obstructive Pulmonary Disease

Patients with COPD have an unambiguously increased perioperative risk for complications, and COPD is perhaps the most frequently cited risk factor for PPCs.[3,13,18] The incidence of PPCs may be as high as 18% among patients with COPD undergoing general surgery operations, and the risk increases with disease severity.[13,18] If possible, surgery should be delayed in patients who present preoperatively with an acute exacerbation.

Empiric antibiotics are not indicated in COPD, but all patients should be screened for acute exacerbations and those with increased secretions should receive a short course of oral antibiotics.[18,129] In cases of persistent symptoms, corticosteroids should also be considered.[130] Preoperative pulmonary rehabilitation with muscle training improves muscle fiber remodeling as well as overall perioperative pulmonary function.[89,131]

Bronchodilator therapy should be maintained throughout the perioperative period in patients with COPD, as their daily use maintains postoperative respiratory function.[132,133] Other measures to reduce PPCs in patients with COPD are similar to those in patients with asthma; avoid airway trauma and medications that may induce bronchospasm.

Pulmonary Hypertension

PH is defined by the World Health Organization as a mean pulmonary artery pressure greater than 25 mm Hg at rest or greater than 30 mm Hg during exercise. Patients with PH are unable to accommodate for physiologic alterations in preload and afterload that occur during surgery and are at greater risk for PPCs.[36] Patients with PH have an increased risk of overall morbidity and mortality when undergoing noncardiac surgery.[134,135] Specifically, the risk of respiratory failure is more common in patients with PH and is the most frequent complication.[24,135]

Perioperative management is focused on prevention of systemic hypotension and acute elevations in pulmonary artery pressure, both of which can be detrimental to the right ventricle.[36] Patients with PH require careful monitoring both during and after an operation.

Smoking

Smokers who undergo noncardiac surgery experience up to a 4-fold increase in PPCs compared with nonsmokers.[32] The rate of PPCs in smokers varies somewhat related to the underlying condition of the lung. Smokers with normal spirometry have only a

4% risk of PPCs, whereas in heavy smokers this rate is as high as 43%.[136,137] Smokers are also more likely to develop pneumonia, fail to wean from a ventilator, require reintubation, and have a higher overall mortality after major surgery.[138]

Smoking impairs tracheobronchial clearance by damaging cilia and increasing mucous secretion and consistency.[139] It also increases the susceptibility to alveolar collapse, leading to increased rates of infection and prolonged mechanical ventilation.[140] Smokers are nearly twice as likely to develop specific respiratory complications such as reintubation, bronchospasm, laryngospasm, aspiration, and hypoxemia when compared with nonsmokers.[141]

Smoking cessation decreases the risk for PPCs by 20%[142] and is particularly important for patients with COPD.[53,132] The benefit of smoking cessation depends on the extent of life-time smoking, length of abstinence, and age at the time of cessation.[2] A review of smoking cessation found an overall postoperative complication risk reduction of 41%; this risk reduction was improved with each additional week of cessation.[142]

A transient increase in sputum production may actually increase risk for PPCs in the first several weeks after smoking cessation.[143–146] Therefore, abstinence should be recommended for a period of at least 4 weeks preoperatively to be beneficial.[147–150]

After smoking cessation, physiologic recovery is as follows[139]:

1 Week—ciliary activity recovers
2 Weeks—airway reactivity is reduced
6 Weeks—sputum volume returns to normal
3 Months—tracheobronchial clearance begins to return to normal
6 Months—marked improvement in small airway narrowing is noted

Smoking cessation 8 weeks before surgery may reduce the risk of PPCs to that of nonsmokers.[61,151]

SUMMARY

PPCs occur frequently among general surgical patients. The spectrum of illness is broad and includes preventable causes of morbidity and death. Careful preoperative evaluation can identify undiagnosed and undertreated illness and allow for preoperative intervention. Optimization of patient, surgical, and anesthetic factors are crucial in the prevention of PPCs.

REFERENCES

1. Canet J, Gallart L. Predicting postoperative pulmonary complications in the general population. Curr Opin Anaesthesiol 2013;26(2):107–15.
2. Canet J, Mazo V. Postoperative pulmonary complications. Minerva Anestesiol 2010;76(2):138–43.
3. Canet J, Gallart L, Gomar C, et al. Prediction of postoperative pulmonary complications in a population-based surgical cohort. Anesthesiology 2010;113(6):1338–50.
4. Smetana GW. Postoperative pulmonary complications: an update on risk assessment and reduction. Cleve Clin J Med 2009;76(Suppl 4):S60–5.
5. Shander A, Fleisher LA, Barie PS, et al. Clinical and economic burden of postoperative pulmonary complications: patient safety summit on definition, risk-reducing interventions, and preventive strategies. Crit Care Med 2011;39(9):2163–72.

6. Thompson DA, Makary MA, Dorman T, et al. Clinical and economic outcomes of hospital acquired pneumonia in intra-abdominal surgery patients. Ann Surg 2006;243(4):547–52.
7. Manku K, Bacchetti P, Leung JM. Prognostic significance of postoperative in-hospital complications in elderly patients. I. Long-term survival. Anesth Analg 2003;96(2):583–9 Table of contents.
8. Sweitzer BJ, Smetana GW. Identification and evaluation of the patient with lung disease. Anesthesiol Clin 2009;27(4):673–86.
9. Coussa M, Proietti S, Schnyder P, et al. Prevention of atelectasis formation during the induction of general anesthesia in morbidly obese patients. Anesth Analg 2004;98(5):1491–5 Table of contents.
10. Sachdev G, Napolitano LM. Postoperative pulmonary complications: pneumonia and acute respiratory failure. Surg Clin North Am 2012;92(2):321–44, ix.
11. Fernandez-Perez ER, Sprung J, Afessa B, et al. Intraoperative ventilator settings and acute lung injury after elective surgery: a nested case control study. Thorax 2009;64(2):121–7.
12. Blum JM, Stentz MJ, Dechert R, et al. Preoperative and intraoperative predictors of postoperative acute respiratory distress syndrome in a general surgical population. Anesthesiology 2013;118(1):19–29.
13. Smetana GW, Lawrence VA, Cornell JE, American College of Physicians. Preoperative pulmonary risk stratification for noncardiothoracic surgery: systematic review for the American College of Physicians. Ann Intern Med 2006;144(8): 581–95.
14. Bapoje SR, Whitaker JF, Schulz T, et al. Preoperative evaluation of the patient with pulmonary disease. Chest 2007;132(5):1637–45.
15. Arozullah AM, Daley J, Henderson WG, et al. Multifactorial risk index for predicting postoperative respiratory failure in men after major noncardiac surgery. The National Veterans Administration Surgical Quality Improvement Program. Ann Surg 2000;232(2):242–53.
16. Arozullah AM, Khuri SF, Henderson WG, et al. Participants in the National Veterans Affairs Surgical Quality Improvement Program. Development and validation of a multifactorial risk index for predicting postoperative pneumonia after major noncardiac surgery. Ann Intern Med 2001;135(10):847–57.
17. Sheer AJ, Heckman JE, Schneider EB, et al. Congestive heart failure and chronic obstructive pulmonary disease predict poor surgical outcomes in older adults undergoing elective diverticulitis surgery. Dis Colon Rectum 2011;54(11): 1430–7.
18. Cook MW, Lisco SJ. Prevention of postoperative pulmonary complications. Int Anesthesiol Clin 2009;47(4):65–88.
19. Qaseem A, Snow V, Fitterman N, et al. Risk assessment for and strategies to reduce perioperative pulmonary complications for patients undergoing noncardiothoracic surgery: a guideline from the American College of Physicians. Ann Intern Med 2006;144(8):575–80.
20. Gupta H, Gupta PK, Fang X, et al. Development and validation of a risk calculator predicting postoperative respiratory failure. Chest 2011;140(5):1207–15.
21. Dronkers JJ, Chorus AM, van Meeteren NL, et al. The association of preoperative physical fitness and physical activity with outcome after scheduled major abdominal surgery. Anaesthesia 2013;68(1):67–73.
22. Mitchell CK, Smoger SH, Pfeifer MP, et al. Multivariate analysis of factors associated with postoperative pulmonary complications following general elective surgery. Arch Surg 1998;133(2):194–8.

23. Barisione G, Rovida S, Gazzaniga GM, et al. Upper abdominal surgery: does a lung function test exist to predict early severe postoperative respiratory complications? Eur Respir J 1997;10(6):1301–8.
24. Ramachandran SK, Nafiu OO, Ghaferi A, et al. Independent predictors and outcomes of unanticipated early postoperative tracheal intubation after nonemergent, noncardiac surgery. Anesthesiology 2011;115(1):44–53.
25. Gupta PK, Franck C, Miller WJ, et al. Development and validation of a bariatric surgery morbidity risk calculator using the prospective, multicenter NSQIP dataset. J Am Coll Surg 2011;212(3):301–9.
26. McAlister FA, Bertsch K, Man J, et al. Incidence of and risk factors for pulmonary complications after nonthoracic surgery. Am J Respir Crit Care Med 2005; 171(5):514–7.
27. Lawrence VA, Cornell JE, Smetana GW, American College of Physicians. Strategies to reduce postoperative pulmonary complications after noncardiothoracic surgery: systematic review for the American College of Physicians. Ann Intern Med 2006;144(8):596–608.
28. Gibbs J, Cull W, Henderson W, et al. Preoperative serum albumin level as a predictor of operative mortality and morbidity: results from the National VA Surgical Risk Study. Arch Surg 1999;134(1):36–42.
29. Chau EH, Lam D, Wong J, et al. Obesity hypoventilation syndrome: a review of epidemiology, pathophysiology, and perioperative considerations. Anesthesiology 2012;117(1):188–205.
30. Budweiser S, Riedl SG, Jorres RA, et al. Mortality and prognostic factors in patients with obesity-hypoventilation syndrome undergoing noninvasive ventilation. J Intern Med 2007;261(4):375–83.
31. Priou P, Hamel JF, Person C, et al. Long-term outcome of noninvasive positive pressure ventilation for obesity hypoventilation syndrome. Chest 2010;138(1): 84–90.
32. Bluman LG, Mosca L, Newman N, et al. Preoperative smoking habits and postoperative pulmonary complications. Chest 1998;113(4):883–9.
33. Lawrence VA, Dhanda R, Hilsenbeck SG, et al. Risk of pulmonary complications after elective abdominal surgery. Chest 1996;110(3):744–50.
34. Beckles MA, Spiro SG, Colice GL, et al, American College of Chest Physicians. The physiologic evaluation of patients with lung cancer being considered for resectional surgery. Chest 2003;123(1 Suppl):105S–14S.
35. Fuso L, Cisternino L, Di Napoli A, et al. Role of spirometric and arterial gas data in predicting pulmonary complications after abdominal surgery. Respir Med 2000;94(12):1171–6.
36. Minai OA, Yared JP, Kaw R, et al. Perioperative risk and management in patients with pulmonary hypertension. Chest 2013;144(1):329–40.
37. Ford GT, Grant DA, Rideout KS, et al. Inhibition of breathing associated with gallbladder stimulation in dogs. J Appl Physiol (1985) 1988;65(1):72–9.
38. Warner DO. Preventing postoperative pulmonary complications: the role of the anesthesiologist. Anesthesiology 2000;92(5):1467–72.
39. Garcia-Miguel FJ, Serrano-Aguilar PG, Lopez-Bastida J. Preoperative assessment. Lancet 2003;362(9397):1749–57.
40. Brown SR, Goodfellow PB. Transverse verses midline incisions for abdominal surgery. Cochrane Database Syst Rev 2005;(4):CD005199.
41. Weller WE, Rosati C. Comparing outcomes of laparoscopic versus open bariatric surgery. Ann Surg 2008;248(1):10–5.

42. Briez N, Piessen G, Torres F, et al. Effects of hybrid minimally invasive oesophagectomy on major postoperative pulmonary complications. Br J Surg 2012; 99(11):1547–53.
43. Walder B, Schafer M, Henzi I, et al. Efficacy and safety of patient-controlled opioid analgesia for acute postoperative pain. A quantitative systematic review. Acta Anaesthesiol Scand 2001;45(7):795–804.
44. Pansard JL, Mankikian B, Bertrand M, et al. Effects of thoracic extradural block on diaphragmatic electrical activity and contractility after upper abdominal surgery. Anesthesiology 1993;78(1):63–71.
45. Popping DM, Elia N, Marret E, et al. Protective effects of epidural analgesia on pulmonary complications after abdominal and thoracic surgery: a meta-analysis. Arch Surg 2008;143(10):990–9 [discussion: 1000].
46. Mauermann WJ, Shilling AM, Zuo Z. A comparison of neuraxial block versus general anesthesia for elective total hip replacement: a meta-analysis. Anesth Analg 2006;103(4):1018–25.
47. Neuman MD, Silber JH, Elkassabany NM, et al. Comparative effectiveness of regional versus general anesthesia for hip fracture surgery in adults. Anesthesiology 2012;117(1):72–92.
48. Jayr C, Thomas H, Rey A, et al. Postoperative pulmonary complications. Epidural analgesia using bupivacaine and opioids versus parenteral opioids. Anesthesiology 1993;78(4):666–76 [discussion: 22A].
49. Urwin SC, Parker MJ, Griffiths R. General versus regional anaesthesia for hip fracture surgery: a meta-analysis of randomized trials. Br J Anaesth 2000; 84(4):450–5.
50. Park WY, Thompson JS, Lee KK. Effect of epidural anesthesia and analgesia on perioperative outcome: a randomized, controlled Veterans Affairs cooperative study. Ann Surg 2001;234(4):560–9 [discussion: 569–71].
51. Liu SS, Wu CL. Effect of postoperative analgesia on major postoperative complications: a systematic update of the evidence. Anesth Analg 2007;104(3): 689–702.
52. Gross JB, Bachenberg KL, Benumof JL, et al. Practice guidelines for the perioperative management of patients with obstructive sleep apnea: a report by the American Society of Anesthesiologists Task Force on perioperative management of patients with obstructive sleep apnea. Anesthesiology 2006;104(5): 1081–93 [quiz: 1117–88].
53. Rock P, Rich PB. Postoperative pulmonary complications. Curr Opin Anaesthesiol 2003;16(2):123–31.
54. Wahba RW. Perioperative functional residual capacity. Can J Anaesth 1991; 38(3):384–400.
55. Lundquist H, Hedenstierna G, Strandberg A, et al. CT-assessment of dependent lung densities in man during general anaesthesia. Acta Radiol 1995;36(6): 626–32.
56. Tokics L, Hedenstierna G, Strandberg A, et al. Lung collapse and gas exchange during general anesthesia: effects of spontaneous breathing, muscle paralysis, and positive end-expiratory pressure. Anesthesiology 1987;66(2):157–67.
57. Hedley-Whyte J, Laver MB, Bendixen HH. Effect of changes in tidal ventilation on physiologic shunting. Am J Physiol 1964;206:891–7.
58. Imberger G, McIlroy D, Pace NL, et al. Positive end-expiratory pressure (PEEP) during anaesthesia for the prevention of mortality and postoperative pulmonary complications. Cochrane Database Syst Rev 2010;(9):CD007922.

59. Warner DO, Warner MA. Human chest wall function while awake and during halothane anesthesia. II. Carbon dioxide rebreathing. Anesthesiology 1995; 82(1):20–31.
60. Grosse-Sundrup M, Henneman JP, Sandberg WS, et al. Intermediate acting non-depolarizing neuromuscular blocking agents and risk of postoperative respiratory complications: prospective propensity score matched cohort study. BMJ 2012;345:e6329.
61. Guldner A, Pelosi P, de Abreu MG. Nonventilatory strategies to prevent postoperative pulmonary complications. Curr Opin Anaesthesiol 2013;26(2):141–51.
62. Murphy GS, Brull SJ. Residual neuromuscular block: lessons unlearned. Part I: definitions, incidence, and adverse physiologic effects of residual neuromuscular block. Anesth Analg 2010;111(1):120–8.
63. Segredo V, Caldwell JE, Matthay MA, et al. Persistent paralysis in critically ill patients after long-term administration of vecuronium. N Engl J Med 1992;327(8): 524–8.
64. Berg H, Roed J, Viby-Mogensen J, et al. Residual neuromuscular block is a risk factor for postoperative pulmonary complications. A prospective, randomised, and blinded study of postoperative pulmonary complications after atracurium, vecuronium and pancuronium. Acta Anaesthesiol Scand 1997;41(9): 1095–103.
65. The Acute Respiratory Distress Syndrome Network. Ventilation with Lower Tidal Volumes as Compared with Traditional Tidal Volumes for Acute Lung Injury and the Acute Respiratory Distress Syndrome. N Engl J Med 2000;342:1301–8.
66. Schultz MJ, Haitsma JJ, Slutsky AS, et al. What tidal volumes should be used in patients without acute lung injury? Anesthesiology 2007;106(6):1226–31.
67. Michelet P, D'Journo XB, Roch A, et al. Protective ventilation influences systemic inflammation after esophagectomy: a randomized controlled study. Anesthesiology 2006;105(5):911–9.
68. Lee PC, Helsmoortel CM, Cohn SM, et al. Are low tidal volumes safe? Chest 1990;97(2):430–4.
69. Wrigge H, Zinserling J, Stuber F, et al. Effects of mechanical ventilation on release of cytokines into systemic circulation in patients with normal pulmonary function. Anesthesiology 2000;93(6):1413–7.
70. Pelosi P, Ravagnan I, Giurati G, et al. Positive end-expiratory pressure improves respiratory function in obese but not in normal subjects during anesthesia and paralysis. Anesthesiology 1999;91(5):1221–31.
71. Hedenstierna G. Oxygen and anesthesia: what lung do we deliver to the postoperative ward? Acta Anaesthesiol Scand 2012;56(6):675–85.
72. Rusca M, Proietti S, Schnyder P, et al. Prevention of atelectasis formation during induction of general anesthesia. Anesth Analg 2003;97(6):1835–9.
73. Magnusson L, Spahn DR. New concepts of atelectasis during general anaesthesia. Br J Anaesth 2003;91(1):61–72.
74. Rothen HU, Sporre B, Engberg G, et al. Re-expansion of atelectasis during general anaesthesia: a computed tomography study. Br J Anaesth 1993;71(6):788–95.
75. Rothen HU, Neumann P, Berglund JE, et al. Dynamics of re-expansion of atelectasis during general anaesthesia. Br J Anaesth 1999;82(4):551–6.
76. National Heart Lung, Blood Institute Acute Respiratory Distress Syndrome Clinical Trials Network, Wiedemann HP, et al. Comparison of two fluid-management strategies in acute lung injury. N Engl J Med 2006;354(24):2564–75.
77. Doherty M, Buggy DJ. Intraoperative fluids: how much is too much? Br J Anaesth 2012;109(1):69–79.

78. Evans RG, Naidu B. Does a conservative fluid management strategy in the perioperative management of lung resection patients reduce the risk of acute lung injury? Interact Cardiovasc Thorac Surg 2012;15(3):498–504.
79. Atzil S, Arad M, Glasner A, et al. Blood transfusion promotes cancer progression: a critical role for aged erythrocytes. Anesthesiology 2008;109(6):989–97.
80. Spahn DR, Shander A, Hofmann A, et al. More on transfusion and adverse outcome: it's time to change. Anesthesiology 2011;114(2):234–6.
81. Arozullah AM, Khuri SF, Henderson WG, et al, Participants in the National Veterans Affairs Surgical Quality Improvement Program. Development and validation of a multifactorial risk index for predicting postoperative pneumonia after major noncardiac surgery. Ann Intern Med 2001;135(10):847–57.
82. Windsor JA, Hill GL. Risk factors for postoperative pneumonia. The importance of protein depletion. Ann Surg 1988;208(2):209–14.
83. Hall D. Perioperative pulmonary embolism: detection, treatment, and outcomes. Am J Ther 2013;20(1):67–72.
84. Blom JW, Doggen CJ, Osanto S, et al. Malignancies, prothrombotic mutations, and the risk of venous thrombosis. JAMA 2005;293(6):715–22.
85. Gould MK, Garcia DA, Wren SM, et al. Prevention of VTE in nonorthopedic surgical patients: Antithrombotic Therapy and Prevention of Thrombosis, 9th ed: American College of Chest Physicians Evidence-Based Clinical Practice Guidelines. Chest 2012;141(2 Suppl):e227S–77S.
86. Geerts WH, Bergqvist D, Pineo GF, et al. Prevention of venous thromboembolism: American College of Chest Physicians Evidence-Based Clinical Practice Guidelines (8th Edition). Chest 2008;133(6 Suppl):381S–453S.
87. Stanley A, Young A. Primary prevention of venous thromboembolism in medical and surgical oncology patients. Br J Cancer 2010;102(Suppl 1):S10–6.
88. Young T, Tang H, Hughes R. Vena caval filters for the prevention of pulmonary embolism. Cochrane Database Syst Rev 2010;(2):CD006212.
89. Nagarajan K, Bennett A, Agostini P, et al. Is preoperative physiotherapy/pulmonary rehabilitation beneficial in lung resection patients? Interact Cardiovasc Thorac Surg 2011;13(3):300–2.
90. Dindo D, Muller MK, Weber M, et al. Obesity in general elective surgery. Lancet 2003;361(9374):2032–5.
91. do Nascimento P Jr, Modolo NS, Andrade S, et al. Incentive spirometry for prevention of postoperative pulmonary complications in upper abdominal surgery. Cochrane Database Syst Rev 2014;(2):CD006058.
92. Guimaraes MM, El Dib R, Smith AF, et al. Incentive spirometry for prevention of postoperative pulmonary complications in upper abdominal surgery. Cochrane Database Syst Rev 2009;(3):CD006058.
93. Glossop AJ, Shephard N, Bryden DC, et al. Non-invasive ventilation for weaning, avoiding reintubation after extubation and in the postoperative period: a meta-analysis. Br J Anaesth 2012;109(3):305–14.
94. Rennotte MT, Baele P, Aubert G, et al. Nasal continuous positive airway pressure in the perioperative management of patients with obstructive sleep apnea submitted to surgery. Chest 1995;107(2):367–74.
95. El-Solh AA, Aquilina A, Pineda L, et al. Noninvasive ventilation for prevention of post-extubation respiratory failure in obese patients. Eur Respir J 2006;28(3):588–95.
96. Adams JP, Murphy PG. Obesity in anaesthesia and intensive care. Br J Anaesth 2000;85(1):91–108.
97. Bjorntorp P. Obesity. Lancet 1997;350(9075):423–6.

98. Hans GA, Lauwick S, Kaba A, et al. Postoperative respiratory problems in morbidly obese patients. Acta Anaesthesiol Belg 2009;60(3):169–75.
99. Clayton JK, Anderson JA, McNicol GP. Preoperative prediction of postoperative deep vein thrombosis. Br Med J 1976;2(6041):910–2.
100. DeMaria EJ, Murr M, Byrne TK, et al. Validation of the obesity surgery mortality risk score in a multicenter study proves it stratifies mortality risk in patients undergoing gastric bypass for morbid obesity. Ann Surg 2007;246(4):578–82 [discussion: 583–4].
101. American Society for Metabolic and Bariatric Surgery Clinical Issues Committee. ASMBS updated position statement on prophylactic measures to reduce the risk of venous thromboembolism in bariatric surgery patients. Surg Obes Relat Dis 2013;9(4):493–7.
102. Schwartz AR, Gold AR, Schubert N, et al. Effect of weight loss on upper airway collapsibility in obstructive sleep apnea. Am Rev Respir Dis 1991;144(3 Pt 1): 494–8.
103. Smith PL, Gold AR, Meyers DA, et al. Weight loss in mildly to moderately obese patients with obstructive sleep apnea. Ann Intern Med 1985;103(6 (Pt 1)): 850–5.
104. Memtsoudis S, Liu SS, Ma Y, et al. Perioperative pulmonary outcomes in patients with sleep apnea after noncardiac surgery. Anesth Analg 2011;112(1): 113–21.
105. Mador MJ, Goplani S, Gottumukkala VA, et al. Postoperative complications in obstructive sleep apnea. Sleep Breath 2013;17(2):727–34.
106. Liao P, Yegneswaran B, Vairavanathan S, et al. Postoperative complications in patients with obstructive sleep apnea: a retrospective matched cohort study. Can J Anaesth 2009;56(11):819–28.
107. Gali B, Whalen FX, Schroeder DR, et al. Identification of patients at risk for postoperative respiratory complications using a preoperative obstructive sleep apnea screening tool and postanesthesia care assessment. Anesthesiology 2009;110(4):869–77.
108. Hwang D, Shakir N, Limann B, et al. Association of sleep-disordered breathing with postoperative complications. Chest 2008;133(5):1128–34.
109. Chung F, Ward B, Ho J, et al. Preoperative identification of sleep apnea risk in elective surgical patients, using the Berlin questionnaire. J Clin Anesth 2007; 19(2):130–4.
110. Fidan H, Fidan F, Unlu M, et al. Prevalence of sleep apnoea in patients undergoing operation. Sleep Breath 2006;10(3):161–5.
111. Bhateja P, Kaw R. Emerging risk factors and prevention of perioperative pulmonary complications. ScientificWorldJournal 2014;2014:546758.
112. Abrishami A, Khajehdehi A, Chung F. A systematic review of screening questionnaires for obstructive sleep apnea. Can J Anaesth 2010;57(5):423–38.
113. Beal M, Chesson A, Garcia T, et al. A pilot study of quantitative aspiration in patients with symptoms of obstructive sleep apnea: comparison to a historic control group. Laryngoscope 2004;114(6):965–8.
114. Valipour A, Makker HK, Hardy R, et al. Symptomatic gastroesophageal reflux in subjects with a breathing sleep disorder. Chest 2002;121(6):1748–53.
115. Vasu TS, Grewal R, Doghramji K. Obstructive sleep apnea syndrome and perioperative complications: a systematic review of the literature. J Clin Sleep Med 2012;8(2):199–207.
116. Kaw R, Pasupuleti V, Walker E, et al. Postoperative complications in patients with obstructive sleep apnea. Chest 2012;141(2):436–41.

117. Kaw R, Chung F, Pasupuleti V, et al. Meta-analysis of the association between obstructive sleep apnoea and postoperative outcome. Br J Anaesth 2012; 109(6):897–906.
118. Olson AL, Zwillich C. The obesity hypoventilation syndrome. Am J Med 2005; 118(9):948–56.
119. Mokhlesi B. Obesity hypoventilation syndrome: a state-of-the-art review. Respir Care 2010;55(10):1347–62 [discussion: 1363–5].
120. Kessler R, Chaouat A, Schinkewitch P, et al. The obesity-hypoventilation syndrome revisited: a prospective study of 34 consecutive cases. Chest 2001; 120(2):369–76.
121. Berg G, Delaive K, Manfreda J, et al. The use of health-care resources in obesity-hypoventilation syndrome. Chest 2001;120(2):377–83.
122. Nowbar S, Burkart KM, Gonzales R, et al. Obesity-associated hypoventilation in hospitalized patients: prevalence, effects, and outcome. Am J Med 2004; 116(1):1–7.
123. Chouri-Pontarollo N, Borel JC, Tamisier R, et al. Impaired objective daytime vigilance in obesity-hypoventilation syndrome: impact of noninvasive ventilation. Chest 2007;131(1):148–55.
124. Warner DO, Warner MA, Barnes RD, et al. Perioperative respiratory complications in patients with asthma. Anesthesiology 1996;85(3):460–7.
125. Woods BD, Sladen RN. Perioperative considerations for the patient with asthma and bronchospasm. Br J Anaesth 2009;103(Suppl 1):i57–65.
126. Smetana GW, Conde MV. Preoperative pulmonary update. Clin Geriatr Med 2008;24(4):607–24, vii.
127. Silvanus MT, Groeben H, Peters J. Corticosteroids and inhaled salbutamol in patients with reversible airway obstruction markedly decrease the incidence of bronchospasm after tracheal intubation. Anesthesiology 2004;100(5):1052–7.
128. Harding SM. Gastroesophageal reflux: a potential asthma trigger. Immunol Allergy Clin N Am 2005;25(1):131–48.
129. Hong CM, Galvagno SM Jr. Patients with chronic pulmonary disease. Med Clin North Am 2013;97(6):1095–107.
130. Smetana GW. A 68-year-old man with COPD contemplating colon cancer surgery. JAMA 2007;297(19):2121–30.
131. Vogiatzis I, Terzis G, Stratakos G, et al. Effect of pulmonary rehabilitation on peripheral muscle fiber remodeling in patients with COPD in GOLD stages II to IV. Chest 2011;140(3):744–52.
132. Mandra A, Simic D, Stevanovic V, et al. Preoperative considerations for patients with chronic obstructive pulmonary disease. Acta Chir Iugosl 2011;58(2):71–5.
133. Suzuki H, Sekine Y, Yoshida S, et al. Efficacy of perioperative administration of long-acting bronchodilator on postoperative pulmonary function and quality of life in lung cancer patients with chronic obstructive pulmonary disease. Preliminary results of a randomized control study. Surg Today 2010;40(10):923–30.
134. Kaw R, Pasupuleti V, Deshpande A, et al. Pulmonary hypertension: an important predictor of outcomes in patients undergoing non-cardiac surgery. Respir Med 2011;105(4):619–24.
135. Lai HC, Lai HC, Wang KY, et al. Severe pulmonary hypertension complicates postoperative outcome of non-cardiac surgery. Br J Anaesth 2007;99(2): 184–90.
136. Chalon S, Moreno H Jr, Benowitz NL, et al. Nicotine impairs endothelium-dependent dilatation in human veins in vivo. Clin Pharmacol Ther 2000;67(4): 391–7.

137. Kroenke K, Lawrence VA, Theroux JF, et al. Postoperative complications after thoracic and major abdominal surgery in patients with and without obstructive lung disease. Chest 1993;104(5):1445–51.
138. Gajdos C, Hawn MT, Campagna EJ, et al. Adverse effects of smoking on postoperative outcomes in cancer patients. Ann Surg Oncol 2012;19(5):1430–8.
139. Gourgiotis S, Aloizos S, Aravosita P, et al. The effects of tobacco smoking on the incidence and risk of intraoperative and postoperative complications in adults. Surgeon 2011;9(4):225–32.
140. Ngaage DL, Martins E, Orkell E, et al. The impact of the duration of mechanical ventilation on the respiratory outcome in smokers undergoing cardiac surgery. Cardiovasc Surg 2002;10(4):345–50.
141. Schwilk B, Bothner U, Schraag S, et al. Perioperative respiratory events in smokers and nonsmokers undergoing general anaesthesia. Acta Anaesthesiol Scand 1997;41(3):348–55.
142. Mills E, Eyawo O, Lockhart I, et al. Smoking cessation reduces postoperative complications: a systematic review and meta-analysis. Am J Med 2011; 124(2):144–54.e8.
143. Moores LK. Smoking and postoperative pulmonary complications. An evidence-based review of the recent literature. Clin Chest Med 2000;21(1):139–46, ix–x.
144. Vaporciyan AA, Merriman KW, Ece F, et al. Incidence of major pulmonary morbidity after pneumonectomy: association with timing of smoking cessation. Ann Thorac Surg 2002;73(2):420–5 [discussion: 425–6].
145. Warner MA, Offord KP, Warner ME, et al. Role of preoperative cessation of smoking and other factors in postoperative pulmonary complications: a blinded prospective study of coronary artery bypass patients. Mayo Clin Proc 1989;64(6): 609–16.
146. Barrera R, Shi W, Amar D, et al. Smoking and timing of cessation: impact on pulmonary complications after thoracotomy. Chest 2005;127(6):1977–83.
147. Warner DO. Perioperative abstinence from cigarettes: physiologic and clinical consequences. Anesthesiology 2006;104(2):356–67.
148. Lindstrom D, Sadr Azodi O, Wladis A, et al. Effects of a perioperative smoking cessation intervention on postoperative complications: a randomized trial. Ann Surg 2008;248(5):739–45.
149. Moller AM, Villebro N, Pedersen T, et al. Effect of preoperative smoking intervention on postoperative complications: a randomised clinical trial. Lancet 2002; 359(9301):114–7.
150. Nakagawa M, Tanaka H, Tsukuma H, et al. Relationship between the duration of the preoperative smoke-free period and the incidence of postoperative pulmonary complications after pulmonary surgery. Chest 2001;120(3):705–10.
151. Wong J, Lam DP, Abrishami A, et al. Short-term preoperative smoking cessation and postoperative complications: a systematic review and meta-analysis. Can J Anaesth 2012;59(3):268–79.

Perioperative Nutrition

Zachary Torgersen, MD, Marcus Balters, MD*

KEYWORDS

- Perioperative • Nutrition • Enteral • Parenteral • Immunonutrition
- Carbohydrate loading • ERAS

KEY POINTS

- Perioperative nutrition impacts surgical outcomes.
- Prehabilitation prepares patients for surgical stress.
- Carbohydrate loading is beneficial.
- Immunonutrition is promising, but more research is necessary.
- Postoperative early enteral nutrition is optimal.
- Parenteral nutrition should be reserved for patients unable to tolerate enteral feeding.

INTRODUCTION

Perioperative nutrition is a vital yet often overlooked aspect of surgical care. The association between poor nutritional status and surgical outcomes has been clearly, eloquently, and repeatedly demonstrated for decades. That being said, a review of the literature on surgical nutrition reveals a disparity between the recommendations of well-designed studies and the nutritional practices commonly applied to surgical patients. Diversity of surgical specialties, entrenchment of surgical dogma, and a closely monitored outcome-based climate all play substantial roles in the maintenance of this divergence. Surgeons are frequently comfortable with tradition and skeptical of change. Convincing a successful surgeon to alter his or her perioperative management, particularly in ways that run in opposition to time-honored teachings, is not the easiest of tasks. Fortunately, a robust collection of rigorous clinical studies offers high-quality evidence supporting the current recommendations on perioperative nutrition.

Surgical nutrition has been a dynamic and evolving discipline from the start. The initial description of the complex metabolic response to surgical stress paved the way for an understanding of the hypermetabolic postoperative state, which led to research into perioperative replacement of stress-induced nutritional deficits.

Conflicts of interest: Neither author reports any conflicts of interest.

Department of Surgery, Creighton University, 601 North 30th Street, Suite 3700, Omaha, NE 68131, USA
* Corresponding author.
E-mail address: Marcusbalters@creighton.edu

Surg Clin N Am 95 (2015) 255–267
http://dx.doi.org/10.1016/j.suc.2014.10.003
0039-6109/15/$ – see front matter Published by Elsevier Inc.

Parenteral nutrition was thus invented and subsequently improved. The benefits of enteral nutrition then became apparent, and early initiation of gastrointestinal feeding postoperatively was recommended. The idea of attenuating the surgical stress response through optimization of the preoperative state was investigated. Prehabilitation, preoperative carbohydrate loading, and immunonutrition currently pervade any discussion on perioperative care. The risks of inadequate perioperative nutrition are well known and potentially disastrous. The purpose of this article is to provide a concise review of perioperative nutrition while emphasizing the attainable clinical benefits demonstrated in current research.

NUTRITION ASSESSMENT

Nutritional assessment is an important component of the preoperative evaluation of surgical patients. Patients at nutritional risk before surgery have an elevated risk of postoperative complications. The Joint Commission recognizes this and requires a nutrition screening within 24 hours of admission on all inpatients followed by a complete assessment for those considered high risk.[1] The goal of effective preoperative screening is to identify high-risk patients allowing for targeted intervention that ultimately decreases surgical morbidity. To that point, evidence suggests that providing preoperative enteral nutrition to those at high risk reduces major postoperative morbidity by 50%.[1] Unlike cardiac risk assessment, there is no standard algorithm for preoperative nutrition. Thus, the surgeon is often responsible for assessing nutritional risk, frequently relying on individual preferences rather than using a validated stratification strategy.

The goal of the preoperative nutritional assessment is not to correct years of nutritional deficits but to identify and optimize or *prehabilitate* patients at nutritional risk for the stress of surgery.[2] Importantly, malnutrition and nutritional risk are not synonymous.[3] Malnutrition is defined as an inability to match metabolic and nutrient requirements. The American Society for Parenteral and Enteral Nutrition (ASPEN) categorizes malnutrition as starvation related, chronic disease related, or acute disease related.[4] Nutritional requirements vary based on the category of malnutrition and the presence of a disease state. Potential causes of preoperative malnutrition include neoplasm, an inability to swallow, a lack of access to nutrition, or gastrointestinal tract dysfunction.[1] It behooves the clinician to elucidate the cause and tailor preoperative intervention to individual patients.

Preoperative risk assessment should consider the patients' nutritional state, the risk of the proposed surgery, and potential postoperative anatomic alterations.[5] Understandably, accurately assessing risk in the preoperative period can be difficult. Patients undertaking esophageal, pancreatic, abdominal wall reconstruction, or hepatobiliary operations are reported to be at an elevated risk.[3] It has been suggested that the American Heart Association's preoperative cardiac risk stratification be used to estimate nutritional risk, acknowledging intraperitoneal and intrathoracic cases lasting more than 2 hours are inherently higher risk.[3]

The need for an available and facile nutrition assessment tool led to the creation of multiple risk calculators of various design. The Malnutrition Universal Screening Tool, the Nutritional Risk Index, the Nutritional Risk Screening (NRS-2002), the Mini Nutritional Assessment, and the Subjective Global Assessment are all examples of suggested risk stratifiers.[3] Unfortunately, only the Nutritional Risk Screening (NRS-2002) has been validated and supported by level I evidence.[2,5]

Traditional teaching in many surgical textbooks and training programs emphasized the use of albumin as an important marker of nutritional status. Albumin is important in body fluid distribution, acid-base balance, and substrate transport.[6] Additionally, albumin is an excellent prognostic indicator, with values of less than 3 associated with poor surgical outcomes.[7] However, albumin has been found lacking in terms of its utility as a nutritional marker.[2] Although albumin composes more than half of the total human serum protein, its concentration is regulated by multiple factors outside of synthesis and degradation. Inflammation, immobility, and capillary permeability all affect plasma albumin levels.[6] Albumin is also generally understood to be a negative acute phase protein. Hepatic protein production during stress is thought to shift toward the production of acute-phase reactants and immune cells and away from albumin synthesis.[8] These factors make albumin an unreliable nutritional indicator in surgical patients, although it bears mentioning that a recent literature review noted increased albumin synthesis in the postoperative period particularly following nutritional supplementation.[6] Finally, normal albumin levels have been observed in patients dying of starvation, further underscoring that albumin is a suboptimal nutritional parameter.[9]

The serum prealbumin level has also been touted as a marker of nutritional status. Prealbumin has a half-life of 2 days, substantially shorter than the 20-day half-life of albumin. This shortened half-life has led to the suggestion that prealbumin levels reflect a more acute and, therefore, accurate assessment of nutritional status. Unfortunately, prealbumin is also a negative acute-phase protein and, therefore, subject to the same unreliability as albumin.[2,9]

Rather than relying solely on a highly variable serum marker, the North American Surgical Nutrition Summit recommends a multifactorial, broad-based assessment. The clinician should gather details regarding the recent oral intake, body weight, and weight loss. Declining recent oral intake, an actual body weight of less than 90% of the ideal body weight, body mass index (BMI) less than 18.5 or greater than 40, and weight loss greater than 5.0% in 1 month, 7.5% in 3 months, and 10% in 6 months indicate nutritional risk. Biomarkers are not excluded from the recommendations but should be used as a part of a comprehensive preoperative assessment. Serum C-reactive protein, albumin, and glycated hemoglobin (HgbA1C) levels all broaden the assessment.[5] Postponement of major elective surgery is recommended in order to achieve a HgbA1C less than 7.5, attempt weight loss in those with a BMI greater than 35, attempt smoking cessation, and address poor nutrition.[5]

SURGICAL RESPONSE TO STRESS

The response to surgical stress is complex and diverse. An understanding of the physiologic response to stress is integral to providing excellent perioperative care and achieving optimal surgical outcomes. Unsurprisingly, much attention has, therefore, been devoted to understanding the stress response. Sir David Cuthbertson[10] described the metabolic ebb and flow occurring after major trauma in 1942. Less than a decade later, Moore and Ball[11] described the altered metabolism experienced by surgical patients in *The Metabolic Response to Surgery*. In 1959, Moore[12] described the impact of perioperative nutrition in *Metabolic Care of the Surgical Patient*. These foundational works clarified the stress response and launched interest in perioperative nutrition.

The surgical stress response is now understood to involve endocrine and inflammatory arms. Additionally, the stress response correlates with the degree of insult.[13] Injury stimulates the hypothalamic-pituitary-adrenal (HPA) axis that ultimately results in increased secretion of cortisol, epinephrine, glucagon, growth hormone, aldosterone, and antidiuretic hormone.[8] On the other hand, the inflammatory response is mediated via numerous cytokines including tumor necrosis factor-alpha, interleukin-1 (IL-1), and IL-6.[8] Cytokines are largely responsible for the subsequent activation of the immune system and have also been shown to stimulate the HPA axis, thus creating interplay between the inflammatory and endocrine responses.

The above-mentioned mediators ultimately create a catabolic state designed to meet the increased energy demands of stressed patients. Glucose, fatty acids, and protein are all readily available substrates; however, glycogen stores are rapidly depleted and skeletal muscle is then subsequently used for hepatic gluconeogenesis. The role of perioperative nutrition is, therefore, to attenuate the stress response and provide appropriate supplementation to mitigate the effects of postoperative catabolism.

ROUTE OF DELIVERY

The enteral and parenteral routes of delivery are available for perioperative supplementation. Total parenteral nutrition was invented by Dr Stanley Dudrick and revolutionized perioperative care. Parenteral nutrition is undoubtedly capable of providing excellent nutrition; however, there are significant risks with this form of supplementation. First, patients require central venous access creating the potential for line complications. Next, hyperglycemia is frequently encountered and close attention to glycemic control is necessary. Further, standard parenteral formulations in the United States often lack important substrates, such as glutamine.[2] Additionally, lipid formulations frequently include proinflammatory omega-6 rather than antiinflammatory omega-3 fatty acids.[2] Finally, infectious complications overall occur more frequently in comparison to enteral nutrition.[14]

The importance of the gastrointestinal tract to immunity is well recognized and cannot be overstated. The gut is home to the largest source of immune tissue in the body. Gut-associated lymphoid tissue (GALT), a form of mucosa-associated lymphoid tissue, is responsible for 60% to 70% of total immunity.[2,15] GALT plays an important role in both innate and adaptive immunity. Paneth cells secrete nonspecific antimicrobial substrates, whereas microvilli cells present intraluminal antigens to lymphocytes in Peyer patches. These lymphocytes are subsequently sensitized and circulate systemically via rich mesenteric lymphatics. The ultimate result of this process is the production of targeted antibodies. Immunoglobulin A antibodies are of particular importance as they provide intraluminal immunity and prevent bacterial translocation.[15] Finally, the gut provides a physical barrier to infection through the production of mucin and the presence of tight junctions.[15]

Importantly, gut starvation and/or critical illness induce changes to the immune function of the gastrointestinal tract. Lack of enteral feeding causes villous blunting and increased mucosal permeability potentially allowing bacterial translocation and bacteremia.[16] Additionally, gut starvation decreases hepatic and peritoneal immune function.[15] Enteral nutrition attenuates these deleterious effects, and multiple studies have demonstrated improved outcomes with early initiation of enteral feeding.[2,17]

Enteral nutrition is currently recommended over parenteral nutrition by all major nutrition and critical care organizations.[1] According to the North American Surgical Nutrition Summit, contraindications to enteral nutrition include obstruction, ischemia, acute peritonitis, and lack of bowel continuity.[5] Additional relative contraindications may include high-output fistulas and severe malabsorption. Enteral feeding has been shown to be safe in patients with open abdomens and those requiring vasopressors. Additionally, animal studies suggest that early enteral feeding proximal to a gastrointestinal anastomosis actually strengthens the newly joined bowel.[18] In the absence of a definite contraindication, enteral nutrition should be initiated in all patients, preferably within 24 hours of surgery.[2] Parenteral nutrition should be considered as an adjunct for patients unable to meet their full nutrition requirements with enteral nutrition or as a primary modality in patients with a contraindication to enteral feeding.

IMMUNONUTRITION

Immunonutrition is a relatively new aspect of perioperative care and refers to the supplementation of specific nutrients, including arginine, omega-3 fatty acids, nucleotides, and/or glutamine. These nutrients are hypothesized to influence the immune and inflammatory response to surgical stress as well as encourage protein synthesis. Two studies published in the early 2000s demonstrated improved outcomes in patients with cancer receiving perioperative immunonutrition and subsequently ignited interest in this area.[19,20] In the interim, investigation has focused on describing the mechanism of action of these supplements and understanding their overall clinical impact. The following serves as a brief overview of the key components of immunonutrition.

ARGININE

Arginine is considered a conditional amino acid as it is used and depleted during stress. Its biological functions include stimulating immune cells (particularly lymphocytes), promoting wound healing, and acting as a precursor of nitric oxide (NO).[1,14] NO is of particular relevance because of its ability to improve microvascular perfusion through vasodilation. Arginine supplementation was viewed with skepticism in critically ill patients as increased vasodilation was thought to contribute to cardiovascular compromise.[21] However, a meta-analysis of previously published randomized controlled trials found decreased postoperative infectious complications, a shorter length of stay, and no increase in morbidity or mortality with arginine supplementation.[22] Further, the clinical implications of the arginine-to-asymmetric dimethylarginine (ADMA) ratio have recently been described. ADMA acts in opposition to arginine inhibiting NO and, therefore, impairing microvascular perfusion. In critical illness, arginine is depleted creating a relative abundance of ADMA. A reduced arginine-to-ADMA ratio has been shown to correlate with increased mortality in the critically ill.[23,24] The potential clinical benefit of arginine supplementation to correct the arginine/ADMA ratio is under investigation. Overall, the available evidence on arginine supplementation in the perioperative period seems to be favorable.

OMEGA-3 FATTY ACIDS

Omega-3 fatty acids are polyunsaturated fatty acids that play a role in the maintenance of cell membranes and modulation of the inflammatory response.[1,25,26] Importantly, they are relatively less abundant in the Western diet compared with omega-6 fatty acids that are linked to a host of negative health effects. Docosahexaenoic acid (DHA) and eicosapentaenoic acid (EPA) are 2 biologically active omega-3 fatty acids. Recent research indicates that DHA and EPA are converted to resolvins, substances that have potent antiinflammatory and analgesic properties.[26] To date, the clinical potential of this discovery remains unknown.

The results regarding perioperative supplementation of omega-3 fatty acids have been divergent. A meta-analysis of randomized controlled trials in critically ill patients demonstrated a significant reduction in mortality in patients receiving enteral supplementation.[27] However, recent randomized controlled trials comparing omega-3 fatty acid supplementation with conventional perioperative nutrition in patients with colorectal and esophageal cancer failed to demonstrate improved outcomes.[28,29] At least one meta-analysis has demonstrated improved outcomes in those receiving both omega-3 fatty acid and arginine supplementation suggesting the potential for therapeutic interplay.[30] Omega-3 fatty acid supplementation seems safe, but more data are necessary to define the clinical impact.

GLUTAMINE

Like arginine, glutamine is a conditional amino acid and composes 70% of the amino acids mobilized during the stress response.[31] Its biological functions include acting as an antioxidant via its role as a precursor to glutathione, providing energy for enterocytes and, thus, maintaining gut integrity, participating in wound healing, and promoting protein synthesis.[1,31] A recent meta-analysis of 16 randomized controlled trials found that parenteral perioperative supplementation decreased postoperative infections, shortened length of stay, and improved nitrogen balance.[32] Another study demonstrated that perioperative parenteral administration to moderately and severely malnourished patients improved glucose homeostasis, decreased infections, and reduced intensive-care-unit stay.[33] Importantly, this study found a benefit in multivariate analysis in the cohort receiving perioperative glutamine over those supplemented only in the postoperative period. Regarding enteral supplementation, a recent prospective randomized trial of head and neck oncology patients demonstrated improved postoperative fat-free body mass and quality of life in those receiving glutamine.[34] Again, more research is necessary before reaching a definitive conclusion on glutamine supplementation, although the balance of evidence seems favorable, particularly in those at nutritional risk.

To summarize, immunonutrition is clearly a promising area of perioperative nutrition. Four recent meta-analyses attest to improved clinical outcomes.[22,30,35,36] Continued research is necessary to define the precise biochemical mechanisms and ultimately describe the optimal perioperative formula. At present, perioperative immunonutrition should be recommended for all patients undergoing major elective gastrointestinal surgery at risk for infectious complications, particularly in the malnourished.[37] It should be initiated 5 to 7 days preoperatively and continued postoperatively.[5]

PREOPERATIVE NUTRITION

As early as 1936, Studley[38] demonstrated that preoperative weight loss was associated with increased operative mortality. Unfortunately, as mentioned previously, preoperative nutritional optimization is often time consuming and difficult to quantify. Surgeons and patients alike frequently do not have the luxury of optimizing nutritional status over an extended period of time. Even in purely elective surgery, the time required for correction of nutritional deficits is individualized and highly variable. The concept of prehabilitation, or a short-course optimization in preparation for surgery, was created to address these concerns. Prehabilitation represents a preoperative bundle designed to prepare the body for the metabolic insult of the perioperative period. Exercise tolerance and weight, nutrition, and glucose control are all addressed.[2] The benefit of such a regimen has been demonstrated in clinical trials.[39]

The impact of preoperative nutritional supplementation on various surgical subgroups has been investigated. A recent multicenter prospective cohort study of more than 1000 patients investigated preoperative supplementation with either enteral or parenteral nutrition. All patients receiving preoperative nutrition were supplemented for at least 7 days before surgery. Nutritional assessment was performed on all study participants using the NRS-2002 survey. According to the authors of the NRS-2002, a score greater than 3 indicates nutritional risk.[40] In the cohort study, patients with an NRS-2002 score of at least 5 that received preoperative supplementation had a significantly shortened length of stay and a postoperative complication rate of half of the nonsupplemented group.[41] No benefit in the subgroup with an NRS-2002 score of 3 to 4 was noted, although the number of patients was small. This study demonstrates that high-risk patients significantly benefit from preoperative nutrition.

Although the prior study used both enteral and parenteral nutrition, the optimal route of delivery has previously been investigated. In 1991, The Veterans Affairs Total Parenteral Nutrition Cooperative Study Group published a landmark trial on preoperative parenteral nutrition. Patients were again stratified according to nutritional risk. Increased rates of infection without significant benefit were observed in the borderline and mildly malnourished groups receiving parenteral nutrition. There was a benefit to parenteral supplementation in severely malnourished patients, although this subgroup represented less than 5% of the study.[7] The investigators commented that the benefit noted in severely malnourished patients should be viewed with caution because of the small sample size. Nevertheless, the results from this study represented a paradigm shift in clinical practice. As of 2009, ASPEN and the Society of Critical Care Medicine continue to recommend parenteral nutrition for 7 days preoperatively in severely malnourished patients unable to tolerate enteral feeding.[42]

As mentioned earlier, enteral nutrition has a myriad of benefits and is the preferred source of feeding whenever possible. This is no different in the preoperative period. Recently, the idea of preoperative carbohydrate loading has been investigated. Traditionally, patients are made nil per os after midnight the evening before their operation. This practice stems from concerns over aspiration risk in patients receiving monitored or general anesthesia. It is now, however, increasingly recognized that fasting for this length of time depletes glycogen stores before the start of surgery. This depletion creates a situation whereby lean body mass is sacrificed during the actual operation to meet energy demands. In order to attenuate the loss of skeletal muscle, carbohydrate supplements are given before surgery. Preoperative carbohydrate loading often includes taking 800 mL of a 12.6% carbohydrate drink the night before surgery and 400 mL of a similar preparation 2 to 3 hours before induction of anesthesia.[3,43] Contrary to conventional teaching regarding the need for lengthy fasts before surgery, there are now abundant data demonstrating the safety and efficacy of preoperative carbohydrate loading. Since 2010, 3 meta-analyses of randomized controlled trials have found improved insulin resistance, shortened hospital stay, and no increase in pulmonary complications with preoperative carbohydrate loading.[44–46] Additionally, a randomized trial demonstrates preservation of muscle mass with carbohydrate loading, whereas animal data find improved maintenance of the intestinal mucosal barrier and earlier return of oral intake.[43,47] Should concerns over aspiration persist, a Cochrane database review from 2003 established that there was no evidence suggesting oral intake of fluids closer to the induction of anesthesia increases pulmonary complications.[48] From these data, the American Society of Anesthesiologists' guidelines are currently accepting of clear liquids up to 2 hours before the induction of anesthesia.[49]

Preoperative carbohydrate loading is an important component of the Enhanced Recovery After Surgery (ERAS) protocols for perioperative care. ERAS protocols represent another bundle approach to perioperative management that has demonstrated a clinical benefit. Multiple studies confirm improved patient outcomes and satisfaction as well as decreased lengths of stay after implementation of ERAS protocols.[3,43,50–52] ERAS protocols have been intensely investigated in colorectal surgery and are being increasingly applied to wider patient populations.[3] These protocols provide evidenced-based recommendations for preoperative, intraoperative, and postoperative care.

Preoperative supplementation provides a significant benefit in the severely malnourished. The gastrointestinal tract is the preferred route of supplementation, but severely malnourished patients unable to tolerate enteral feeds have drastically improved outcomes with parenteral nutrition. Prehabilitation and ERAS bundles are beneficial and will likely become increasingly incorporated into clinical management. Preoperative carbohydrate loading is safe and effective and should be considered in all patients.

POSTOPERATIVE NUTRITION

Providing adequate postoperative nutrition improves outcomes. Substantial evidence indicates that early enteral nutrition is associated with significant reductions in morbidity and mortality. Multiple meta-analyses have demonstrated the positive clinical impact of beginning enteral nutrition within 24 hours of surgery.[18,53] Early stimulation of the gastrointestinal tract maintains the mucosal barrier and prevents the bacterial translocation described in gut starvation. The significant role of the gut in immune function is again emphasized by a recent study in which infectious complications following liver transplantation decreased drastically in those receiving early enteral nutrition.[54]

Most patients are able to tolerate enteral nutrition without untoward effects. As mentioned earlier, studies have demonstrated that early enteral feeding is advisable in critically ill patients requiring mechanical ventilation or vasopressor support and in trauma patients with open abdomens.[55,56] Trauma patients with open abdomens receiving early enteral nutrition had higher fascial closure rates and decreased mortality. Failure to achieve fascial closure is significant as it can result in long-term debilitating rehabilitation with increased risk of entero-atmospheric fistula formation.

Concern over anastomotic dehiscence has led many surgeons to avoid feeding a fresh anastomosis. Enteral feeding distal to an anastomosis is acceptable and commonly practiced in proximal gastrointestinal surgery. Randomized data indicate that early enteral feeding via a jejunostomy tube is associated with improved outcomes in proximal gastrointestinal cancer resections.[57] Additionally, there is evidence in animal studies that early enteral feeding *proximal* to a fresh gastrointestinal anastomosis promotes healing without increasing the rates of disruption.[18] This finding has yet to be evaluated in a human trial.

Concerns over aspiration with early feeding seem to be overstated. Similar to evidence suggesting routine postoperative reliance on nasogastric decompression is unnecessary, a clinically significant increase in aspiration has not been demonstrated in early enteral feeding.[53,58] To that end, the North American Surgical Nutrition Summit recommends judicious use of enteral nutrition even in the presence of postoperative ileus.[5] Routine gastric residual monitoring may be unnecessary as prospective randomized data in critically ill ventilated patients fail to demonstrate a decrease in pneumonia with this practice.[59,60] To summarize, early enteral nutrition improves outcomes and is indicated in most postoperative patients.

Despite the overwhelming support in favor of aggressive nutrition, many patients' nutritional needs are not met postoperatively for a variety of reasons. Adhering to a few principles can facilitate postoperative enteral nutrition. The ERAS group's recommendations for colorectal surgery emphasize judicious fluid management and multimodal pain management.[50] Preventing fluid overload decreases bowel wall edema, and adequate analgesia facilitates early ambulation. Additionally, oral intake should be resumed early, and there is no reason to await the return of bowel function.[2,50] Finally, the regimented process of initiating a clear liquid diet and sequentially advancing may be unnecessary and delay resumption of adequate nutrition.[3,61]

Although most patients are candidates for enteral nutrition, some must rely on parenteral supplementation. The current recommendations for postoperative parenteral nutrition are based on its necessity preoperatively. Patients receiving parenteral nutrition preoperatively should have it restarted on postoperative day 1.[5] In the absence of preoperative parenteral nutrition, patients expected to have a nonfunctional gastrointestinal tract for 7 days postoperatively should be started on parenteral therapy, although it should be noted that there is little benefit unless supplementation is continued for greater than 7 days.[5] Unlike enteral nutrition, early initiation of parenteral nutrition is not recommended.[14,62] A recent randomized controlled trial of critically ill patients with contraindications to enteral nutrition did not find any benefit to the early initiation of parenteral nutrition.[63]

SUMMARY

The importance of perioperative nutrition cannot be overstated. An abundance of high-quality research provides guidelines regarding safe and efficacious management. Unfortunately, old habits seem to die hard, and antiquated practices continue to permeate surgical culture. Frankly speaking, poor nutrition is associated with poor surgical outcomes. Preoperative nutrition assessment, though often tedious, identifies high-risk patients that benefit dramatically from nutritional supplementation. Preoperative assessment should proceed with an eye toward *prehabilitation* or the preparation of patients for the metabolic onslaught of the perioperative period. Attenuation of the stress response through carbohydrate loading improves outcomes and shortens the length of stay. Fears over increased aspiration with carbohydrate loading have been discredited. Early initiation of enteral feeding within 24 hours of surgery improves outcomes, particularly in the critically ill in whom feeding was previously considered dangerous. There are relatively few contraindications to enteral nutrition, but those who truly cannot receive gastrointestinal feeding benefit from parenteral supplementation. Immunonutrition seems efficacious, although more research into its precise mechanisms is necessary. ERAS protocols have demonstrated clinical utility and will likely continue to expand to broader surgical populations.

Patient care and outcomes are important to every practicing surgeon. In this time of cost control and monitored outcomes, surgeons must remain keenly up to date and open-minded on areas of potential improvement. Surgical nutrition often lags behind the voluminous well-designed studies emphasizing the benefits of aggressive perioperative care. There is room for improvement. Ultimately, it is incumbent on the surgeon to practice the evidence-based recommendations demonstrated to improve outcomes.

REFERENCES

1. Enomoto TM, Larson D, Martindale RG. Patients requiring perioperative nutritional support. Med Clin North Am 2013;97(6):1181–200.
2. Martindale RG, McClave SA, Taylor B, et al. Perioperative nutrition: what is the current landscape? JPEN J Parenter Enteral Nutr 2013;37(5 Suppl):5S–20S.
3. Miller KR, Wischmeyer PE, Taylor B, et al. An evidence-based approach to perioperative nutrition support in the elective surgery patient. JPEN J Parenter Enteral Nutr 2013;37(5 Suppl):39S–50S.

4. White JV, Guenter P, Jensen G, et al. Consensus statement: Academy of Nutrition and Dietetics and American Society for Parenteral and Enteral Nutrition: characteristics recommended for the identification and documentation of adult malnutrition (undernutrition). JPEN J Parenter Enteral Nutr 2012;36(3):275–83.
5. McClave SA, Kozar R, Martindale RG, et al. Summary points and consensus recommendations from the North American Surgical Nutrition Summit. JPEN J Parenter Enteral Nutr 2013;37(5 Suppl):99S–105S.
6. Hulshoff A, Schricker T, Elgendy H, et al. Albumin synthesis in surgical patients. Nutrition 2013;29(5):703–7.
7. Perioperative total parenteral nutrition in surgical patients. The Veterans Affairs Total Parenteral Nutrition Cooperative Study Group. N Engl J Med 1991;325(8): 525–32.
8. Blackburn GL. Metabolic considerations in management of surgical patients. Surg Clin North Am 2011;91(3):467–80.
9. Neel DR, McClave S, Martindale R. Hypoalbuminaemia in the perioperative period: clinical significance and management options. Best Pract Res Clin Anaesthesiol 2011;25(3):395–400.
10. Cuthbertson D. Post-shock metabolic response. Lancet 1942;1(1):433–6.
11. Moore F, Ball M. The metabolic response to surgery. Springfield (IL): Charles C. Thomas; 1949.
12. Moore F. Metabolic care of the surgical patient. Philadelphia: W.B. Saunders; 1959.
13. Ni Choileain N, Redmond HP. Cell response to surgery. Arch Surg 2006;141(11): 1132–40.
14. Abunnaja S, Cuviello A, Sanchez JA. Enteral and parenteral nutrition in the perioperative period: state of the art. Nutrients 2013;5(2):608–23.
15. Fukatsu K, Kudsk KA. Nutrition and gut immunity. Surg Clin North Am 2011;91(4): 755–70, vii.
16. van der Hulst RR, von Meyenfeldt MF, van Kreel BK, et al. Gut permeability, intestinal morphology, and nutritional depletion. Nutrition 1998;14(1):1–6.
17. Jayarajan S, Daly JM. The relationships of nutrients, routes of delivery, and immunocompetence. Surg Clin North Am 2011;91(4):737–53, vii.
18. Osland E, Yunus RM, Khan S, et al. Early versus traditional postoperative feeding in patients undergoing resectional gastrointestinal surgery: a meta-analysis. JPEN J Parenter Enteral Nutr 2011;35(4):473–87.
19. Braga M, Gianotti L, Nespoli L, et al. Nutritional approach in malnourished surgical patients: a prospective randomized study. Arch Surg 2002;137(2): 174–80.
20. Gianotti L, Braga M, Nespoli L, et al. A randomized controlled trial of preoperative oral supplementation with a specialized diet in patients with gastrointestinal cancer. Gastroenterology 2002;122(7):1763–70.
21. Suchner U, Heyland DK, Peter K. Immune-modulatory actions of arginine in the critically ill. Br J Nutr 2002;87(Suppl 1):S121–32.
22. Drover JW, Dhaliwal R, Weitzel L, et al. Perioperative use of arginine-supplemented diets: a systematic review of the evidence. J Am Coll Surg 2011;212(3):385–99, 399.e1.
23. Visser M, Vermeulen MA, Richir MC, et al. Imbalance of arginine and asymmetric dimethylarginine is associated with markers of circulatory failure, organ failure and mortality in shock patients. Br J Nutr 2012;107(10):1458–65.
24. Gough MS, Morgan MA, Mack CM, et al. The ratio of arginine to dimethylarginines is reduced and predicts outcomes in patients with severe sepsis. Crit Care Med 2011;39(6):1351–8.

25. Calder PC. Mechanisms of action of (n-3) fatty acids. J Nutr 2012;142(3): 592S–9S.
26. Ji RR, Xu ZZ, Strichartz G, et al. Emerging roles of resolvins in the resolution of inflammation and pain. Trends Neurosci 2011;34(11):599–609.
27. Chen W, Jiang H, Zhou ZY, et al. Is omega-3 fatty acids enriched nutrition support safe for critical ill patients? A systematic review and meta-analysis. Nutrients 2014;6(6):2148–64.
28. Sorensen LS, Thorlacius-Ussing O, Schmidt EB, et al. Randomized clinical trial of perioperative omega-3 fatty acid supplements in elective colorectal cancer surgery. Br J Surg 2014;101(2):33–42.
29. Sultan J, Griffin SM, Di Franco F, et al. Randomized clinical trial of omega-3 fatty acid-supplemented enteral nutrition versus standard enteral nutrition in patients undergoing oesophagogastric cancer surgery. Br J Surg 2012;99(3):346–55.
30. Marik PE, Zaloga GP. Immunonutrition in high-risk surgical patients: a systematic review and analysis of the literature. JPEN J Parenter Enteral Nutr 2010;34(4): 378–86.
31. Pollock GR, Van Way CW 3rd. Immune-enhancing nutrition in surgical critical care. Mo Med 2012;109(5):388–92.
32. Yue C, Tian W, Wang W, et al. The impact of perioperative glutamine-supplemented parenteral nutrition on outcomes of patients undergoing abdominal surgery: a meta-analysis of randomized clinical trials. Am Surg 2013;79(5):506–13.
33. Mercadal Orfila G, Llop Talaveron JM. Effectiveness of perioperative glutamine in parenteral nutrition in patients at risk of moderate to severe malnutrition. Nutr Hosp 2011;26(6):1305–12.
34. Azman M, MohdYunus MR, Sulaiman S, et al. Enteral glutamine 0.3-0.4mg/kg/day supplementation in surgical patients with head and neck malignancy: a randomized controlled trial. Head Neck 2014. [Epub ahead of print].
35. Cerantola Y, Hubner M, Grass F, et al. Immunonutrition in gastrointestinal surgery. Br J Surg 2011;98(1):37–48.
36. Marimuthu K, Varadhan KK, Ljungqvist O, et al. A meta-analysis of the effect of combinations of immune modulating nutrients on outcome in patients undergoing major open gastrointestinal surgery. Ann Surg 2012;255(6):1060–8.
37. Braga M, Wischmeyer PE, Drover J, et al. Clinical evidence for pharmaconutrition in major elective surgery. JPEN J Parenter Enteral Nutr 2013;37(5 Suppl): 66S–72S.
38. Studley HO. Percentage of weight loss: a basic indicator of surgical risk in patients with chronic peptic ulcer. 1936. Nutr Hosp 2001;16(4):141–3 [discussion: 140–1].
39. Li C, Carli F, Lee L, et al. Impact of a trimodal prehabilitation program on functional recovery after colorectal cancer surgery: a pilot study. Surg Endosc 2013;27(4):1072–82.
40. Kondrup J, Rasmussen HH, Hamberg O, et al, Ad Hoc ESPEN Working Group. Nutritional risk screening (NRS 2002): a new method based on an analysis of controlled clinical trials. Clin Nutr 2003;22(3):321–36.
41. Jie B, Jiang ZM, Nolan MT, et al. Impact of preoperative nutritional support on clinical outcome in abdominal surgical patients at nutritional risk. Nutrition 2012;28(10):1022–7.
42. McClave SA, Martindale RG, Vanek VW, et al. Guidelines for the provision and assessment of nutrition support therapy in the adult critically ill patient: Society of Critical Care Medicine (SCCM) and American Society for Parenteral and Enteral Nutrition (A.S.P.E.N. JPEN J Parenter Enteral Nutr 2009;33(3): 277–316.

43. Yuill KA, Richardson RA, Davidson HI, et al. The administration of an oral carbohydrate-containing fluid prior to major elective upper-gastrointestinal surgery preserves skeletal muscle mass postoperatively–a randomised clinical trial. Clin Nutr 2005;24(1):32–7.
44. Awad S, Varadhan KK, Ljungqvist O, et al. A meta-analysis of randomised controlled trials on preoperative oral carbohydrate treatment in elective surgery. Clin Nutr 2013;32(1):34–44.
45. Bilku DK, Dennison AR, Hall TC, et al. Role of preoperative carbohydrate loading: a systematic review. Ann R Coll Surg Engl 2014;96(1):15–22.
46. Li L, Wang Z, Ying X, et al. Preoperative carbohydrate loading for elective surgery: a systematic review and meta-analysis. Surg Today 2012;42(7):613–24.
47. Luttikhold J, Oosting A, van den Braak CC, et al. Preservation of the gut by preoperative carbohydrate loading improves postoperative food intake. Clin Nutr 2013;32(4):556–61.
48. Brady M, Kinn S, Stuart P. Preoperative fasting for adults to prevent perioperative complications. Cochrane Database Syst Rev 2003;(4):CD004423.
49. American Society of Anesthesiologists Committee. Practice guidelines for preoperative fasting and the use of pharmacologic agents to reduce the risk of pulmonary aspiration: application to healthy patients undergoing elective procedures: an updated report by the American Society of Anesthesiologists Committee on Standards and Practice Parameters. Anesthesiology 2011;114(3):495–511.
50. Lassen K, Soop M, Nygren J, et al. Consensus review of optimal perioperative care in colorectal surgery: Enhanced Recovery After Surgery (ERAS) Group recommendations. Arch Surg 2009;144(10):961–9.
51. Gustafsson UO, Scott MJ, Schwenk W, et al. Guidelines for perioperative care in elective colonic surgery: Enhanced Recovery After Surgery (ERAS(R)) Society recommendations. World J Surg 2013;37(2):259–84.
52. Ren L, Zhu D, Wei Y, et al. Enhanced Recovery After Surgery (ERAS) program attenuates stress and accelerates recovery in patients after radical resection for colorectal cancer: a prospective randomized controlled trial. World J Surg 2012;36(2):407–14.
53. Lewis SJ, Andersen HK, Thomas S. Early enteral nutrition within 24 h of intestinal surgery versus later commencement of feeding: a systematic review and meta-analysis. J Gastrointest Surg 2009;13(3):569–75.
54. Ikegami T, Shirabe K, Yoshiya S, et al. Bacterial sepsis after living donor liver transplantation: the impact of early enteral nutrition. J Am Coll Surg 2012;214(3):288–95.
55. Khalid I, Doshi P, DiGiovine B. Early enteral nutrition and outcomes of critically ill patients treated with vasopressors and mechanical ventilation. Am J Crit Care 2010;19(3):261–8.
56. Burlew CC, Moore EE, Cuschieri J, et al. Who should we feed? Western Trauma Association multi-institutional study of enteral nutrition in the open abdomen after injury. J Trauma Acute Care Surg 2012;73(6):1380–7 [discussion: 1387–8].
57. Barlow R, Price P, Reid TD, et al. Prospective multicentre randomised controlled trial of early enteral nutrition for patients undergoing major upper gastrointestinal surgical resection. Clin Nutr 2011;30(5):560–6.
58. Nelson R, Edwards S, Tse B. Prophylactic nasogastric decompression after abdominal surgery. Cochrane Database Syst Rev 2007;(3):CD004929.
59. Poulard F, Dimet J, Martin-Lefevre L, et al. Impact of not measuring residual gastric volume in mechanically ventilated patients receiving early enteral feeding: a prospective before-after study. JPEN J Parenter Enteral Nutr 2010;34(2):125–30.

60. Reignier J, Mercier E, Le Gouge A, et al. Effect of not monitoring residual gastric volume on risk of ventilator-associated pneumonia in adults receiving mechanical ventilation and early enteral feeding: a randomized controlled trial. JAMA 2013; 309(3):249–56.
61. Jeffery KM, Harkins B, Cresci GA, et al. The clear liquid diet is no longer a necessity in the routine postoperative management of surgical patients. Am Surg 1996; 62(3):167–70.
62. Heyland DK, Montalvo M, MacDonald S, et al. Total parenteral nutrition in the surgical patient: a meta-analysis. Can J Surg 2001;44(2):102–11.
63. Doig GS, Simpson F, Sweetman EA, et al. Early parenteral nutrition in critically ill patients with short-term relative contraindications to early enteral nutrition: a randomized controlled trial. JAMA 2013;309(20):2130–8.

Prophylactic Antibiotics and Prevention of Surgical Site Infections

Peter A. Najjar, MD, Douglas S. Smink, MD, MPH*

KEYWORDS

- Surgical site infection • Prophylactic antibiotics • Perioperative infection control

KEY POINTS

- Surgical site infections (SSIs) are the most common type of healthcare-associated infection in the United States, affecting more than 500,000 patients annually. Studies suggest that 40% to 60% of these infections may be preventable.
- Patients diagnosed with SSI face a 2 to 11 times increase in mortality along with prolonged hospital stays, treatment-associated risks, and potential long-term sequelae.
- Nationwide efforts to improve SSI rates include monitoring compliance with preventive guidelines via the Surgical Care Improvement Program (SCIP) along with reporting of risk-adjusted infection rates via the National Healthcare Safety Network (NHSN) and the American College of Surgeons National Surgical Quality Improvement Program (ACS-NSQIP).
- Preoperative prophylaxis with appropriately selected procedure-specific antibiotics administered 1 hour before skin incision is a mainstay of SSI prevention; excess prophylactic antibiotic use either through poor selection or continuation postoperatively is a major driver of increased multidrug-resistant organism isolates.
- Adjunctive measures, such as surgical safety checklists, minimally invasive surgical techniques, and maintenance of perioperative homeostasis, can help further reduce the burden of SSI.

INTRODUCTION

Healthcare-associated infections (HAIs) present a significant source of preventable morbidity and mortality. More than 30% of all HAIs are represented by surgical site infections (SSIs), making them the most common subtype.[1,2] Between 1.9% and

---

Conflict of Interest: None.
Department of Surgery, Brigham and Women's Hospital, Harvard Medical School, 75 Francis Street, Boston, MA 02115, USA
* Corresponding author.
E-mail address: dsmink@partners.org

Surg Clin N Am 95 (2015) 269–283
http://dx.doi.org/10.1016/j.suc.2014.11.006 surgical.theclinics.com
0039-6109/15/$ – see front matter

2.7% of all surgical patients, more than 500,000 per year, are diagnosed with an SSI leading to an estimated 8000 annual deaths.[3–6]

Studies suggest that 40% to 60% of these infections are preventable.[7] Despite this, many hospitals have yet to implement evidence-based best practices.[3,8] This article reviews the impact of SSIs, describes their measurement and reporting, and most importantly provides perioperative strategies for their prevention with a focus on the appropriate use of prophylactic antibiotics.

SURGICAL SITE INFECTION METRICS

Clinical and Social Costs

SSIs represent a significant clinical and financial burden. Those diagnosed with an SSI face a 2 to 11 times increase in mortality.[9,10] Although most survive their infection, prolonged hospital stays and secondary risks associated with treatment are common.[11] Even when patients recover, many find their overall quality of life is significantly impacted over the long term.[12] In addition to these clinical concerns, associated costs can range from $400 for superficial SSI to upward of $30,000 for organ/space SSIs leading to system-wide excess costs of more than $7 billion per year.[13,14]

Scope of the Problem

- 500,000 SSIs per year
- 8000 annual deaths
- 40%–60% preventable
- $7 billion in excess cost

Tracking Surgical Site Infections: Outcomes

The impact of SSIs and their preventability have spurred national efforts to measure and reduce their incidence. The Centers for Disease Control and Prevention (CDC) has made hospital infections a priority, establishing the National Nosocomial Infections Surveillance system in the 1970s to monitor US acute care hospital infection rates.[15] This system, known today as the National Healthcare Safety Network (NHSN), is still the most widely used HAI tracking mechanism. More than 12,000 medical facilities including acute-care hospitals, long-term acute-care hospitals, and ambulatory surgery centers report SSIs and other HAIs to the NHSN.[16]

More recently, the American College of Surgeons National Surgical Quality Improvement Program (ACS-NSQIP) and the Veterans Affairs Surgical Quality Improvement Program that preceded it have also made strides in SSI tracking at participating acute-care hospitals nationwide.

Tracking Surgical Site Infections: Process Measures

Initiated by the Centers for Medicare and Medicaid Services and the CDC, the Surgical Care Improvement Project (SCIP) is a multistakeholder partnership to reduce surgical complications including SSI. Since 2005, several process metrics around SSI have been developed, implemented, and revised with hospital performance being publically reported and sometimes tied to reimbursement (**Table 1**). Despite their widespread use, adherence to SCIP measures has not been convincingly linked to a reduction in SSI rates.[7]

Table 1
SCIP inpatient quality measures

ID#	Measure Name
SCIP-Inf-1	Prophylactic antibiotic received within 1 h before surgical incision
SCIP-Inf-2	Appropriate prophylactic antibiotic selection for surgical patients
SCIP-Inf-3	Prophylactic antibiotics discontinued within 24 (48 for cardiac surgery) h after surgery end time
SCIP-Inf-4	Cardiac surgery patients with controlled postoperative blood glucose
SCIP-Inf-6	Surgery patients with appropriate hair removal
SCIP-Inf-9	Urinary catheter removal on postoperative day 1 or 2
SCIP-Inf-10	Surgery patients with perioperative temperature management

Adapted from Surgical Care Improvement Project Core Measure Set Effective for Discharges January 1, 2014. Surgical Care Improvement Project. The Joint Commission. Available at: http://www.jointcommission.org/assets/1/6/SCIP-Measures-012014.pdf. Accessed June 1, 2014.

Classifying Wounds

Critical to SSI tracking is risk adjusting for the level of wound contamination. The clean, clean-contaminated, contaminated, and dirty or infected wound classifications provided by the CDC in **Box 1** are currently in widest use.[17]

Box 1
Criteria for classifying surgical wounds

Clean

An uninfected operative wound in which no inflammation is encountered and the respiratory, alimentary, genital, or uninfected urinary tracts are not entered. In addition, clean wounds are primarily closed and, if necessary, drained with closed drainage. Operative incisional wounds that follow nonpenetrating (blunt) trauma should be included in this category if they meet the criteria.

Clean-Contaminated

Operative wounds where the respiratory, alimentary, genital, or urinary tracts are entered under controlled conditions and without unusual contamination. Specifically, operations involving the biliary tract, appendix, vagina, and oropharynx are included in this category, provided no evidence of infection or major break in technique is encountered.

Contaminated

Open, fresh, accidental wounds. In addition, operations with major breaks in sterile technique (eg, open cardiac massage) or gross spillage from the gastrointestinal tract, and incisions in which acute, nonpurulent inflammation is encountered including necrotic tissue without evidence of purulent drainage (eg, dry gangrene) are included in this category.

Dirty or Infected

Includes old traumatic wounds with retained devitalized tissue and those that involve existing clinical infection or perforated viscera. This definition suggests that the organisms causing postoperative infection were present in the operative field before the operation.

Adapted from April 2013 CDC/NHSN protocol corrections, clarification, and additions. Available at: http://www.cdc.gov/nhsn/PDFs/pscManual/9pscSSIcurrent.pdf. Accessed May 30, 2014.

Classifying Surgical Site Infections

The CDC defines an SSI as an infection related to an operative procedure that occurs within 30 or 90 days postoperatively depending on the procedure.[17] NSQIP and Veterans Affairs Surgical Quality Improvement Program definitions are largely based on the CDC model.[18] SSIs are further classified by the CDC based on their anatomic involvement relative to the surgical wound as in **Fig. 1** and **Box 2**.[19]

SURGICAL SITE INFECTION PREVENTION STRATEGIES: PREOPERATIVE

Antibiotic Prophylaxis

Appropriately selected antibiotic prophylaxis can protect patients from postoperative infection by reducing the bacterial load present within the surgical site at the time of operation.[20] In addition to specific risks to patients, however, the increasing burden of fungal and antibiotic-resistant organisms highlights the importance of evidence-based practice and antibiotic stewardship.[21,22]

Antibiotic Selection

Evidence-based guidelines should direct antibiotic selection guided by the organisms most commonly linked to SSI following the operative procedure. Selection based on local antibiograms may supersede the national recommendations listed (**Table 2**).

Timing

In addition to appropriate selection, timing of antibiotic administration and redosing play important roles (**Table 3**). Preoperative dosing within 1 hour or less of incision is an important factor in prophylactic efficacy in addition to appropriate antibiotic

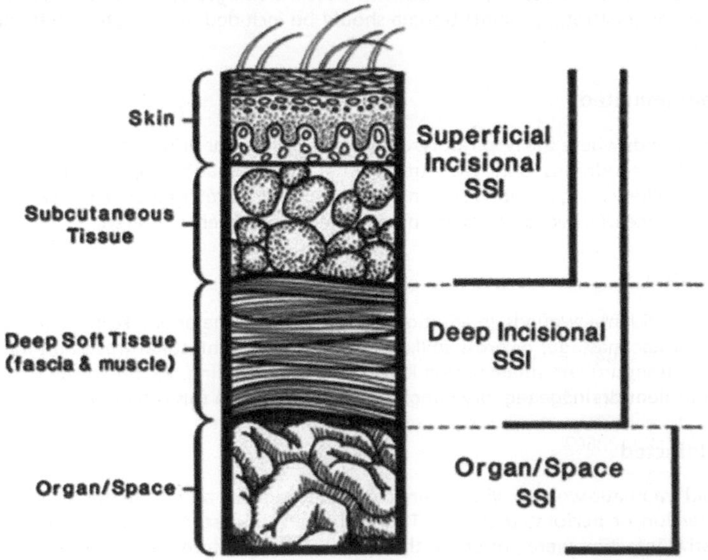

Fig. 1. Anatomic SSI classifications. (*From* Horan TC, Gaynes RP, Martone WJ, et al. CDC definitions of nosocomial surgical site infections, 1992: a modification of CDC definitions of surgical wound infections. Infect Control Hosp Epidemiol 1992;13(10):607.)

Box 2
Criteria for defining a SSI

Superficial incisional SSI

Infection occurs within 30 days after the operation and infection involves only skin or subcutaneous tissue of the incision and at least one of the following:

- Purulent drainage, with or without laboratory confirmation, from the superficial incision.
- Organisms isolated from an aseptically obtained culture of fluid or tissue from the superficial incision.
- At least one of the following signs or symptoms of infection: pain or tenderness, localized swelling, redness, or heat and superficial incision is deliberately opened by surgeon, unless incision is culture-negative.
- Diagnosis of superficial incisional SSI by the surgeon or attending physician.

Deep incisional SSI

Infection occurs within 30 days after the operation if no implant is left in place or within 1 year if implant is in place and the infection seems to be related to the operation and infection involves deep soft tissues (eg, fascial and muscle layers) of the incision and at least one of the following:

- Purulent drainage from the deep incision but not from the organ/space component of the surgical site.
- A deep incision spontaneously dehisces or is deliberately opened by a surgeon when the patient has at least one of the following signs or symptoms: fever (>38°C), localized pain, or tenderness, unless site is culture-negative.
- An abscess or other evidence of infection involving the deep incision is found on direct examination, during reoperation, or by histopathologic or radiologic examination.
- Diagnosis of a deep incisional SSI by a surgeon or attending physician.

Organ/space SSI

Infection occurs within 30 days after the operation if no implant is left in place or within 1 year if implant is in place and the infection seems to be related to the operation and infection involves any part of the anatomy (eg, organs or spaces), other than the incision, which was opened or manipulated during an operation and at least one of the following:

- Purulent drainage from a drain that is placed through a stab wound into the organ/space.
- Organisms isolated from an aseptically obtained culture of fluid or tissue in the organ/space.
- An abscess or other evidence of infection involving the organ/space that is found on direct examination, during reoperation, or by histopathologic or radiologic examination.
- Diagnosis of an organ/space SSI by a surgeon or attending physician.

From Horan TC, Gaynes RP, Martone WJ, et al. CDC definitions of nosocomial surgical site infections, 1992: a modification of CDC definitions of surgical wound infections. Infect Control Hosp Epidemiol 1992;13(10):607.

selection.[23,24] Administration within 120 minutes of incision is acceptable for vancomycin and fluoroquinolones requiring prolonged infusion times. Redosing should be based on antibiotic half-life or extensive blood loss.[23,25] Redose for blood loss greater than 1500 mL or procedures greater than two half-lives long.

Table 2
Antibiotic prophylaxis recommendations

Type of Procedure	Recommended Agents	Alternatives for β-Lactam Allergy
Cardiac/coronary artery bypass	Cefazolin, cefuroxime	Clindamycin, vancomycin
Cardiac device insertion procedures (eg, pacemaker implantation)	Cefazolin, cefuroxime	Clindamycin, vancomycin
Ventricular-assist devices	Cefazolin, cefuroxime	Clindamycin, vancomycin
Thoracic procedures including lobectomy, pneumonectomy, lung resection, and thoracotomy	Cefazolin, ampicillin-sulbactam	Clindamycin, vancomycin
Gastroduodenal procedures involving entry into lumen of gastrointestinal tract (bariatric, pancreaticoduodenectomy)	Cefazolin	Clindamycin or vancomycin + aminoglycoside or aztreonam or fluoroquinolone
Procedures without entry into gastrointestinal tract (antireflux, highly selective vagotomy) for high-risk patients	Cefazolin	Clindamycin or vancomycin + aminoglycoside or aztreonam or fluoroquinolone
Biliary tract, open procedure	Cefazolin, cefoxitin, cefotetan, ceftriaxone, ampicillin-sulbactam	Clindamycin or vancomycin + aminoglycoside or aztreonam or fluoroquinolone Metronidazole + aminoglycoside or fluoroquinolone
Elective laparoscopic procedure in low-risk patients	None	None
Elective laparoscopic procedure in high-risk patients	Cefazolin, cefoxitin, cefotetan, ceftriaxone, ampicillin-sulbactam	Clindamycin or vancomycin + aminoglycoside or aztreonam or fluoroquinolone Metronidazole + aminoglycoside or fluoroquinolone

Appendectomy for uncomplicated appendicitis	Cefoxitin, cefotetan, cefazolin + metronidazole	Clindamycin + aminoglycoside or aztreonam or fluoroquinolone Metronidazole + aminoglycoside or fluoroquinolone
Small bowel surgery in nonobstructed patients	Cefazolin	Clindamycin + aminoglycoside or aztreonam or fluoroquinolone
Small bowel surgery in obstructed patients	Cefazolin + metronidazole, cefoxitin, cefotetan	Metronidazole + aminoglycoside or fluoroquinolone
Hernia repair (hernioplasty and herniorrhaphy)	Cefazolin	Clindamycin, vancomycin
Colorectal surgery	Cefazolin + metronidazole, cefoxitin, cefotetan, ampicillin-sulbactam Ceftriaxone + metronidazole Ertapenem	Clindamycin + aminoglycoside or aztreonam or fluoroquinolone Metronidazole + aminoglycoside or fluoroquinolone
Clean-contaminated cancer surgery	Cefazolin + metronidazole, cefuroxime + metronidazole, ampicillin-sulbactam	Clindamycin
Vascular surgery	Cefazolin	Clindamycin, vancomycin
Heart, lung, or heart-lung transplantation	Cefazolin	Clindamycin, vancomycin
Liver transplantation	Piperacillin-tazobactam, cefotaxime + ampicillin	Clindamycin or vancomycin + aminoglycoside or aztreonam or fluoroquinolone
Pancreas and pancreas-kidney transplantation	Cefazolin, fluconazole (for patients at high risk of fungal infection, such as those with enteric drainage of the pancreas)	Clindamycin or vancomycin + aminoglycoside or aztreonam or fluoroquinolone
Plastic surgery: clean with risk factors or clean-contaminated	Cefazolin, ampicillin-sulbactam	Clindamycin, vancomycin

Adapted from Bratzler DW, Dellinger EP, Olsen KM, et al. Clinical practice guidelines for antimicrobial prophylaxis insurgery. Am J Health Syst Pharm 2013;70:195–283.

Table 3
Antibiotic dosing guidelines

Antimicrobial	Recommended Adult Dose	Half-Life (h) in Adults with Normal Renal Function	Recommended Redosing Interval
Ampicillin-sulbactam	3 g (ampicillin 2 g/ sulbactam 1 g)	0.8–1.3	2
Ampicillin	2 g	1–1.9	2
Aztreonam	2 g	1.3–2.4	4
Cefazolin	2 g, 3 g for pts weighing ≥120 kg	1.2–2.2	4
Cefuroxime	1.5 g	1–2	4
Cefotaxime	1 g	0.9–1.7	3
Cefoxitin	2 g	0.7–1.1	2
Cefotetan	2 g	2.8–4.6	6
Ceftriaxone	2 g	5.4–10.9	NA
Ciprofloxacin	400 mg	3–7	NA
Clindamycin	900 mg	2–4	6
Ertapenem	1 g	3–5	NA
Fluconazole	400 mg	30	NA
Gentamicin	5 mg/kg based on dosing weight (single dose)	2–3	NA
Levofloxacin	500 mg	6–8	NA
Metronidazole	500 mg	6–8	NA
Moxifloxacin	400 mg	8–15	NA
Piperacillin-tazobactam	3.375 g	0.7–1.2	2
Vancomycin	15 mg/kg	4–8	NA
Erythromycin base	1 g	0.8–3	NA
Metronidazole	1 g	6–10	NA
Neomycin	1 g	2–3 (3% absorbed under normal gastrointestinal conditions)	NA

Redosing in the operating room is recommended at an interval of approximately two times the half-life of the agent in patients with normal renal function. Recommended redosing intervals marked as "not applicable" (NA) are based on typical case length; for unusually long procedures, redosing may be needed.

Adapted from Bratzler DW, Dellinger EP, Olsen KM, et al. Clinical practice guidelines for antimicrobial prophylaxis insurgery. Am J Health Syst Pharm 2013;70:195–283.

Mechanical Bowel Preparation

Preventing SSI after colorectal surgery is especially challenging given the significant bacterial colonization of the large intestine. Reducing this burden using oral antibiotics and bowel preparations designed to evacuate the large bowel has been the subject of controversy. A recent Cochrane review along with a propensity-matched cohort of 2000 patients did show improvement in SSI rates in patients receiving intravenous (IV) and oral antibiotics along with a mechanical bowel preparation over patients receiving IV antibiotics alone; effect size, however, was small and studies evaluating specific regimens with respect to one another are challenged by heterogeneity and sample size concerns.[26,27] Both Cochrane and Agency for Healthcare Research and Quality reviews of oral mechanical bowel preparation versus enema or no preparation including more than 5000 patients showed no significant outcome differences.[28,29]

ADDITIONAL PREOPERATIVE SURGICAL SITE INFECTION PREVENTION STRATEGIES

Surgical Safety Checklists

Checklist use has been associated with improved compliance with antibiotic administration guidelines and significantly lower SSI rates in several global trials.[30,31] However, implementation factors loom large. Buy-in from front-line providers is critical, because large-scale mandatory implementation without extensive training likely mitigates impact.[32]

Skin Decontamination

Preoperative patient-applied chlorhexidine scrubs may decrease SSI rates as compared with no bathing; however, a significant benefit over bathing with regular soap has not been demonstrated.[33] The costs associated with specialized scrubs make it wise to limit their use to procedures associated with the highest risks associated with SSI, such as colorectal surgery, cardiac surgery, or orthopedic surgery for prostheses.[34,35]

Preoperative skin preparation with chlorhexidine-alcohol has shown benefit over povidine-iodine solutions. A prospective, randomized trial including 849 patients with clean-contaminated wounds showed significant decreases in superficial (4.2% vs 8.6%) and deep SSIs (1% vs 3%) with preoperative cleansing using chlorhexidine-alcohol versus povidone-iodine.[36]

Nasal decontamination with mupirocin has been shown to decrease SSI rates in several randomized controlled trials for colonized cardiac surgery patients. Routine decontamination of all patients has not been conclusively shown to be effective and should not be used because of concerns around promoting resistance.[37]

Hair Removal

Hair removal is a common preoperative practice; however, a meta-analysis of 11 randomized controlled trials reveals little evidence to support hair removal as strategy for SSI prophylaxis. If hair is removed, however, electric clippers should be used; razors have been linked to increased SSI rates.[38]

Surgical Scrubs

Modern "dry scrub" alcohol rubs are equivalent to traditional aqueous surgical scrubs when used as directed. Chlorhexidine scrubs are more effective and long-lasting than iodine in decreasing bacterial counts; however, it is unclear if this impacts SSI rates.[39]

INTRAOPERATIVE CONSIDERATIONS

Irrigation

Several studies over the past three decades have evaluated wound and intracavity irrigation with regard to SSI rates. The secular effects of increased evidence-based antibiotic prophylaxis make studies difficult to interpret; however, there seems to be little evidence in support of irrigation to prevent SSI in current practice.[40]

Laparoscopy

Laparoscopy is generally associated with decreased SSI rates in virtually all procedures in which it is a viable technique.[41–44] In light of this, some authors have suggested that minimally invasive surgery should be viewed as an important component in the SSI reduction toolbox.[45,46]

Incision and Closure

The use of electrocautery has no discernable impact on SSI rates relative to traditional scalpels for skin incision.[47] In two recent meta-analyses, however, triclosan-coated sutures significantly decreased SSI in abdominal surgery, but not breast or cardiac surgery.[48,49] As with other high-cost prevention strategies with marginal benefit, it is important to limit use to the highest-risk procedures if at all.

Maintenance of Homeostasis

In addition to the obvious importance of maintaining stable hemodynamics throughout the perioperative period, goal-directed intraoperative hemodynamic control significantly decreases SSI rates.[50]

Maintenance of normothermia is also critical. Even mild intraoperative hypothermia is associated with more than two times the risk of SSI in two randomized studies.[51,52]

Adequate oxygenation is a basic tenet of perioperative management; supraphysiologic oxygenation, however, may have a role to play in certain procedures. High fraction of inspired oxygen may be beneficial in high-SSI-risk procedures, such as colorectal surgery; it is unclear how to balance this against concerns over the potential toxicity associated with prolonged hyperoxygenation.[53,54] Accordingly, CDC recommends maintaining a fraction of inspired oxygen of 50% intraoperatively and in the immediate postoperative period for selected procedures.

Local Antibiotics

Some studies have shown a benefit to the local application of antibiotics in selected procedures, such as impregnated cement in orthopedic surgery and antibiotic irrigation in breast augmentation.[55] Recent in vitro data suggest that soaking synthetic mesh in an antibiotic solution increases bacterial clearance after contamination.[56] There is not yet convincing clinical evidence to support local or topical antibiotic use in general, however, and certainly not in lieu of IV antibiotics when indicated.

POSTOPERATIVE CONSIDERATIONS

Antibiotic Prophylaxis

The routine use of postoperative antibiotics for infection prophylaxis beyond 24 hours has not been shown to decrease SSI rates in general surgery.[57] In light of adverse effects including antibiotic-associated diarrhea and the development of multidrug-resistant organisms, postoperative antibiotic prophylaxis should not be used in patients without evidence of infection or significant contamination intraoperatively.[25] A growing awareness of antibiotic overuse has led to the development of SCIP measures, listed in **Table 1**, to combat the practice.

Blood Transfusion

The relationship between blood transfusion and SSI is complicated. Although several studies show a strong positive correlation, it is unclear whether allogeneic blood is causative or merely indicates increased infection risk. Nevertheless, there is currently no evidence to support withholding blood products as a strategy to reduce SSI.[58–60]

Glucose Control

Poorly controlled diabetes and stress-induced hyperglycemia ($>$200 mg/dL) are recognized risk factors for SSI. Careful management of perioperative blood sugar, especially in patients with diabetes, can reduce postoperative infections. There is no convincing evidence, however, that strict glycemic control beyond usual care ($<$200 mg/dL) is protective against SSI.[61]

Wound Management

For clean wounds, although silver-impregnated dressings may provide some benefit in high-risk cases, postoperative dressings likely have little role to play in SSI prevention.[62] A recent Cochrane review showed no appreciable difference between various wound dressings and wounds open to air, although interpretation of these results was limited by small studies and heterogeneity.[63]

A randomized controlled clinical trial has shown a benefit to daily probing of contaminated wounds, however, with reductions in SSI rates, pain, and length of stay in the intervention group.[64]

SUMMARY

SSIs are the most common type of HAI in the United States, affecting more than 500,000 patients annually.[4] Patients diagnosed with SSI, some 40% to 60% of which may be preventable, face a 2 to 11 times increase in mortality along with prolonged hospital stays, treatment-associated risks, and potential long-term sequelae.[7,9,10,12]

The widespread impact of SSI has led to nationwide efforts to improve infection rates by monitoring compliance with preventive guidelines via the SCIP along with reporting of risk-adjusted infection rates via the NHSN and the ACS-NSQIP.

Preoperative prophylaxis with appropriately selected procedure-specific antibiotics administered 1 hour before skin incision is a mainstay of SSI prevention.[23] Excess prophylactic antibiotic use either through poor selection or continuation postoperatively is a major driver of increased multidrug-resistant organism isolates.[21,22]

Adjunctive measures, such as surgical safety checklists, minimally invasive surgical techniques, and maintenance of perioperative homeostasis, can help further reduce the burden of SSI.[30,31,42,44,48]

REFERENCES

1. April 2013 CDC/NHSN protocol corrections, clarification, and additions. Available at: http://www.cdc.gov/nhsn/PDFs/pscManual/9pscSSIcurrent.pdf. Accessed May 28, 2014.
2. Magill SS, Hellinger W, Cohen J, et al. Prevalence of healthcare-associated infections in acute care hospitals in Jacksonville, Florida. Infect Control Hosp Epidemiol 2012;33(3):283–91.
3. Meeks DW, Lally KP, Carrick MM, et al. Compliance with guidelines to prevent surgical site infections: as simple as 1-2-3? Am J Surg 2011;201:76–83.
4. CDC. Data from the National Hospital Discharge Survey. 2010. Available at: http://www.cdc.gov/nchs/data/nhds/4procedures/2010pro_numberpercentage.pdf. Accessed May 28, 2014.
5. Mu Y, Edwards JR, Horan TC, et al. Improving risk-adjusted measures of surgical site infection for the national healthcare safety network. Infect Control Hosp Epidemiol 2011;32(10):970–86.

6. Klevens RM, Edwards JR, Richards CL Jr, et al. Estimating health care-associated infections and deaths in U.S. hospitals. Public Health Rep 2007; 122(2):160–6.
7. Hawn M, Vick CC, Richman J, et al. Surgical site infection prevention. Ann Surg 2011;8:494–501.
8. Anthony T, Murray B, Sum-Ping W, et al. Evaluating an evidence-based bundle for preventing surgical site infection: a randomized trial. Arch Surg 2011;146(3): 263–9.
9. Astagneau P, Rioux C, Golliot F, et al, INCISO Network Study Group. Morbidity and mortality associated with surgical site infections: results from the 1997–1999 INCISO surveillance. J Hosp Infect 2001;48(4):267–74.
10. Anderson DJ, Kaye KS, Classen D, et al. Strategies to prevent surgical site infections in acute care hospitals. Infect Control Hosp Epidemiol 2008;29: S51–61.
11. Kirkland KB, Briggs JP, Trivette SL, et al. The impact of surgical-site infections in the 1990s: attributable mortality, excess length of hospitalization, and extra costs. Infect Control Hosp Epidemiol 1999;20(11):725–30.
12. Anthony T, Long J, Hynan LS, et al. Surgical complications exert a lasting effect on disease-specific health-related quality of life for patients with colorectal cancer. Surgery 2003;134(2):119–25.
13. Urban JA. Cost analysis of surgical site infections. Surg Infect (Larchmt) 2006; 7(Suppl I):S19.
14. Stone PW, Braccia D, Larson E. Systematic review of economic analyses of health care-associated infections. Am J Infect Control 2005;33:501–9.
15. Healthcare associated infections: surgical site infections. Centers for Disease Control and Prevention. Available at: http://www.cdc.gov/HAI/ssi/ssi.html. Accessed July 3, 2014.
16. CDC. About the National Healthcare Safety Network, 2014. Available at: http://www.cdc.gov/nhsn/about.html. Accessed May 30, 2014.
17. April 2013 CDC/NHSN protocol corrections, clarification, and additions. Available at: http://www.cdc.gov/nhsn/PDFs/pscManual/9pscSSIcurrent.pdf. Accessed May 30, 2014.
18. American College of Surgeons. National Surgical Quality Improvement Program Operations Manual. Effective Jan. 1 2014 – June 30 2014.
19. Horan TC, Gaynes RP, Martone WJ, et al. CDC definitions of nosocomial surgical site infections, 1992: a modification of CDC definitions of surgical wound infections. Infect Control Hosp Epidemiol 1992;13(10):606–8.
20. Bratzler DW, Hunt DR. The surgical infection prevention and surgical care improvement projects: national initiatives to improve outcomes for patients having surgery. Clin Infect Dis 2006;43:322.
21. Jarvis WR. Epidemiology of nosocomial fungal infections, with emphasis on *Candida* species. Clin Infect Dis 1995;20:1526.
22. Hidron AI, Edwards JR, Patel J, et al. NHSN annual update: antimicrobial-resistant pathogens associated with healthcare-associated infections: annual summary of data reported to the National Healthcare Safety Network at the Centers for Disease Control and Prevention, 2006–2007. Infect Control Hosp Epidemiol 2008;29:996.
23. Classen DC, Evans RS, Pestotnik SL, et al. The timing of prophylactic administration of antibiotics and the risk of surgical-wound infection. N Engl J Med 1992; 326:281.
24. Hawn MT, Richman JS, Vick CC, et al. Timing of surgical antibiotic prophylaxis and the risk of surgical site infection. JAMA Surg 2013;148:649–57.

25. Steinberg JP, Braun BI, Hellinger WC, et al. Timing of antimicrobial prophylaxis and the risk of surgical site infection: results from the trial to reduce antimicrobial prophylaxis errors. Ann Surg 2009;250:10–6.
26. Nelson RL, Glenny AM, Song F. Antimicrobial prophylaxis for colorectal surgery. Cochrane Database Syst Rev 2009;(1):CD001181.
27. Englesbe MJ, Brooks L, Kubus J, et al. A statewide assessment of surgical site infection following colectomy: the role of oral antibiotics. Ann Surg 2010;252:514–20.
28. Guenaga KF, Matos D, Wille-Jorgensen P. Mechanical bowel preparation for elective colorectal surgery. Cochrane Database Syst Rev 2011;(9):CD001544.
29. Dahabreh IJ, Steele DW, Shah N, et al. Oral mechanical bowel preparation for colorectal surgery. Comparative effectiveness review No. 128. (Prepared by the Brown University Evidence-Based Practice Center under Contract No. 290-2012-00012-I.). Rockville (MD): Agency for Healthcare Research and Quality; 2014. AHRQ Publication No. 14-EHC018-EF.
30. Haynes AB, Weiser TG, Berry WR, et al. A surgical safety checklist to reduce morbidity and mortality in a global population. N Engl J Med 2009;360:491–9.
31. de Vries EN, Dijkstra L, Smorenburg SM, et al. The SURgical PAtient Safety System (SURPASS) checklist optimizes timing of antibiotic prophylaxis. Patient Saf Surg 2010;4:6.
32. Urbach DA, Govindarajan A, Saskin R, et al. Introduction of surgical safety checklists in Ontario, Canada. N Engl J Med 2014;370:1029–38.
33. Webster J. Preoperative bathing or showering with skin antiseptics to prevent surgical site infection. Cochrane Database Syst Rev 2007;(2):CD004985.
34. Lynch W, Davey PG, Malek M, et al. Cost-effectiveness analysis of the use of chlorhexidine detergent in preoperative whole-body disinfection in wound infection prophylaxis. J Hosp Infect 1992;21:179–91.
35. Kapadia BH, Johnson AJ, Issa K, et al. Economic evaluation of chlorhexidine cloths on healthcare costs due to surgical site infections following total knee arthroplasty. J Arthroplasty 2013;28(7):1061.
36. Darouiche RO, Wall MJ Jr, Itani KM, et al. Chlorhexidine-alcohol versus povidone-iodine for surgical-site antisepsis. N Engl J Med 2010;362(1):18–26.
37. Hebert C, Robicsek A. Decolonization therapy in infection control. Curr Opin Infect Dis 2010;23:340.
38. Tanner J, Woodings D, Moncaster K. Preoperative hair removal to reduce surgical site infection. Cochrane Database Syst Rev 2006;(3):CD004122.
39. Tanner J, Swarbrook S, Stuart J. Surgical hand antisepsis to reduce surgical site infection. Cochrane Database Syst Rev 2008;(1):CD004288.
40. National Institute for Health and Care Excellence. Surgical site infection: Evidence Update June 2013. Available at: https://www.evidence.nhs.uk/evidence-update-43. Accessed June 1, 2014.
41. Golub R, Siddiqui F, Pohl D. Laparoscopic versus open appendectomy: a meta-analysis. J Am Coll Surg 1998;186:545–53.
42. Centers for Disease Control and Prevention. National Nosocomial Infections Surveillance (NNIS) System Report, data summary from January 1992 through June 2003, issued August 2003. Am J Infect Control 2003;31(8):481–98.
43. Phatak UR, Pedroza C, Millas SG, et al. Revisiting the effectiveness of interventions to decrease surgical site infections in colorectal surgery: a Bayesian perspective. Surgery 2012;152(2):202–11.
44. Shabanzadeh DM, Sørensen LT. Laparoscopic surgery compared with open surgery decreases surgical site infection in obese patients: a systematic review and meta-analysis. Ann Surg 2012;256(6):934–45.

45. Gandaglia G, Ghani KR, Sood A, et al. Effect of minimally invasive surgery on the risk for surgical site infections: results from the national surgical quality improvement program (NSQIP) database. JAMA Surg 2014;149:1039–44.
46. Kim SP, Smaldone MC. Is a minimally invasive approach the solution for reducing surgical site infections? JAMA Surg 2014;149:1044.
47. Charoenkwan K, Chotirosniramit N, Rerkasem K. Scalpel versus electrosurgery for abdominal incisions. Cochrane Database Syst Rev 2012;(6):CD005987.
48. Edmiston CE, Daoud FC, Leaper DJ. Is there an evidence-based argument for embracing an antimicrobial (triclosan)-coated suture technology to reduce the risk for surgical-site infections?: a meta- analysis. Surgery 2013;154:89–100.
49. Wang ZX, Jiang CP, Cao Y, et al. Systematic review and meta-analysis of triclosan-coated sutures for the prevention of surgical-site infection. Br J Surg 2013;100:465–73.
50. Dalfino L, Giglio MT, Puntillo F, et al. Haemodynamic goal-directed therapy and postoperative infections: earlier is better. A systematic review and meta-analysis. Crit Care 2011;15(3):R154.
51. Kurz A, Sessler DI, Lenhardt R. Perioperative normothermia to reduce the incidence of surgical-wound infection and shorten hospitalization. Study of Wound Infection and Temperature Group. N Engl J Med 1996;334(19): 1209–15.
52. Melling AC, Ali B, Scott EM, et al. Effects of preoperative warming on the incidence of wound infection after clean surgery: a randomised controlled trial. Lancet 2001;358:876.
53. Togioka B, Galvagno S, Sumida S, et al. The role of perioperative high inspired oxygen therapy in reducing surgical site infection: a meta-analysis. Anesth Analg 2012;114(2):334–42.
54. Munoz-Price LS, Sands L, Lubarsky DA. Effect of high perioperative oxygen supplementation on surgical site infections. Clin Infect Dis 2013;57:1465.
55. McHugh SM, Collins CJ, Corrigan MA, et al. The role of topical antibiotics used as prophylaxis in surgical site infection prevention. J Antimicrob Chemother 2011; 66(4):693–701.
56. Sadava EE, Krpata DM, Gao Y, et al. Does presoaking synthetic mesh in antibiotic solution reduce mesh infections? An experimental study. J Gastrointest Surg 2013;17(3):562–8.
57. McDonald M, Grabsch E, Marshall C, et al. Single-versus multiple-dose antimicrobial prophylaxis for major surgery: a systematic review. Aust N Z J Surg 1998;68:388.
58. Vamvakas EC, Carven JH, Hibberd PL. Blood transfusion and infection after colorectal cancer surgery. Transfusion 1996;36:1000–8.
59. Vamvakas EC, Carven JH. Transfusion of white-cell-containing allogeneic blood components and postoperative wound infection: effect of confounding factors. Transfus Med 1998;8:29–36.
60. Talbot TR, D'Agata EM, Brinsko V, et al. Perioperative blood transfusion is predictive of poststernotomy surgical site infection: marker for morbidity or true immunosuppressant? Clin Infect Dis 2004;38:1378–82.
61. Kao LS, Meeks D, Moyer VA, et al. Peri-operative glycaemic control regimens for preventing surgical site infections in adults. Cochrane Database Syst Rev 2009;(3):CD006806.
62. Krieger BR, Davis DM, Sanchez JE, et al. The use of silver nylon in preventing surgical site infections following colon and rectal surgery. Dis Colon Rectum 2011;54:1014–9.

63. Dumville JC, Walter CJ, Sharp CA, et al. Dressings for the prevention of surgical site infection. Cochrane Database Syst Rev 2011;(7):CD003091.
64. Towfigh S, Clarke T, Yacoub W, et al. Significant reduction of wound infections with daily probing of contaminated wounds: a prospective randomized clinical trial. Arch Surg 2011;146(4):448–52.

Deep Venous Thrombosis and Venous Thromboembolism Prophylaxis

Keely L. Buesing, MD*, Barghava Mullapudi, MD,
Kristin A. Flowers, MD

KEYWORDS

- Venous thromboembolism • Deep venous thrombosis • Risk factors
- Management strategies • Prophylaxis

KEY POINTS

- Venous thromboembolism (VTE) affects up to 25% of hospitalized patients, with up to 30% of those experiencing complications.
- Risk stratification is important in choosing therapy for prevention and management of VTE.
- Management of VTE depends on precipitating factors and future risk of VTE progression versus bleeding.
- Low-molecular-weight heparin is the preferred anticoagulant for initial treatment of VTE.

Venous thromboembolism (VTE), which includes deep venous thrombosis (DVT) and pulmonary embolism (PE), remains an all too familiar risk for surgical patients, occurring in up to 25% of those hospitalized.[1] These patients are a unique population who possess all 3 components of Virchow triad (stasis, hypercoagulability, and endothelial injury), completing the triad known to be the cause of thrombus formation. Despite validated guidelines, the problem is frequently left inappropriately addressed, leaving patients at risk for a process that can lead to significant morbidity and mortality. Fifty percent of all DVTs are asymptomatic, but approximately 30% will have additional complications.[2]

For some patients, a DVT is a transient episode (ie, the symptoms resolve once the disease is successfully treated). For others, it can lead to a PE, which occurs in more than one-third of patients with DVT.[1,2] PE causes sudden death in up to 34% of patients,[3] particularly when one or more of the larger pulmonary arteries are completely blocked by clot. Most of those who survive do not have any lasting effects; however, if the embolus in the lung fails to completely dissolve, chronic pulmonary

Disclosure statement: The authors have nothing to disclose.
Division of Trauma & Surgical Critical Care, Department of General Surgery, University of Nebraska Medical Center, 983280 Nebraska Medical Center, Omaha, NE 68198-3280, USA
* Corresponding author.
E-mail address: keely.buesing@unmc.edu

Surg Clin N Am 95 (2015) 285–300
http://dx.doi.org/10.1016/j.suc.2014.11.005 surgical.theclinics.com

hypertension may eventually occur, causing chronic shortness of breath and varying degrees of heart failure.

The Surgeon General's First Call to Action to Prevent Deep Vein Thrombosis and Pulmonary Embolism came in 2008 and estimated 350,000 to 600,000 Americans each year have a DVT and/or PE. Furthermore, at least 100,000 deaths are attributed to DVT/PE each year.[3] Of those who survive, many go on to have complications with serious and negative impacts on quality of life. DVT and PE are estimated to be the number one preventable cause of death in hospitalized patients. To offset this risk, the Surgical Care Improvement Project states in its guidelines that all surgical patients should have thromboprophylaxis ordered and administered within 24 hours of an operation. The Joint Commission also requires that all surgical patients receive anticoagulation, reflecting measures adopted by the Centers for Medicare and Medicaid Services, starting May 1st, 2009.[4]

Despite initiatives and mandates, VTE prophylaxis is underutilized in the United States. A 2009 analysis by Franklin Michota,[5] citing data from a study by Brigham and Women's Hospital in 2000, revealed that only 34% of high-risk patients receive appropriate prophylaxis. An article published in 2014 by the *Journal of the American College of Surgeons* about adopting mandatory VTE risk stratification and administration similarly revealed that only 58.5% of surgical patients at risk received VTE prophylaxis.[4] Why? The reasons cited are as follows:

1. There is a fear of anticoagulant-associated bleeding.
2. There is a lack of awareness regarding VTE.
3. It is thought that guidelines are based on risks and benefits of prophylaxis in clinical trials that exclude recommendations for certain subsets of patients.
4. Individual risk assessment is necessary, making a protocol difficult to reinforce.

The following sections are intended to address each of these cited reasons individually.

BLEEDING RISK

The International Medical Prevention Registry on Venous Thromboembolism investigators developed a scoring system to calculate the risk of bleeding in medical patients.[6] **Table 1** shows the bleeding risk factors identified for purposes of this study.

Scores greater than or equal to 7.0 were associated with a 7.9% risk of any bleeding and a 4.1% risk of major bleeding.[6] If the risk of bleeding is greater than the risk of VTE, then chemical prophylaxis can be avoided.

The ninth edition of the American College of Chest Physicians' (ACCP) guidelines, revised and published in 2012, includes a consideration of the bleeding risk in patients receiving anticoagulants. They did not assess how the risk of bleeding would influence every recommendation because it would be unlikely to change the recommendation, there are few data assessing outcomes in patients with differing risks of bleeding, and because of the lack of validated tools for stratifying bleeding risk. For extended-duration anticoagulation, recommendations are based on 4 primary risk groups for VTE and 3 risk groups for major bleeding (**Table 2**). The estimated total of recurrent VTE versus major bleeding for each of the 12 combinations is shown in **Table 3**.[7]

LACK OF AWARENESS REGARDING VENOUS THROMBOEMBOLISM

Table 4 is a reproduction of the Venous Thromboembolism Update by Joseph Caprini, MD, and summarizes the incidence and percent of complications of VTE in an attempt to underscore the significance of VTE and associated complications.[8]

Table 1
Factors at admission associated with bleeding risk

Bleeding Risk Factors	Points
Moderate renal failure; GFR 30–59 vs >60 mL/min/m^2	1
Male vs female	1
Age: 40–84 y vs <40 y old	1.5
Current cancer	2
Rheumatic disease	2
Central venous catheter	2
ICU/CCU	2.5
Severe renal failure; GFR <30 vs >60 mL/min/m^2	2.5
Hepatic failure (INR >1.5)	2.5
Age: >85 y vs <40 y	3.5
Platelet count <50 × 10^9 cells/L	4
Bleeding within 3 mo before admission	4
Active gastroduodenal ulcer	4.5

Scores greater than or equal to 7.0 were associated with 7.9% risk of any bleeding and a 4.1% risk of major bleeding.

Abbreviations: CCU, critical care unit; GFR, glomerular filtration rate; ICU, intensive care unit; INR, international normalized ratio.

From Decousus H, Tapson VF, Bergmann JF, et al. Factors at admission associated with bleeding risk in medical patients. Findings from the IMPROVE investigators. Chest 2011;139(1):75; with permission.

Table 2
Rates of recurrent VTE and major bleeding events with long-term anticoagulation

	Outcomes After 5 y of Treatment	Risk of Bleeding: Low	Intermediate	High
First VTE provoked by surgery	Recurrent VTE reduction %	2.6 (2.2–2.9) (0.1 fatal)	2.6 (2.2–2.9) (0.1 fatal)	2.6 (2.2–2.9) (0.1 fatal)
	Major bleeding increase %	2.4 (0–8.7) (0.3 fatal)	4.9 (0.1–17.3) (0.5 fatal)	19.6 (0.2–69.2) (2.2 fatal)
First VTE provoked by a nonsurgical factor/first unprovoked distal DVT	Recurrent VTE reduction %	13.2 (11.3–14.2) (0.5 fatal)	13.2 (11.3–14.2) (0.5 fatal)	13.2 (11.3–14.2) (0.5 fatal)
	Major bleeding increase %	2.4 (0–8.7) (0.3 fatal)	4.9 (0.1–17.3) (0.5 fatal)	19.6 (0.2–69.2) (2.2 fatal)
First unprovoked proximal DVT or PE	Recurrent VTE reduction %	26.4 (22.5–28.5) (1 fatal)	26.4 (22.5–28.5) (1 fatal)	26.4 (22.5–28.5) (1 fatal)
	Major bleeding increase %	2.4 (0–8.7) (0.3 fatal)	4.9 (0.1–17.3) (0.5 fatal)	19.6 (0.2–69.2) (2.2 fatal)
Second unprovoked VTE	Recurrent VTE reduction %	39.6 (33.7–42.7) (1.4 fatal)	39.6 (33.7–42.7) (1.4 fatal)	39.6 (33.7–42.7) (1.4 fatal)
	Major bleeding increase%	2.4 (0–8.7) (0.3 fatal)	4.9 (0.1–17.3) (0.5 fatal)	19.6 (0.2–69.2) (2.2 fatal)

Data from Kearon C, Akl EA, Comerota AJ, et al. Antithrombotic therapy and prevention of thrombosis, 9th ed: American College of Chest Physicians evidence-based clinical practice guidelines. Chest 2012;141(2 Suppl):e419S–94S.

Table 3 Complications of VTE	
PE	• There is a 1%–5% incidence in patients with 4 or more risk factors for VTE. • 16% mortality at 3 mo is caused by PE (30–80,000 patients); 34% of these patients present as sudden death.
Pulmonary hypertension	• 4% of patients with a PE develop chronic pulmonary hypertension.
Clinical VTE	• It involves drugs, testing, wearing hose, and changes in lifestyle. ◦ Risk of phlegmasia alba and cerulea dolens ◦ Risk of venous gangrene with limb loss
Silent VTE	Risk of subsequent event is 2 × the control population; the greatest risk is in the following 2 y.[9,11]
Embolic stroke	• There is a 20%–30% patent foramen ovale rate. ◦ 50% of patients with embolic stroke are disabled. ◦ 20% of patients with embolic stroke die. ◦ 30% of patients with embolic stroke recover.

Adapted from Caprini JA. Venous thromboembolism update. Available at: http://web2.facs.org/download/Caprini.pdf.

Symptomatic patients with a PE have a higher risk of recurrent VTE than those with symptomatic VTE alone. There is a higher recurrence rate of VTE in men than women (20% vs 6%, relative risk 3.6).[2,9] Sometimes, lifestyle-altering vigilance is required to avoid and/or manage the potential impact of other risk factors (prolonged air travel, further surgery, trauma, and so forth).

Chronic venous insufficiency (CVI) may develop after DVT. CVI is also known as postthrombotic syndrome (PTS), which can occur months to years following a thrombotic event in up to 30% of patients. CVI results from a thrombus injuring or destroying one or more of the venous valves in deep veins of the leg, resulting in leg pain and edema with prolonged standing, accompanied by mild to extensive varicose veins, skin breakdown, ulceration, and eventually skin pigmentation changes. These patients may also develop chronic venous stasis ulcers, which provide a complicated problem to clinically manage.[9–11]

GUIDELINES NOT APPLICABLE TO MY PATIENT

The ninth edition of the ACCP's guidelines and the Caprini score (see the discussion on individual risk assessment later) include patient populations from orthopedics, plastic

Table 4
VTE prophylaxis based on Caprini score and risk group

Risk	Caprini Score	VTE Incidence[a] (%)	Prophylaxis
Very low	0	0.5	Early ambulation
Low	1–2	1.5	IPCDs
Moderate	3–4	3.0	LMWH or UFH, ± IPCDs
High	5+	6.0	LMWH or UFH, *plus* IPCDs or GCS

Abbreviations: GCS, graduated compression stockings; IPCD, intermittent pneumatic compression device.

[a] Estimated baseline risk in the absence of prophylaxis.

Data from Gould MK, Garcia DA, Wren S, et al. Prevention of VTE in nonorthopedic surgical patients: antithrombotic therapy and prevention of thrombosis, 9th ed: American College of Chest Physicians evidence-based clinical practice guidelines. Chest 2012;141(2 Suppl):e227S–77S.

and reconstructive surgery, otolaryngology, and vascular and general surgery. Validation studies were conducted using plastic surgery, otolaryngology and general surgery patients. Both the bleeding risk and VTE risk scores identify patients with a clinically relevant risk, allowing the surgeon to determine the risk-to-benefit ratio in an objective, standardized fashion.

NEED FOR INDIVIDUALIZED RISK ASSESSMENT

The Caprini score is a validated scoring system that shows an increased DVT incidence rate by risk level.[12–14] Scores greater than 2 are deemed moderate risk and scores greater than 5 are high risk for VTE, with an incidence of 3.0% and 6.5%, respectively.[15] The Caprini score uses risk factors for VTE to assign points, resulting in a score with which the surgeon can weigh the risk of bleeding against the risk of VTE to determine what prophylaxis is appropriate for an individual patient. There is a direct correlation between an increased risk score and the development of clinically relevant VTE over a wide variety of surgical subspecialties.[13] The Caprini score "avoids blanket prophylaxis with anticoagulants since those with low scores have a risk of thrombosis that is lower than the bleeding risks with anticoagulation."[9] **Fig. 1** is an example of a sheet used to calculate the Caprini risk score and notes the appropriate pharmacologic or mechanical prophylaxis for each risk group. It also lists risk factors for DVT as identified by Caprini.

In summary, a Caprini score greater than 8 increases the risk of VTE about 20-fold, whereas scores of 7 to 8 are at a 5- to 10-fold increase when compared with low-risk patients across surgical subspecialties.[14,16]

A summary of general DVT prophylaxis based on the ACCP's guidelines, which incorporate the Caprini scoring system, can be seen in **Table 5**. Prophylaxis for specific patient groups is discussed later.

MANAGEMENT OF UNCOMPLICATED VENOUS THROMBOEMBOLISM

It is important to avoid both extension and recurrence of DVT in order to reduce the risk of PE and the occurrence of PTSs. Treatment guidelines recommend that patients with uncomplicated DVT be initially treated using low-molecular-weight heparin (LMWH), unfractionated heparin (UFH), fondaparinux, or a hirudin derivative. LMWH or fondaparinux are suggested rather than intravenous (IV) or subcutaneous UFH. Once-daily administration of LMWH is recommended over twice-daily regimens. The addition of an oral vitamin K antagonist (VKA) is warranted for at least 3 months or longer if certain factors (discussed earlier) are identified placing a patient at high risk for recurrence.[7,17] This treatment should be started the same day as parenteral therapy, and the continuation of parenteral therapy should span a minimum of 5 days and until the international normalized ratio (INR) is 2.0 or more for at least 24 hours.

The following is a discussion of treatment guidelines in relation to the location of VTE, based on the ninth edition of the ACCP's guidelines.

Lower Extremity Deep Venous Thrombosis

Proximal deep venous thrombosis

Up to 50% of patients who have a proximal lower extremity DVT develop a PE[7]; therefore, attenuation of the thrombotic process is of utmost importance. In patients with a proximal DVT of the leg provoked by surgery, anticoagulation is recommended for 3 months. In patients with a proximal DVT provoked by a nonsurgical transient risk factor, anticoagulation for only 3 months is recommended, even if the bleeding risk is low or moderate. In patients with an unprovoked DVT, extended anticoagulant therapy

Deep Vein Thrombosis (DVT)
Prophylaxis Orders
(For use in Elective General Surgery Patients)

BIRTHDATE
NAME
CPI No.
SEX M F VISIT No. ________

Thrombosis Risk Factor Assessment
(Choose all that apply)

Each Risk Factor Represents 1 Point

- ☐ Age 41-60 years
- ☐ Acute myocardial infarction
- ☐ Swollen legs (current)
- ☐ Congestive heart failure (<1 month)
- ☐ Varicose veins
- ☐ Medical patient currently at bed rest
- ☐ Obesity (BMI >25)
- ☐ History of inflammatory bowel disease
- ☐ Minor surgery planned
- ☐ History of prior major surgery (<1 month)
- ☐ Sepsis (<1 month)
- ☐ Abnormal pulmonary function (COPD)
- ☐ Serious Lung disease including pneumonia (<1 month)
- ☐ Oral contraceptives or hormone replacement therapy
- ☐ Pregnancy or postpartum (<1 month)
- ☐ History of unexplained stillborn infant, recurrent spontaneous abortion (≥ 3), premature birth with toxemia or growth-restricted infant
- ☐ Other risk factors________

Subtotal:

Each Risk Factor Represents 2 Points

- ☐ Age 61-74 years
- ☐ Central venous access
- ☐ Arthroscopic surgery
- ☐ Major surgery (>45 minutes)
- ☐ Malignancy (present or previous)
- ☐ Laparoscopic surgery (>45 minutes)
- ☐ Patient confined to bed (>72 hours)
- ☐ Immobilizing plaster cast (<1 month)

Subtotal:

Each Risk Factor Represents 3 Points

- ☐ Age 75 years or older
- ☐ Family History of thrombosis*
- ☐ History of DVT/PE
- ☐ Positive Prothrombin 20210A
- ☐ Positive Factor V Leiden
- ☐ Positive Lupus anticoagulant
- ☐ Elevated serum homocysteine
- ☐ Heparin-induced thrombocytopenia (HIT) (Do not use heparin or any low molecular weight heparin)
- ☐ Elevated anticardiolipin antibodies
- ☐ Other congenital or acquired thrombophilia

If yes: Type________

* most frequently missed risk factor

Subtotal:

Each Risk Factor Represents 5 Points

- ☐ Stroke (<1 month)
- ☐ Multiple trauma (<1 month)
- ☐ Elective major lower extremity arthroplasty
- ☐ Hip, pelvis or leg fracture (<1 month)
- ☐ Acute spinal cord injury (paralysis) (<1 month)

Subtotal:

TOTAL RISK FACTOR SCORE:

FACTORS ASSOCIATED WITH INCREASED BLEEDING

Patient may not be a candidate for anticoagulant therapy & SCDs should be considered.

Active Bleed, Ingestion of Oral Anticoagulants, Administration of glycoprotein IIb/IIIa inhibitors, History of heparin induced thrombocytopenia

CLINICAL CONSIDERATIONS FOR THE USE OF SEQUENTIAL COMPRESSION DEVICES (SCD)

Patient may not be a candidate for SCDs & alternative prophylactic measures should be considered.

Patients with Severe Peripheral Arterial Disease, CHF, Acute Superficial DVT

Total Risk Factor Score	Risk Level	Prophylaxis Regimen
0	VERY LOW	☐ Early ambulation
1-2	LOW	☐ Sequential Compression Device (SCD)
3-4	MODERATE	Choose ONE of the following medications +/- compression devices: ☐ Sequential Compression Device (SCD) - Optional ☐ Heparin 5000 units SQ TID ☐ Enoxaparin/Lovenox: ☐ 40mg SQ daily (WT < 150kg, CrCl > 30mL/min) ☐ 30mg SQ daily (WT < 150kg, CrCl = 10-29mL/min) ☐ 30mg SQ BID (WT > 150kg, CrCl > 30mL/min) (Please refer to Dosing Guidelines on the back of this form)
5 or more	HIGH	Choose ONE of the following medications PLUS compression devices: ☐ Sequential Compression Device (SCD) ☐ Heparin 5000 units SQ TID (Preferred with Epidurals) ☐ Enoxaparin/Lovenox (Preferred): ☐ 40mg SQ daily (WT < 150kg, CrCl > 30mL/min) ☐ 30mg SQ daily (WT < 150kg, CrCl = 10-29mL/min) ☐ 30mg SQ BID (WT > 150kg, CrCl > 30mL/min) (Please refer to Dosing Guidelines on the back of this form)

☐ Ambulatory Surgery - No orders for venous thromboembolic prophylaxis required
☐ VTE Prophylaxis Contraindicated, Reason: ________

Joseph A. Caprini, MD, MS, FACS, RVT
VTE Risk Factor Assessment Tool

Physician Signature	Dr. #	Date	Time
Processed By:	Date/Time:		

Fig. 1. Example of Caprini score sheet used to individualize VTE risk assessment and guide VTE prophylaxis. BMI, body mass index; CHF, congestive heart failure; COPD, chronic obstructive pulmonary disease. (*From* Caprini JA, Arcelus JI, Hasty JH, et al. Clinical assessment of venous thromboembolic risk in surgical patients. Semin Thromb Hemost 1991;17(Suppl 3):304–12; with permission.)

greater than 3 months is recommended if the bleeding risk is low to moderate. After 3 months of therapy, these patients should be evaluated for the risk-to-benefit ratio of extended therapy; for low to moderate risk, therapy should be extended past 3 months. In case of a high bleeding risk, only 3 months of therapy is recommended. For a second unprovoked DVT, extended anticoagulant therapy over 3 months is

Table 5
VTE prophylaxis for specific laparoscopic procedures

Procedure	Risk Factors	Recommendation
Lap chole	0 or 1	None, PCDs, UFH, or LMWH
Lap chole	2 or more	PCDs, UFH, or LMWH
Lap appy	0 or 1	None, PCDs, UFH, or LMWH
Lap appy	2 or more	PCDs, UFH, or LMWH
Diagnostic lap	2 or more	PCDs, UFH, or LMWH
Lap inguinal hernia	2 or more	PCDs, UFH, or LMWH
Lap Nissen	0 or 1	PCDs, UFH, or LMWH
Lap Nissen	2 or more	PCDs *and* UFH or LMWH
Splenectomy	0 or 1	PCDs, UFH, or LMWH
Splenectomy	2 or more	PCDs *and* UFH or LMWH
Other major lap procedures: Roux-Y, and so forth	0 or more	PCDs *and* UFH or LMWH

Abbreviations: appy, appendectomy; chole, cholecystectomy; Lap, laparoscopic; PCD, pneumatic compression device; UFH, unfractionated heparin.

Adapted from Society of American Gastrointestinal and Endoscopic Surgeons (SAGES) Guidelines Committee. Guidelines for deep venous thrombosis prophylaxis during laparoscopic surgery. Surg Endosc 2007;21:1007–9; with permission.

recommended for patients with a low to moderate bleeding risk. For those with a high risk of bleeding, only 3 months of therapy is used.[7]

Isolated distal deep venous thrombosis

Of patients who develop a distal (below the knee) lower extremity DVT, 10% to 20% will have extension to more proximal veins. In patients with acute distal DVT of the leg and without severe symptoms or risk factors for extension, guidelines suggest serial imaging of the deep veins for 2 weeks to monitor for extension rather than initial anticoagulation. If the thrombus does not extend to more proximal leg veins (above the level of the knee), no anticoagulation is recommended. If the thrombus extends, then anticoagulation should be initiated and follows the same pathway as for acute proximal DVT. If patients are managed initially with anticoagulation because of symptoms or a high risk for extension, the same approach as with proximal DVT is used.[7]

For both proximal and distal (symptomatic or extending) acute DVT of the leg, in patients with cancer, extended anticoagulant therapy greater than 3 months is recommended. LMWH is recommended over VKA for patients with cancer; for those not treated with LMWH, VKA is recommended over dabigatran or rivaroxaban for long-term therapy. In all patients, the extended use of anticoagulant should be reevaluated at regular intervals (ie, annually). If using a VKA, a therapeutic INR range of 2.0 to 3.0 (target 2.5) is recommended. The use of compression stockings is suggested for all patients with acute symptomatic DVT and should be worn for 2 years.

Upper Extremity Deep Venous Thrombosis

In patients with acute upper extremity DVT (UEDVT) that involves the axillary or more proximal veins, initial parenteral anticoagulation (with LMWH or fondaparinux, preferably) is recommended followed by therapy for at least 3 months. If the DVT is associated with a central venous catheter, it is recommended that the catheter not be removed if it is functional and there is an ongoing need; anticoagulation should be continued as long as the catheter is in place. If the catheter is removed, 3 months of anticoagulation is recommended. The use of compression sleeves or vasoactive medications is not suggested.

Splanchnic Vein Thrombosis

In patients with symptomatic splanchnic vein thrombosis (hepatic, portal, mesenteric, and/or splenic vein thromboses), anticoagulation is recommended. In patients with incidentally detected splanchnic vein thrombosis, no anticoagulation is recommended unless certain factors are present, such as progression, lack of cavernous formation, and ongoing cancer therapy. Esophageal varices secondary to acute portal vein thrombosis are not necessarily a contraindication to therapy because such treatment may improve portal hypertension.[7]

LOW-MOLECULAR-WEIGHT HEPARIN VERSUS UNFRACTIONATED HEPARIN FOR THE INITIAL TREATMENT OF DEEP VENOUS THROMBOSIS

Several meta-analyses have summarized the trials addressing this question. The evidence suggests that LMWH is associated with decreased mortality, lower recurrence of VTE, and decreased incidence of major bleeding compared with IV UFH.[7] However, the quality of this evidence is low because of the high risk of bias in the primary studies and evidence of publication bias in favor of LMWH. It does have the advantage of easier administration without need for monitoring and lower incidence of heparin-induced thrombocytopenia. These advantages need to be weighed against the risk of accumulation in patients with renal failure.

ADJUNCTS TO ANTICOAGULATION

Compression stockings should be initiated immediately on recognition of DVT to decrease the risk of PTS and continued as long as patients have swelling, usually for at least 2 years.[7]

Inferior vena cava (IVC) filters have been shown to lower the risk of fatal PE in patients with a DVT who are unable to be anticoagulated and in those who failed therapy (ie, PE despite adequate anticoagulation). When the bleeding risk resolves, a conventional course of anticoagulation is still recommended. In most instances, IVC filters should not be used in patients without a DVT or PE as a prophylactic measure alone, regardless of the risk factors, including trauma, surgery, or even cancer.[18]

MANAGEMENT OF COMPLICATIONS OF DEEP VENOUS THROMBOSIS

Pulmonary Embolism

Unless contraindicated, full-dose anticoagulation should be started when a PE is diagnosed and even in cases of high suspicion until imaging studies prove otherwise. Treatment should be initiated preferentially with weight-based full-dose LMWH. As an alternative, either continuous IV UFH titrated to an activated partial thromboplastin time of 60 to 80 seconds or fondaparinux can be used, according to both the ACCP and European Society of Cardiology's guidelines.[7,17]

In patients with acute PE, early initiation of VKA (same day as parenteral therapy) over delayed initiation and continuation of parenteral anticoagulation for a minimum of 5 days and until the INR is 2.0 or more for at least 24 hours is recommended.[7]

In case of unstable PE or massive PE with significant right heart strain on echocardiography, either catheter-directed or systemic thrombolysis should be the treatment of choice. Systemically, tissue plasminogen activator 10 mg bolus followed by a continuous infusion of the remaining 90 mg over 2 hours is administered when not contraindicated. This treatment may acutely avoid cardiogenic shock and death or, later, development of chronic thromboembolic pulmonary hypertension.[17]

After immediate anticoagulation, long-term anticoagulation should be established with a VKA for 3 months if PE is attributed to an isolated or acquired cause or continued for life if the PE is attributed to a permanent or recurrent cause.[7]

Phlegmasia Cerulea Dolens and Phlegmasia Alba Dolens

Phlegmasia syndromes historically had amputation rates of 20% to 50% and PE rates of 12% to 40% before the advent of thrombolytic therapies.[19] Phlegmasia syndromes that are associated with acute iliac and femoral vein thrombosis have been successfully treated by catheter-directed fibrinolysis.[20,21] If patients are not candidates for fibrinolysis, then open surgical venous thrombectomy and creation of an arteriovenous fistula is necessary to obtain rapid venous decompression and decrease the risk of PTS.[22,23] If compartment syndrome is suspected, then fasciotomies should be promptly performed. In case of microvascular thrombosis without extension to the iliac or femoral veins and unlikely to benefit from thrombolysis, fasciotomies may still be necessary to salvage the limb. Morbidity in the setting of compartment syndrome and fasciotomies is high, with up to 65% of patients experiencing subsequent major or minor complications, such as amputation, superficial perineal nerve injury, need for further muscle debridement, wound complications, and death.[23]

DEEP VENOUS THROMBOSIS SECONDARY TO ANATOMIC CAUSES

Paget-Schroetter syndrome, or effort thrombosis, is usually found in young athletes who perform repetitive motion (eg, baseball, volleyball, swimming), secondary to hypertrophy and/or lateral insertion of the subclavius muscle, which compresses the subclavian vein and causes thrombosis. This syndrome was historically treated with anticoagulation alone with a high rate of chronic pain and swelling, but now the treatment has evolved to be multimodal. The current suggested regimen includes early anticoagulation, endovascular thrombolysis and balloon venoplasty of the narrowed segment.[24]

Iliac vein compression syndrome and secondary thrombosis, known as May-Thurner syndrome, occurs when there is an obstruction or thrombosis of the lower extremity venous outflow as a result of compression by the overlying right iliac artery. This syndrome most commonly presents in young females in the left iliac vein who may or may not have intrinsic risk factors for DVT, such as factor V Leiden or the use of oral contraceptives.[25,26] Historically, these were treated with anticoagulation, but now several series have shown that use of anticoagulation along with catheter-directed thrombolysis and placement of a stent at the area of stenosis has been shown to improve PTS and patency.[7,27] The latest randomized multicenter trials (the Acute venous Thrombosis: Thrombus Removal with Adjunctive Catheter-Directed Thrombolysis and the European Catheter-Directed Venous Thrombolysis in Acute Iliofemoral Vein Thrombosis studies) reflect significantly improved patency and reduced incidence of PTS in patients who receive catheter-directed thrombolysis.[28,29]

VENOUS THROMBOEMBOLISM PREVENTION IN SPECIFIC PATIENT POPULATIONS

The information presented to follow reflects the most recent version of the ACCP's guidelines on VTE prevention for specific surgical specialties. It is intended as a concise summary of the rationale and final recommendations taking into account the unique characteristics of each patient population.

Minimally Invasive Surgery

In 2007, the Society of American Gastrointestinal Endoscopic Surgeons', published their guidelines and recommendations for VTE prophylaxis in laparoscopic surgery.[30] Intended to be flexible, the guidelines are meant to be adjusted according to individual patient characteristics while maintaining the goals set for open procedures. Where published data are lacking, expert opinion was used to augment the final recommendations. Risk stratification follows the factors known for open procedures, and the committee makes specific mention that not enough evidence exists to suggest that body position alters risk.

Table 5 lists prophylaxis recommendations for specific laparoscopic procedures along with a listing of the associated levels of evidence.

Malignancy

In a recent study, patients with cancer with VTE had an approximate 3-fold increase in hospitalizations (1.38 vs 0.55) and incurred higher total health care costs than similar patients without VTE ($74,959 vs $41,691 per patient; $P<.0001$).[31] Other publications have shown that the number of VTE events are significantly increased in patients with cancer over 12 months following initiation of chemotherapy versus control groups (12.6% vs 1.4%, $P<.0001$). Incidence varied by cancer type, from 8.2% (bladder) to as high as 19.2% (pancreas).[32]

Because of the high incidence of VTE in this patient population, a unique risk score was developed by Khorana, which has been endorsed by multiple guidelines, including those from the American Society of Clinical Oncology and the National Comprehensive Cancer Network (NCCN),[33,34] and is shown in **Table 6**.

The NCCN revised and published their recommendations for VTE prophylaxis in 2014. In summary, inpatients who have no contraindication to anticoagulation should receive prophylactic anticoagulation and/or intermittent pneumatic compression devices (IPCDs) and/or graduated compression stockings (GCS). Those with contraindications to anticoagulation should receive IPC and/or GCS. After discharge, it is recommended that patients who underwent an operation receive anticoagulation for up to 4 weeks postoperatively. For medical oncology patients, those with multiple myeloma receiving thalidomide or lenalidomide who are at high risk (see **Table 6**) should receive VTE prophylaxis with either LMWH 40 mg every 24 hours or warfarin (to a target INR of 2–3). Low-risk patients with myeloma should receive 81 to

Table 6
Risk scoring in patients with cancer

Patient Characteristics	Risk Score[a]
Site of Cancer	
Very high risk (stomach, pancreas)	2
High risk (lung, lymphoma, gynecologic, bladder, testicular)	1
Prechemotherapy platelet count $\geq 350 \times 10^9$/L	1
Hemoglobin level <10 g/dL or use of red cell growth factors	1
Prechemotherapy leukocyte count >11,000/mm^3	1
Body mass index ≥ 35 kg/m^2	1

[a] High-risk score, ≥3; intermediate-risk score, 1–2; low-risk score, 0.

Adapted from Khorana AA, Kuderer NM, Culakova E, et al. Development and validation of a predictive model for chemotherapy-associated thrombosis. Blood 2008;111:4902–7.

325 mg aspirin per day. For all other patients who have not undergone an operation, no routine VTE prophylaxis is recommended.[34]

Bariatrics

To date, no consensus exists regarding VTE prophylaxis in morbidly obese patients. A 2013 survey of practice patterns among 385 bariatric surgeons revealed the majority agreed on what qualifies a patient as high risk and use VTE chemoprophylaxis preoperatively. VTE screening and duration of therapy, however, varied widely among practitioners. Most of the surgeons surveyed routinely performed bariatric surgery laparoscopically (98.7%).[35]

Risk factors thought to qualify a patient as high risk for VTE included history of DVT, known hypercoagulable status, severe immobility, body mass index exceeding 55 kg/m^2, and Pa_{O_2} less than 60 mm Hg. More than half of the surgeons routinely performed preoperative DVT screening (56%), either by clinical examination alone (33.1%) or routine ultrasound (20.9%). Preoperative VTE prophylaxis was used by 92.4% of respondents, with 48.0% using unfractionated heparin, 33.4% using enoxaparin sodium (Lovenox), 2.6% using fondaparinux, and 8.3% using another agent. Retrievable IVC filters have also been used in the past with this patient population, and 28.1% continue to routinely use them preoperatively.[35]

Sequential compression devices were used by most of the respondents, both intraoperatively and postoperatively (96.3% and 91.6%, respectively). Postoperative chemical prophylaxis was also used routinely (97%), starting on postoperative day 0 in most (70%). Lovenox was the most commonly used agent (49.5%), followed by heparin (33%), other agents (9.1%), and fondaparinux (5.4%). Chemical prophylaxis was discontinued at discharge in most cases (48.5%). If continued after discharge (as with 43.8% of respondents), the most common duration of therapy was 2 to 4 weeks (40.1%) with Lovenox (39.7%). If a retrievable IVC filter was used, it was most commonly removed 30 to 90 days postoperatively (55.2%).[35] The wide range of practice patterns among bariatric surgeons reflects the need for validated studies regarding this subset of patients.

Orthopedics

In patients undergoing total hip or knee arthroplasty, the ACCP's ninth edition guidelines recommend use of 10 to 14 days of one of the following antithrombotic agents: LMWH, fondaparinux, apixaban, dabigatran, rivaroxaban, low-dose UFH, VKA, aspirin, or IPCDs worn for a minimum of 18 hours per day. For patients undergoing repair of hip fractures, they recommend a minimum of 10 to 14 days of LMWH, fondaparinux, UFH, VKA, aspirin, or IPCDs worn for a minimum of 18 hours per day. For the aforementioned patients receiving LMWH, they recommend starting either 12 hours or more preoperatively or 12 hours or more postoperatively. For all patients, LMWH is preferred to other agents.[36]

For patients undergoing major orthopedic surgery, they recommend extending VTE prophylaxis for up to 35 days from the day of surgery. For those with an increased risk of bleeding, they suggest using IPCDs or no prophylaxis rather than anticoagulation. For patients who decline or are uncooperative with injections or IPCDs, they recommend using one of the oral agents rather than alternative forms. They do not recommend using IVC filters for primary prevention in patients with an increased bleeding risk or contraindications to both pharmacologic and mechanical prophylaxis. Screening Doppler or duplex ultrasound postoperatively before discharge is not recommended. For patients with isolated lower leg injuries requiring immobilization, they suggest no prophylaxis. Finally, for patients undergoing knee arthroscopy without a prior VTE history, they suggest no thromboprophylaxis.[36]

Trauma

Trauma patients' risk of DVT can vary from 5% to 63%, depending on risk factors, prophylaxis modality, and methods of detection.[37,38] Coagulopathy in trauma patients is multifactorial, thought to be caused by consumption of clotting factors, acidosis, hypothermia, dilution from IV fluids and blood product administration, immobility, and shock itself and its systemic activation of anticoagulant and fibrinolytic pathways.[39] Greenfield and colleagues[40] developed a risk assessment profile (RAP) to identify the factors associated with an increased incidence of DVT, which was validated in a study by Gearhart and colleagues.[41] In this study, patients with an RAP score of 5 or more were 3 times more likely to develop VTE than patients with an RAP score less than 5. **Table 7** depicts the RAP score developed by Greenfield and colleagues.[40]

The ninth edition of the ACCP's guidelines recommend the use of LMWH for major trauma patients as soon as it is safe to do so, with an acceptable alternative of LMWH plus optimal use of a mechanical method, such as IPCDs. If there exists a

Table 7
RAP in trauma patients

	Points
Underlying Condition	
Obesity	2
Malignancy	2
Abnormal coagulation	2
History of VTE	3
Iatrogenic factors	
Femoral venous line	2
Transfusion >4 units	2
Operation >2 h	2
Major venous repair	3
Injury-related factors	
Chest AIS >2	2
Abdomen AIS >2	2
Head AIS >2	2
Spinal fractures	3
Glasgow coma score <8	3
Severe lower extremity fracture	4
Pelvic fracture	4
Spinal cord injury	4
Age (y)	
40–59	2
60–74	3
≥75	4

Abbreviation: AIS, abbreviated injury score.

From Gearhart MM, Luchette FA, Proctor MC, et al. The risk assessment profile score identifies trauma patients at risk for deep vein thrombosis. Surgery 2000;128(4):631–40; with permission.

Table 8
EAST guidelines for VTE prophylaxis in trauma patients

Prophylaxis	Level I Recom	Level II Recom	Level III Recom
LDH	None	There is little evidence to support benefit in trauma patients.	An individual decision should be made.
LMWH	None	It is recommended in pelvic fractures, complex lower extremity fractures, and spinal cord injury.	Patients with an ISS >9 should receive LMWH primarily.
A-V foot pump	None	None	It can be used as a substitute in high-risk patients who cannot wear IPCDs.
IPCDs	None	None	It may have some benefit in isolated studies in traumatic brain injury.
IVC filters	None	None	It can be used in very high-risk patients who cannot receive anticoagulation.

Abbreviations: A-V, arteriovenous; LDH, low-density heparin; ISS, injury severity score; Recom, recommendations.

Adapted from Rogers FB, Cipolle MD, Velmahos G, et al. Practice management guidelines for the prevention of venous thromboembolism in trauma patients: the EAST practice management guidelines work group. J Trauma 2002;53(1):142–64.

contraindication to LMWH, mechanical prophylaxis alone is recommended with either IPCDs or GCS. For major trauma patients with impaired mobility, the ACCP recommends VTE prophylaxis until the time of discharge. The ACCP does not recommend IVC filters as prophylaxis for patients with spinal cord injury; instead, they recommend LMWH or, alternatively, IPCDs with low-dose heparin or LMWH. If anticoagulant therapy is contraindicated, the use of IPCDs and/or compression stockings is recommended.

The Eastern Association for the Surgery of Trauma (EAST) has developed evidence-based guidelines for VTE prophylaxis, last published in 2002. A summary of their recommendations can be found in **Table 8**.[42]

SUMMARY

The development of VTE remains a high risk in hospitalized surgical patients, leading to complications in up to 30%. The stratification of patient risk factors and subsequent utilization of a validated prophylaxis and treatment regimen is, therefore, of utmost importance. Familiarity with the current guidelines and recommendations ultimately results in decreased morbidity, mortality, and health care costs.

REFERENCES

1. Silverstein MD, Heit JA, Mohr DN, et al. Trends in the incidence of deep vein thrombosis and pulmonary embolism: a 25-year population-based study. Arch Intern Med 1998;158(6):585–93.
2. Heit JA, Silverstein MD, Mohr DN, et al. Predictors of survival after deep vein thrombosis and pulmonary embolism: a population-based, cohort study. Arch Intern Med 1999;159(5):445–53.

3. Office of the Surgeon General (US), National Heart, Lung, and Blood Institute (US). The Surgeon General's call to action to prevent deep vein thrombosis and pulmonary embolism. Rockville (MD): Office of the Surgeon General (US); 2008. References. Available at: http://www.ncbi.nlm.nih.gov/books/NBK44183/.
4. Cassidy M, Rosenkranz P, McAneny D. Reducing postoperative venous thromboembolism complications with a standardized risk-stratified prophylaxis protocol and mobilization program. J Am Coll Surg 2014;218(6):1095–104.
5. Michota FA. Bridging the gap between evidence and practice in venous thromboembolism prophylaxis: the quality improvement process. J Gen Intern Med 2007;22(12):1762–70.
6. Spyropouloos AC, Anderson FA Jr, Fitzgerald G, et al. Predictive and associative models to identify hospitalized medical patients at risk for VTE. Chest 2011; 139(1):69–79.
7. Kearon C, Akl EA, Comerota AJ, et al. Antithrombotic therapy and prevention of thrombosis, 9th ed: American College of Chest Physicians evidence-based clinical practice guidelines. Chest 2012;141(2 Suppl):e419S–94S.
8. Available at: http://web2.facs.org/download/Caprini.pdf. Accessed date June 24, 2014.
9. Prandoni P, Lensing AW, Cogo A, et al. The long-term clinical course of acute deep venous thrombosis. Ann Intern Med 1996;125(1):1–7.
10. Mohr DN, Silverstein MD, Heit JA, et al. The venous stasis syndrome after deep venous thrombosis or pulmonary embolism: a population-based study. Mayo Clin Proc 2000;75(12):1249–56.
11. Heit JA, Mohr DN, Silverstein MD, et al. Predictors of recurrence after deep vein thrombosis and pulmonary embolism: a population-based cohort study. Arch Intern Med 2000;160(6):761–8.
12. Caprini JA, Arcelus JI, Hasty JH, et al. Clinical assessment of venous thromboembolic risk in surgical patients. Semin Thromb Hemost 1991;17(Suppl 3): 304–12.
13. Bahl V, Hu H, Henke PK, et al. A validation study of a retrospective venous thromboembolism risk scoring method. Ann Surg 2010;251:344–5.
14. Caprini JA. Risk assessment as a guide for the prevention of the many faces of venous thromboembolism. Am J Surg 2010;199(Suppl):S3–10.
15. Gould MK, Garcia DA, Wren S, et al. Prevention of VTE in nonorthopedic surgical patients: antithrombotic therapy and prevention of thrombosis, 9th ed: American College of Chest Physicians evidence-based clinical practice guidelines. Chest 2012;141(2 Suppl):e227S–77S.
16. Shuman AG, Hu HM, Pannucci CJ, et al. Stratifying the risk of venous thromboembolism in otolaryngology. Otolaryngol Head Neck Surg 2012;146:719–24.
17. Torbicki A, Perrier A, Konstantinides S, et al. Guidelines on the diagnosis and management of acute pulmonary embolism: the task force for the diagnosis and management of acute pulmonary embolism of the European Society of Cardiology (ESC). Eur Heart J 2008;29:2276–315.
18. Streiff MB. Diagnosis and initial treatment of venous thromboembolism in patients with cancer. J Clin Oncol 2009;27:4889–94.
19. Perkins JM, Magee TR, Galland RB. Phlegmasia caerulea dolens and venous gangrene. Br J Surg 1996;83:19–23.
20. Tardy B, Moulin N, Mismetti P, et al. Intravenous thrombolytic therapy in patients with phlegmasia caerulea dolens. Haematologica 2006;91:281–2.
21. Tung CS, Soliman PT, Walace MJ, et al. Successful catheter-directed venous thrombolysis in phlegmasia cerulean dolens. Gynecol Oncol 2007;107:140–2.

22. Einarsson E, Albrechtsson U, Eklof B. Thrombectomy and temporary AV-fistula in iliofemoral vein thrombosis. Technical considerations and early results. Int Angiol 1986;5:65–72.
23. Plate G, Einarsson E, Ohlin P, et al. Thrombectomy with temporary AV fistula: the treatment of choice in acute iliofemoral venous thrombosis. J Vasc Surg 1984;1: 867–76.
24. AbuRahma AF, Robinson PA. Effort subclavian vein thrombosis: evolution of management. J Endovasc Ther 2000;7:302–8.
25. De Bast Y, Dahin L. May-Thurner syndrome will be completed? Thromb Res 2009; 123:498–502.
26. Murphy EH, Davis EM, Journeycake JM, et al. Symptomatic iliofemoral DVT after onset of oral contraceptive use in women with previously undiagnosed May-Thurner syndrome. J Vasc Surg 2009;49:697–703.
27. Knipp BS, Ferguson E, Williams DM, et al. Factors associated with outcome after interventional treatment of symptomatic iliac vein compression syndrome. J Vasc Surg 2007;46:743–9.
28. Comerota AJ. The ATTRACT trial: rationale for early intervention for iliofemoral DVT. Perspect Vasc Surg Endovasc Ther 2009;21:221–4 [quiz: 224–5].
29. Enden T, Sandvik L, Klow NE, et al. Catheter-directed venous thrombolysis in acute iliofemoral vein thrombosis-the CaVenT study: rationale and design of a multicenter, randomized, controlled, clinical trial (NCT00251771). Am Heart J 2007;154:808–14.
30. Society of American Gastrointestinal and Endoscopic Surgeons (SAGES) Guidelines Committee. Guidelines for deep venous thrombosis prophylaxis during laparoscopic surgery. Surg Endosc 2007;21:1007–9.
31. Khorana AA, Dalal MR, Lin J, et al. Health care costs associated with venous thromboembolism in selected high-risk ambulatory patients with solid tumors undergoing chemotherapy in the United States. Clinicoecon Outcomes Res 2013;5:101–8.
32. Khorana AA, Dalal MR, Lin J, et al. Incidence and predictors of venous thromboembolism (VTE) among ambulatory high-risk cancer patients undergoing chemotherapy in the United States. Cancer 2013;119(3):648–55.
33. Lyman GH, Khorana AA, Kuderer NM, et al. Venous thromboembolism prophylaxis and treatment in patients with cancer: American Society of Clinical Oncology clinical practices update. J Clin Oncol 2013;31(17):2189–204.
34. Streiff MB, Bockenstedt PL, Cataland SR, et al. Venous thromboembolic disease. J Natl Compr Canc Netw 2013;11(11):1402–29.
35. Pryor HI 2nd, Singleton A, Lin E, et al. Practice patterns in high-risk bariatric venous thromboembolism prophylaxis. Surg Endosc 2013;27(3):843–8.
36. Falck-Ytter Y, Francis CW, Johanson NA, et al. Prevention of VTE in orthopedic surgery patients: antithrombotic therapy and prevention of thrombosis, 9th ed: American College of Chest Physicians evidence-based clinical practice guidelines. Chest 2012;141(2 Suppl):e278S–325S.
37. Bendinelli C, Balogh Z. Postinjury thromboprophylaxis. Curr Opin Crit Care 2008; 14(6):673–8.
38. Dunbar NM, Chandler WL. Thrombin generation in trauma patients. Transfusion 2009;49(12):2652–60.
39. Toker S, Hak DJ, Morgan SJ. Deep vein thrombosis prophylaxis in trauma patients. Thrombosis 2011;2011:505373.
40. Greenfield LJ, Proctor MC, Rodriguez JL, et al. Posttrauma thromboembolism prophylaxis. J Trauma 1997;42:100–3.

41. Gearhart MM, Luchette FA, Proctor MC, et al. The risk assessment profile score identifies trauma patients at risk for deep vein thrombosis. Surgery 2000;128(4):631–40.
42. Rogers FB, Cipolle MD, Velmahos G, et al. Practice management guidelines for the prevention of venous thromboembolism in trauma patients: the EAST practice management guidelines work group. J Trauma 2002;53(1):142–64.

Postoperative Pain Control

Jessica Lovich-Sapola, MD, MBA[a], Charles E. Smith, MD[a],
Christopher P. Brandt, MD[b,*]

KEYWORDS

• Postoperative pain • Multimodal analgesia • Opioids • Nerve blocks
• Local anesthetics

KEY POINTS

- Inadequate treatment of postoperative pain may lead to worse outcomes and persistent postoperative pain.
- A multimodal approach to pain management (including preemptive and preventative analgesia) lessens the dependence on any given medication and improves outcome.
- Local anesthetics can be administered via multiple routes (eg, wound infiltration, epidural, peripheral nerve blocks) to improve analgesia and decrease opioid requirements and opioid-related side effects.
- Despite multiple adverse effects, opioids remain the mainstay of surgical pain control.

INTRODUCTION

Pain is defined by the International Association for the Study of Pain as "an unpleasant sensory and emotional experience associated with actual or potential tissue damage, or described in terms of such damage."[1] Effective control and management of postoperative pain are clearly of primary concern to the patient and also of importance to the surgeon, because of potential adverse effects of the physiologic response to pain from surgery. Inadequate treatment of postoperative pain continues to be an important clinical problem, not only leading to worse outcomes in the immediate postoperative period but also an increased risk for persistent postoperative pain. Persistent postsurgical pain, pain that lasts beyond the typical healing period of 1 to 2 months, has become increasingly recognized as a significant issue after surgery and may exceed 30% after some operations, particularly amputations, thoracotomy, mastectomy, and inguinal hernia repairs.[2]

The authors have no disclosures.
[a] Department of Anesthesiology, MetroHealth Medical Center, Case Western Reserve University, 10900 Euclid Ave, Cleveland, OH 44106, USA; [b] Department of Surgery, MetroHealth Medical Center, Case Western Reserve University, 2500 MetroHealth Dr., Cleveland, OH 44109, USA
* Corresponding author.
E-mail address: cbrandt@metrohealth.org

Surg Clin N Am 95 (2015) 301–318
http://dx.doi.org/10.1016/j.suc.2014.10.002 surgical.theclinics.com

Inadequate pain relief occurs secondary to multiple factors, including insufficient knowledge of the care providers, fear of medication side effects, and inadequate patient preparation. Optimal management of postoperative pain requires an understanding of the pathophysiology of pain, methods used for assessment of pain in individual patients, and awareness of the various options available for pain control. Key factors to consider are type of surgical procedure, skills of the surgeon and anesthesiologist, concerns of the patient, and the experience and cooperation of nursing and other health care providers. Based on this foundation of understanding, use of a procedure-specific, multimodal perioperative pain management provides a rational basis for enhanced postoperative recovery and reduction of morbidity.[3–5]

PATHOPHYSIOLOGY OF POSTOPERATIVE PAIN

Acute postoperative pain is a normal response to surgical intervention and is a cause of delayed recovery and discharge after surgery as well as increased risk of wound infection and respiratory/cardiovascular complications.[6] Untreated acute pain leads to reduced patient satisfaction and increased morbidity and mortality and also places a burden on the patient and health system finances. Acute pain that becomes intractable and persists is referred to as chronic postsurgical pain (CPSP). CPSP can have a significant impact on the patient's quality of life and daily activities, including disturbances of sleep and affective mood.[2,6] Pain lasting more than 1 month after surgery occurs in 10% to 50% of individuals after common procedures, and 2% to 10% of these patients continue on to experience severe chronic pain.[7] Risk factors for the development of CPSP are outlined in **Box 1**.

Acute postsurgical pain occurs secondary to inflammation from tissue trauma or direct nerve injury and can be classified as nociceptive or neuropathic (**Table 1**). Tissue trauma releases local inflammatory mediators, which can produce hyperalgesia (increased sensitivity to stimuli in the area surrounding an injury) or allodynia (misperception of pain to nonnoxious stimuli). Other mechanisms contributing to hyperalgesia and allodynia include sensitization of the peripheral pain receptors (primary hyperalgesia) and increased excitability of central nervous system neurons (secondary hyperalgesia).[8]

It is increasingly recognized that genetic factors should be considered within the context of the interacting physiologic, psychological, and environmental factors that influence responses to pain and analgesia.[1] Genetic factors regulating opioid pharmacokinetics (metabolizing enzymes, transporters) and pharmacodynamics (receptors and signal transduction elements) contribute to a large interpatient variability in postoperative opioid requirements. Specific examples include genetic polymorphisms, which affect plasma concentrations of active metabolites of codeine and tramadol as well as plasma concentrations of methadone.[1]

Pain control has traditionally used opioid analgesia to target central mechanisms involved in the perception of pain. A multimodal approach recognizing the pathophysiology of surgical pain uses several agents to decrease pain receptor activity and diminish the local hormonal response to injury.[8,9] This approach lessens the dependence on a given medication and mechanism. For example, local anesthetics can directly block pain receptor activity, antiinflammatory agents can decrease the hormonal response to injury, and drugs such acetaminophen, ketamine, clonidine, dexmedetomidine, gabapentin, and pregabalin can produce analgesia by targeting specific neurotransmitters.[8] Nonopioid agents used for management of postoperative pain are outlined in **Table 2**.

Box 1
Risk factors for chronic postsurgical pain

- Pain, moderate to severe, lasting more than 1 month
- Repeat surgery
- Catastrophizing[a]
- Anxiety
- Female gender
- Younger age (adults)
- Workers' compensation
- Genetic predisposition
- Surgical approach with risk of nerve damage
- Moderate to severe postoperative pain
- Radiation therapy to area
- Neurotoxic chemotherapy
- Depression
- Neuroticism

[a] Refers to giving greater weight to the worst possible outcome, however unlikely, or experiencing a situation as unbearable or impossible when it is just uncomfortable.

Adapted from Macintyre PE, Scott DA, Schug SA, et al. Acute pain management: scientific evidence [Systematic reviews and meta-analyses]. 3rd edition. 2010. Available at: http://www.anzca.edu.au/resources/college-publications/pdfs/Acute%20Pain%20Management/books-and-publications/acutepain.pdf. Accessed June 25, 2014; and Kehlet H, Rathmell JP. Persistent postsurgical pain. Anesthesiology 2010;112:514–5.

Table 1
Types of pain

Nociceptive Pain	• Normal processing of stimuli that damages normal tissues • Responds to opioids
Somatic	• Pain arises from bone, joint, muscle, skin, or connective tissue • Aching, throbbing • Localized
Visceral	• Arises from visceral organs • Tumor: localized pain • Obstruction of hollow viscus: poorly localized
Neuropathic Pain	• Abnormal processing of sensory input by PNS or CNS
Centrally generated	• Deafferentation pain: injury to PNS or CNS (eg, phantom pain) • Sympathetically maintained pain: dysregulation of autonomic nervous system (eg, complex regional pain syndrome I and II)
Peripherally generated	• Painful polyneuropathies: pain is felt along the distribution of many peripheral nerves (eg, diabetic neuropathy) • Painful mononeuropathies: associated with a known peripheral nerve injury (eg, nerve root compression, trigeminal neuralgia)

Abbreviations: CNS, central nervous system; PNS, peripheral nervous system.

Data from Pasero C, McCaffery M. Pain assessment and pharmacologic management. (MO): Elsevier/Mosby; 2011.

Table 2
Nonopioid medications to reduce postoperative pain

Drug	Comment
Acetaminophen (paracetamol)	• Effective analgesic for acute pain • Incidence of adverse effects comparable with placebo • Reduces opioid consumption • Available IV
Nonselective NSAIDs (eg, ibuprofen, ketorolac, naproxen)	• Effective in treatment of acute postoperative pain • Reduces opioid consumption and incidence of nausea, vomiting, and sedation • Incidence of perioperative renal impairment is low[a] • Risk of gastropathy increased when ketorolac use exceeds 5 d • Patients should be well hydrated and without significant kidney disease • Ketorolac and ibuprofen available IV
COX-2 inhibitors	• Effective in treatment of acute postoperative pain • Reduce opioid consumption, and increase patient satisfaction • Do not result in a decrease in opioid-related side effects • Do not impair platelet function
Aspirin	• Increases bleeding after tonsillectomy
Ketamine: subanesthetic doses	• Acts primarily as noncompetitive antagonist of NMDA receptor • Effective adjuvant for pain associated with central sensitization (eg, severe acute pain, neuropathic pain, opioid-resistant pain) • May reduce CPSP and opioid-induced tolerance/ hyperalgesia • Opioid sparing; reduces incidence of nausea and vomiting • Safe and effective analgesic for painful procedures in pediatrics
Antidepressants and selective serotonin reuptake inhibitors	• Useful for acute neuropathic pain
Anticonvulsants (Gabapentin and pregabalin)	• Reduce postoperative pain, opioid requirements, and incidence of vomiting, pruritus, and urinary retention, but increase risk of sedation • May be useful for acute neuropathic pain (based on experience with chronic neuropathic pain)
IV lidocaine infusion	• Opioid sparing; reduced pain scores, nausea, vomiting and duration of ileus up to 72 h after abdominal surgery • May be useful agent to treat acute neuropathic pain
α_2 Agonists (clonidine, dexmedetomidine)	• Improves perioperative opioid analgesia. Decreased opioid requirements and opioid side effects • Side effects: sedation, hypotension

Abbreviations: COX-2, cyclooxygenase 2; IV, intravenous; NMDA, *N*-methyl-D-aspartate receptor; NSAIDs, nonsteroidal antiinflammatory drugs.

[a] Risk of adverse renal effects of nonselective NSAIDs and COX-2 inhibitors is increased in the presence of preexisting renal impairment, hypovolemia, hypotension, use of other nephrotoxic agents, and angiotensin-converting enzyme inhibitors.

Adapted from Macintyre PE, Schug SA, Scott DA, et al. APM: SE Working Group of the Australian and New Zealand College of Anaesthetists and Faculty of Pain Medicine (2010), Acute Pain Management: Scientific Evidence (3rd edition), ANZCA & FPM, Melbourne; and Solomon DH. NSAIDs: therapeutic use and variability of response in adults. In: Furst DE, editor. UpToDate. Waltham (MA): UpToDate; 2014.

PREOPERATIVE MANAGEMENT

Preprocedure Evaluation

The management of surgical pain begins with the preprocedure evaluation. The anesthesia and surgical team should work closely before, during, and after the surgical procedure to optimize the patient's entire perioperative experience.[2]

The goal of the preoperative examination is to identify patients at risk for complications, along with any comorbidities that can be optimized. This is a good time to evaluate and determine information about previous and ongoing pain issues, as well as pain control methods that have worked or have failed to work in the past. It is also a time to assess for risk factors for postoperative pain.[10] A baseline pain assessment is an important part of any preoperative evaluation; however, standardization of the pain measurement can be difficult because of the subjective nature of the assessment. Because pain is a subjective experience modulated by factors such as previous events, culture, prognosis, coping strategies, fear, and anxiety, most measures of pain are based on self-report.[10]

Self-report measures are influenced by mood, sleep disturbance, and drugs. Postoperatively, it may not be possible to obtain reliable self-reports, because of impaired consciousness, cognitive dysfunction, extremes of age, and language barriers.[10] Some patients may be unable to understand a pain scale or may be unwilling to cooperate (eg, severe anxiety).[10] Pain scales presently used fall into multiple categories: single-dimension scales (visual analog and numerical rating scales) and multidimensional scales (McGill Pain Questionnaire).[10] It is important to assess not only a level of pain but the specific location of the pain and its character, duration, intensity, and frequency.

Patient Education

Patients are often concerned about their perioperative pain control, and the preoperative evaluation is an important opportunity to discuss the plan. A large part of patient education is setting the correct expectations of pain control in the perioperative period. The expectation should never be that the patient will have no pain.[2] Cognitive and psychological factors play a significant role in the severity of reported postsurgical pain, and evidence shows that psychological factors such as anxiety, depression, neuroticism, and catastrophizing are key determinants in the experience of pain (see **Table 1**).[1,6] The standard approach to provider education on pain emphasizes processes at the subcellular and cellular scale, with little attention given to the social component of pain, such as suffering, isolation, and pain behavior. Many physicians are therefore poorly prepared to deal with the social and psychological issues involved in treating postoperative pain in everyday clinical practice. Studies affirm that a dysphoric social dimension, isolation, withdrawal, distress, and the stigma of chronic pain contribute to the patient's multidimensional experience of pain almost as much as the physical nociception.[11] Failure to address this social dimension of pain can often render most standard pain management practices futile.

Preemptive and Preventative Analgesia Plan

Preemptive analgesia occurs when preoperative treatment is more effective than the identical treatment administered after incision or surgery. The only difference is the timing of administration. Preventative analgesia occurs when the intervention exceeds the expected duration of action of the intervention. The intervention may or may not be initiated before surgery.

The efficacy of preemptive analgesic interventions, such as epidural analgesia, local anesthetic wound infiltration, and use of nonsteroidal antiinflammatory drugs (NSAIDs), has been shown in a variety of settings.[1] Preventative analgesic interventions such as *N*-methyl-D-aspartate receptor antagonist drugs (ketamine and dextromethorphan) (see **Table 2**) and epidural analgesia have also been shown to have a salutary effect on postoperative pain.[1]

Choice of analgesia is highly dependent on the specific surgical procedure being performed, in terms of analgesic efficacy, potential side effects, and effects on recovery. The Prospect Working Group, composed of surgeons and anesthesiologists, has developed recommendations for pain management for a variety of adult elective surgeries, such as hemorrhoidectomy, inguinal hernia repair, laparoscopic cholecystectomy, noncosmetic breast cancer surgery, radical prostatectomy, open thoracotomy, primary total hip arthroplasty, and total knee arthroplasty. The recommendations follow a detailed methodology and are formulated based on evidence, with expert interpretation in the context of clinical practice. The evidence and recommendations for specific analgesia plans are freely accessible on the Internet.[3]

INTRAOPERATIVE MANAGEMENT

The surgical stress response is characterized by neuroendocrine, metabolic, and inflammatory changes, which can adversely affect organ function and perioperative outcomes and result in increased postoperative pain.[2] These responses are increased with the degree of surgical stimulation and magnified by hypothermia and psychological stress. Intraoperative surgical stress can be ameliorated with deeper planes of anesthesia, neural blockade, and reduction in the degree of surgical invasiveness, resulting in decreased postoperative pain. Specific methods used to decrease intraoperative stress include intravenous (IV) lidocaine, β-blockers, α_2 agonists, and regional anesthesia using local anesthetics.

Intravenous Medications

IV lidocaine with a bolus of 100 mg followed by an infusion of 2 to 3 mg/h has analgesic, antihyperalgesic, and antiinflammatory properties.[2] For colorectal and radical retropubic prostate surgeries, IV lidocaine has been shown to decrease the opioid requirements and facilitate early return of bowel function.[2]

β-Blockers have been used to blunt the sympathetic response to tracheal intubation and attenuate the surgical stress response of surgery. They reduce the requirement for volatile anesthetic agents and also have an opioid sparing effect.[2]

The α_2 agonists clonidine and dexmedetomidine have anesthetic and analgesic properties, which decrease postoperative pain and reduce opioid consumption and opioid-related side effects.[2] Dexmedetomidine is more selective than clonidine for the α_2 effects, with a half-life of about 2 hours. Unlike clonidine, dexmedetomidine can be given IV. Dexmedetomidine causes hyperpolarization of locus ceruleus neurons, which results in decreased activity in ascending noradrenergic pathway, inhibition of sympathetic-mediated pain at peripheral nociceptors, inhibition of substance P and glutamate release at primary afferent neurons, and inhibition of firing at second-order neurons.[12] Side effects include sedation and hypotension. The use of α_2 agonists consistently improves opioid analgesia, but the side effects may limit their clinical usefulness.[1] Dexmedetomidine should not be used in patients with advanced heart block, severe ventricular dysfunction, and shock, and clearance is lower in patients with hepatic impairment. Dexmedetomidine is used only in a monitored setting (eg, operating room, intensive care unit [ICU]). Unlike opioids, dexmedetomidine is associated with minimal to no respiratory depression.

Neuraxial Techniques

Neuraxial blockade of nociceptive stimuli by an epidural or spinal anesthetic can blunt the metabolic and neuroendocrine stress response to surgery.[2] The epidural blockade should be provided with a solution of local anesthetic and low-dose opioid and established before surgical incision and continued postoperatively. Neuraxial techniques not only provide excellent analgesia but can also facilitate mobilization and physical therapy postoperatively.[13] They have also been associated with a decreased incidence and severity of ileus.[2] A thoracic epidural is recommended for surgeries including but not limited to open colorectal, thoracic, esophageal, aortic, and renal surgery. A lumbar epidural is usually not recommended for most abdominal surgery, because of questionable adequate segmental analgesia, high degree of urinary retention, and lower limb motor and sensory blockade, all of which delay mobilization.[2]

Contraindications to neuraxial anesthesia include patient refusal, bleeding diathesis, severe hypovolemia, increased intracranial pressure, and infection at the site of injection. Relative contraindications include severe aortic or mitral stenosis, severe left ventricular outflow obstruction, the presence of sepsis or bacteremia, and patients with dementia, psychosis, or emotional instability, which may make catheter placement more difficult.[2] Complications of neuraxial blockade include inadequate analgesia, intravascular injection, total spinal anesthesia, subdural injection, backache, postdural puncture headache, neurologic injury, epidural hematoma, meningitis, epidural abscess, and shearing of the catheter.[2]

Transversus Abdominus Plane Blocks

The transversus abdominus plane (TAP) block is a peripheral nerve block that anesthetizes the abdominal wall and can be an effective adjunct to multimodal postoperative analgesia after abdominal surgical procedures.[14] The TAP block is most often used to provide surgical anesthesia for minor, superficial procedures of the lower abdominal wall and postoperative pain control for procedures below the umbilicus.[2] The use of this block may decrease need for opioid therapy, thereby reducing the incidence of respiratory depression.[15] Main disadvantages of the TAP block are the limited duration of action with a single shot of local anesthetic and the sparing of the upper thoracic dermatomes.[15]

Peripheral Nerve Blocks

Continuous peripheral nerve blocks affect the afferent nociceptive pathways and are an excellent way to decrease the required doses of opioids.[2,16] Specific types of peripheral blocks are noted in **Tables 3–5**. Contraindications and risks of peripheral nerve blockade include inability of the patient to cooperate, bleeding disorders, pharmacologic anticoagulation, infection at the site, preexisting nerve damage, and allergy to local anesthetics.[2]

Wound Infiltration Anesthesia

Local anesthesia may be accomplished by infiltration of the wound with lidocaine or bupivacaine.[17] Onset of action is rapid after intradermal or subcutaneous administration and epinephrine prolongs the duration of anesthesia.[18] The dose of local anesthetic required depends on the extent of the area to be anesthetized and the expected duration of the surgical procedure. In patients undergoing colorectal

Table 3
Upper extremity blocks

Type	Nerves Blocked	Indication/Procedure Site	Contraindication
Interscalene brachial plexus	C5–7	• Shoulder and upper arm	• Severe pulmonary disease • Preexisting contralateral phrenic nerve palsy
Supraclavicular	Brachial plexus	• At or below the elbow • Ideal for catheter placement	• Severe pulmonary disease • Preexisting contralateral phrenic nerve palsy
Infraclavicular	Brachial plexus	• Distal to the elbow	• Vascular catheters in this region • Ipsilateral pacemaker
Axillary	Brachial plexus	• Distal to the elbow	

Data from Butterworth J, Mackey D, Wasnick J. Morgan and Mikhail's clinical anesthesiology. New York (NY): Lange/McGraw-Hill; 2013.

surgery, local anesthetic wound infiltration techniques reduced opioid requirements and pain scores and improved recovery compared with placebo/routine analgesia.[19] However, diverse study design is a major limitation of this analysis. Liposomal bupivacaine (Exparel) has been developed to allow for a prolonged duration of effect, because significant bupivacaine plasma concentrations can remain up to 96 hours after single-dose administration. A pooled analysis of several studies evaluating the effect of liposomal bupivacaine[20] showed decreased postoperative pain after 72 hours

Table 4
Lower extremity blocks

Type	Nerves Blocked	Indication/Procedure Site	Contraindication
Lumbar plexus	L1–4	• Anterior thigh and medial leg	
Sacral plexus	L4–5 and S1–4	• Posterior thigh and most of leg and foot	
Femoral		• Hip, thigh, knee, and saphenous nerve of the ankle	• Previous vascular grafting • Local adenopathy
Lateral femoral cutaneous	L2–3	• Lateral thigh	
Obturator		• Complete anesthesia of the knee	
Saphenous	Most medial branch of the femoral nerve	• Medial leg and ankle	
Sciatic	L4–5 and S1–3	• Hip, thigh, knee, lower leg and foot	
Ankle	1. Saphenous nerve 2. Deep peroneal 3. Superficial peroneal 4. Posterior tibial 5. Sural	• Foot	

Data from Butterworth J, Mackey D, Wasnick J. Morgan and Mikhail's clinical anesthesiology. New York (NY): Lange/McGraw-Hill; 2013.

Table 5
Blocks of the trunk

Type	Nerves Blocked	Indication	Risks
Superficial cervical plexus	C1–4	• Cutaneous analgesia to the neck, anterior shoulder, and clavicle	
Intercostal	Individual injection at the vertebral level required	• Analgesia after thoracic and upper abdominal surgery • Rib fracture • Herpes zoster • Cancer	• Highest complication risk of any block • Results in highest blood levels of local anesthetic per volume injected of any block • Pneumothorax
Paravertebral	Individual injection at the vertebral level required	• Procedures of the thoracic and abdominal wall • Mastectomy • Inguinal or abdominal hernia • Nephrectomy	• Sympathectomy • Pneumothorax

Data from Butterworth J, Mackey D, Wasnick J. Morgan and Mikhail's clinical anesthesiology. New York (NY): Lange/McGraw-Hill; 2013.

and a decrease in opioid consumption when compared with nonliposomal bupivacaine. There are still only a few comparative studies using liposomal bupivacaine, and its use may be limited by the significant difference in cost compared with bupivacaine hydrochloride. Dosing and duration of action for selected local anesthetics are shown in **Table 6**.

Tumescent Anesthesia

Tumescent anesthesia refers to subcutaneous injection of large volumes of dilute local anesthetic in combination with epinephrine and other agents.[18] The doses of lidocaine range from 35 to 55 mg/kg and are associated with plasma concentrations that may peak at more than 8 to 12 hours after the procedure. This technique of local anesthesia is most frequently used by plastic surgeons during liposuction surgery. Although generally safe with proper use, cases of high local anesthetic concentrations and cardiac arrest and death have been reported with this technique.

Topical Local Anesthesia

Local anesthetic formulations have been developed to penetrate intact skin. EMLA is a eutectic mixture of 2.5% lidocaine and 2.5% prilocaine base. It can be used for

Table 6
Local anesthetic dosing for infiltration anesthesia

Drug	Maximum Dose* (mg) Plain	Duration (min) Plain	Maximum Dose* (mg) with Epinephrine	Duration (min) with Epinephrine
Lidocaine	300	30–60	500	120
Bupivacaine	175	120–240	200	180–240

* For an average 70 kg adult.

Data from Gandhi G, Baratta JL, Heitz JW, et al. Acute pain management in the postanesthesia care unit. Anesthesiol Clin 2012;30(3):1–15.

venipuncture, IV cannulation, skin grafting, and circumcision. EMLA is applied under an occlusive bandage for 45 to 60 minutes to obtain effective cutaneous anesthesia. There is a risk of methemoglobinemia from prilocaine.[18]

Topical anesthesia can also be applied through cut skin to facilitate suturing of lacerations in pediatrics (eg, lidocaine-epinephrine-tetracaine and tetracaine-phenylephrine) and for mucosal analgesia and vasoconstriction (eg, oxymetazoline or phenylephrine and lidocaine).

POSTOPERATIVE MANAGEMENT

Opioids

Opioids remain the cornerstone of the management of surgical pain, despite their potential side effects (**Table 7**), and can be given through IV, intramuscular, oral, or transdermal routes. IV opioids provide rapid and effective analgesia for patients with moderate to severe pain. Morphine is the prototypical opioid agonist and the standard for management of acute pain. It has moderate analgesic potency, slow onset, and intermediate duration of action. The half-life is 2 hours, and its duration of action is about 5 hours. The metabolites of morphine are excreted by the kidney, and, therefore, the sedating effects can be prolonged in patients with renal failure.[21]

Hydromorphone is a semisynthetic opioid, which is 4 to 6 times more potent than morphine. The onset of action is more rapid than morphine, but the duration of action is shorter. It is a better choice for patients with renal failure and has a lower incidence of pruritus and sedation than morphine. It is particularly useful in patients who are opioid tolerant.[21]

Fentanyl is a synthetic opioid, which is 50 to 80 times more potent than morphine. It has a rapid onset of within 5-7 minutes, with a short duration of only about 1 hour. IV

Table 7
Adverse effects of opioids

Adverse Effect	Comment
Respiratory depression	• Dose related. Decreased central CO_2 responsiveness → hypoventilation, increased arterial CO_2 levels, decreased respiratory rate, and oxygen saturation • Best early clinical indicator is increasing sedation
Nausea and vomiting	• Dose related • Significantly reduced by droperidol, dexamethasone, and ondansetron
Impaired gastrointestinal motility	• Opioids impair return of bowel function after surgery • May be reversed by peripheral acting opioid antagonists
Urinary retention	• Reversed by naloxone
Pruritus	• Can be effectively treated with naloxone, naltrexone, nalbuphine, and droperidol
Delirium and cognitive dysfunction	• Increased risk of delirium with meperidine
Tolerance and hyperalgesia	• Tolerance = desensitization of antinociceptive pathways to opioids • Opioid-induced hyperalgesia = sensitization of pronociceptive pathways → pain hypersensitivity

Data from Macintyre PE, Schug SA, Scott DA, et al. APM:SE Working Group of the Australian and New Zealand College of Anaesthetists and Faculty of Pain Medicine (2010), Acute Pain Management: Scientific Evidence (3rd edition), ANZCA & FPM, Melbourne.

fentanyl can be particularly effective when rapid analgesia is needed, such as in the postanesthesia care unit or ICU. Transdermal fentanyl is an alternative to sustained-release oral morphine and oxycodone preparations. These patches have a drug reservoir, which is separated from the skin by a microporous rate-limiting membrane, and provide medication that last for 2 to 3 days.[2] Fentanyl absorption lasts for several hours, even once the patch is removed. Disadvantages of the transdermal route include the slow rate of onset and the inability to rapidly change dosage, as blood levels of fentanyl increase and plateau at 12 to 40 hours. Safety alerts have been issued warning against use of fentanyl patches in opioid-naive patients, and potentially dangerous increases in serum fentanyl levels occur with increased body temperature or exposure of patches to external heat sources.[2,22]

Meperidine lowers seizure threshold, has a dysphoric effect, and is not recommended for postoperative pain control. In addition, meperidine has a slower rate of metabolism in the elderly and in patients with hepatic and renal impairment, leading to accumulation of meperidine and its active metabolite normeperidine, and consequent risk for seizures.[1]

Oxycodone is a potent opioid agonist, which is metabolized in the liver. In an experimental pain model, oxycodone was more effective than morphine for pain related to mechanical and thermal stimulation of the esophagus, suggesting that it could be more effective than morphine for visceral pain.[1]

Tramadol is an effective analgesic for mild to moderate pain and neuropathic pain. The risk of respiratory depression is less compared with other opioids, and significant respiratory depression has been reported only in patients with severe renal failure.[1]

Patient-Controlled Analgesia

Patient-controlled analgesia (PCA) provides better pain control, greater patient satisfaction, and fewer opioid side effects when compared with on-request opioids.[21] The PCA is based on the idea of a negative feedback loop.[23] When the patients experience pain, they self-administer medication, and once the pain is reduced, they stop giving themselves medication.[23] Patients should be given a loading dose of opioid until a reported pain score of 4 out of 10 is achieved or a respiratory rate of fewer than 12 breaths per minute, before the PCA is begun.[21] The PCA is then programmed as a bolus dose, which the patients receive each time they press the button. The maximum number of doses is limited per hour. There is also a lockout interval of time, which limits how closely consecutive doses can be given. The PCA is usually used with morphine or hydromorphone. Fentanyl PCA is often restricted to hospital units with continuous monitoring, such as the ICU, secondary to the increased risk of respiratory depression. Sufentanil is another potent opioid that can be used for PCA. Sublingual sufentanil 15 μg microtablets (sufentanil nanotab PCA system; AcelRx Pharmaceuticals, Inc., Redwood City, CA) has recently been shown to provide an alternative to IV PCA for adult inpatients after major open abdominal or orthopedic surgery.[24] However, the nanotab oral/transmucosal delivery system is not approved for clinical use.

NONOPIOID ANALGESICS

Nonsteroidal Antiinflammatory Drugs

NSAIDs such as ibuprofen, ketorolac, naproxen, and cyclooxygenase 2 (COX-2) inhibitors are effective analgesics in a variety of acute pain states and have a broad spectrum of antiinflammatory and antipyretic effects (see **Table 2**).[1] IV ketorolac is widely used during the perioperative period for short-term treatment of acute pain and as an adjunct to opioids for the treatment of moderate to severe postoperative pain. Maximal benefit occurs when the NSAID is continued for 3 to 5 days postoperatively.[25] The addition of NSAIDs to systemic opioids diminishes postoperative pain intensity, reduces opioid requirements, and decreases opioid side effects, such as postoperative nausea and vomiting and respiratory depression.[2] NSAIDs are the key components of multimodal analgesia but are generally inadequate as the sole analgesic agent in control of severe postoperative pain. When used in combination with opioids, NSAIDs improve analgesia, decrease opioid consumption, and decrease incidence of opioid-related adverse effects, such as postoperative nausea, vomiting, and sedation.[1]

NSAIDs increase the risk of gastrointestinal bleeding and postoperative bleeding, decreased kidney function, impaired wound healing, and risk of anastomotic leakage.[2] Their use should therefore be guided by the type of surgery being performed and by consultation between the surgical and anesthesia teams. COX-2 inhibitors also reduce postoperative pain, with less risk of NSAID-related platelet dysfunction and bleeding, but are associated with cardiovascular risk in the perioperative period.[2] The risk of adverse renal effects of nonselective NSAIDs and COX-2 inhibitors is increased in the presence of preexisting renal impairment, hypovolemia, hypotension, and use of other nephrotoxic agents and angiotensin-converting enzyme inhibitors.

Acetaminophen

Oral, rectal, and parenteral acetaminophen (paracetamol) can be an effective component of multimodal anesthesia. Acetaminophen significantly reduces pain intensity and spares opioid consumption after abdominal surgery. The analgesic effect is 30% less than that of NSAIDs, but side effects are fewer.[2] Acetaminophen can also be used in conjunction with an NSAID to improve postoperative analgesia and as an adjunct to PCA opioids to reduce morphine requirements.[26,27] The primary concern with use of acetaminophen is hepatotoxicity, which is most concerning in the elderly and patients who chronically consume alcohol.[22]

Antidepressants

Antidepressants are useful for patients with neuropathic pain, even when depression is not a diagnosis of the patient. The analgesic effects occur at lower doses than needed for antidepressant activity. Older tricyclic agents, such as amitriptyline and nortriptyline, which block the reuptake of serotonin and norepinephrine, seem to be more effective than selective serotonin reuptake inhibitors.[2] The onset of pain relief is usually not immediate and may take weeks to have a complete effect. Antidepressants work best for pain from nerve damage secondary to diabetes, peripheral neuropathy, spinal cord injury, stroke, and radiculopathy.[2]

Anticonvulsants

Anticonvulsant medications are useful for patients with neuropathic pain as well as for suppressing postoperative pain.[28] The most commonly used agents include gabapentin, phenytoin, carbamazepine, and clonazepam. Pregabalin is a newer agent, which has been approved for all forms of neuropathic pain.[2] The synergism between gabapentin and opioids results in an opioid sparing effect.[28] Procedures in which gabapentin use for postoperative pain relief has been studied include breast surgery, hysterectomy, spinal surgery, postamputation, orthopedic surgery, and postthoracotomy.[28]

Corticosteroids

Corticosteroids when used as an adjuvant decrease opioid consumption and help reduce postoperative pain.[25] Dexamethasone is the preferred corticosteroid, because it also reduces postoperative nausea and vomiting.

Ketamine

Ketamine can be used as an antihyperalgesic in the perioperative period.[7] Although traditionally used intraoperatively, low-dose ketamine has increasingly been given for postoperative analgesia.[23] Perioperative subanesthetic doses have been shown to decrease the opioid requirements and decrease the reported pain intensity.[23] At the low doses used in the postoperative period, ketamine does not result in the hallucinations or cognitive impairment that are often seen with high doses.[23]

Local Anesthetics

The lidocaine patch is primarily used for relief of allodynia (painful hypersensitivity) and chronic pain in postherpetic neuralgia. Onset is approximately 4 hours. Absorption is dependent on dose, application site, and duration of exposure. The time to peak effect of 5% transdermal lidocaine is approximately 11 hours after application of 3 patches. Lidocaine patches have been used successfully for the treatment of pain secondary to rib fractures, back pain, and orthopedic surgeries. On-Q is a system that uses a catheter temporarily implanted in an incision, allowing for continuous release and infiltration of local anesthetic agents. Studies have suggested clinical benefit with use of this system after abdominal, gynecologic, and thoracic surgeries.[1,29,30] A meta-analysis of studies using the system after colorectal surgery via laparotomy[31] showed a reduction in pain with movement and decrease in total opioid consumption, but no decrease in length of stay or ileus. Definitive conclusions about the overall benefit of this approach await further study.

Transcutaneous Electrical Nerve Stimulation

Transcutaneous electrical nerve stimulation (TENS) produces analgesia by stimulating large afferent fibers.[2] Although not commonly used, TENS has been shown to decrease postoperative pain, with little if any risk to the patient, and can be used to treat mild to moderate acute pain.[2,25]

MULTIMODAL

The best treatment plan for a patient's postsurgical pain is the multimodal approach. By using a combination of the medications and techniques discussed in this article, the physician is able to create a personalized treatment plan that takes into account the patient's personal and medical needs. Multimodal pain management combines the use of different pharmacologic mechanisms of action and additive or synergistic effects, which work by acting at different sites within the central and peripheral nervous system.[25] The goal is to provide optimal pain control, limit the amount of opioids required after surgery, and therefore, decrease their associated adverse effects.

Once the multimodal plan is established, the patient must be followed to determine whether the plan is meeting the patient's needs or if any changes need to be made. This follow-up includes routine monitoring of vital signs and oxygenation. The nursing staff should closely monitor for and report any side effects (**Table 8**). However, successful management of acute postoperative pain requires close liaison with all personnel involved in the care of the patient. Many institutions now have an acute pain service (APS), which can be called on to deal with complex pain management issues such as acute on chronic pain, acute pain after major trauma, opioid-tolerant patients, and specific patient populations. There is daily clinical participation of anesthesiologists, together with input from other physicians and staff, leading to

Table 8
Monitoring for potential side effects of postoperative analgesia

System	Side Effect
Cardiovascular	• Hypertension/hypotension • Bradycardia/tachycardia
Respiratory	• Hypoventilation • Hypoxia
Gastrointestinal	• Nausea • Vomiting • Ileus
Urinary	• Urinary retention
Neurologic	• Change in mental status • Sensory or motor block
Hematologic	• Hematoma at neuraxial catheter/peripheral nerve catheter site (impaired neurologic function as well)
Skin	• Rash • Pruritus

maximum patient benefit. Implementation of an APS may improve pain relief and reduce the incidence of side effects.

SPECIAL CONSIDERATIONS

Ambulatory Surgery

The number of outpatient surgical procedures continues to increase. With this increase, the complexity of the procedure and patient comorbidity are also increasing. Inadequate pain control is one of the leading causes of prolonged stays and readmission after outpatient surgery.[23] Despite advances in surgical technique, the incidence of moderate to severe postoperative pain on discharge is still about 25% to 35%.[25]

The traditional reliance on opioid-based pain management may not be ideal in the ambulatory setting, because many of the side effects may delay discharge. Using nonopioid techniques with different mechanisms of action, such as acetaminophen, NSAIDs, local anesthetics, nerve blocks, tissue infiltration, wound instillation, or topical anesthetics, may give improved pain management, with fewer side effects.

Pediatrics

Undertreatment of acute pain is common with children.[23] In addition to anatomic, physiologic, pharmacodynamic, and pharmacokinetic differences, there are unique barriers to the treatment of postoperative pain in children. One of the myths is that children and infants do not feel pain or that the pain is not remembered, and therefore, there is no consequence of experiencing the pain. This theory is false, and poor pain control has been associated with increased morbidity and mortality.[23] Pediatric patients often have difficulty communicating their pain, and special scales are available to assist in self-reporting.

Children as young as 4 years old have been reported to have the cognitive and physical ability to use an IV PCA device.[23] For the child who is unable to use PCA, intermittent boluses are recommended. With the exception of the child with sleep apnea, respiratory depression after opioids is rare in children, compared with adults. The use of NSAIDs or acetaminophen may improve the overall analgesia and reduce the opioid use. Peripheral and neuraxial techniques can be used in the pediatric population as well.[23]

The Elderly

The elderly population will continue to increase in the next several decades. The elderly have changes in their physiology, pharmacokinetics, pharmacodynamics, and nociceptive processing, which influence the effectiveness of the standard pain management techniques. In addition, the elderly may present with other barriers, such as communication, social, and cognitive issues, which may limit effective postoperative pain control. The elderly are at increased risk of postoperative complications, especially in the presence of severe or uncontrolled pain.[23]

As a patient ages, there are reported decreases in the intensity of pain perception and symptoms. This change was documented in studies of myocardial infarctions lacking in angina symptoms. Studies have shown a decrease in Aδ and C fiber nociceptive function, delay in central sensitization, increase in pain thresholds, and decreased sensitivity to low-intensity noxious stimuli.[23] However, these studies have also shown that the elderly had an increased response to high-intensity stimuli, decreased pain tolerance, and decreased descending modulation, which may explain the high incidence of elderly patients reporting chronic postoperative pain.[23] Physiologic changes in the elderly patient include longer circulation times and longer duration of action secondary to reduced clearance of medications, and analgesic requirements tend to decrease with increasing age.[23] IV PCA is appropriate in the elderly, because it allows the patient to compensate for individual variability. Use of patient-controlled epidural analgesia has been reported to improve postoperative outcomes, such as gastrointestinal function after abdominal surgery, decreased incidence of myocardial infarction, decreased pain scores, and decreased pulmonary complications.[23]

Delirium is one of the most significant complications in elderly patients after surgery and is associated with increased mortality and prolonged hospital stays. Delirium is multifactorial, but uncontrolled pain may be a contributor to its development, because higher pain scores have been associated with a decline in mental status and development of postoperative delirium.[23] Opioids other than meperidine have not been associated with the development of delirium.

Obesity and Obstructive Sleep Apnea

Patients with obstructive sleep apnea (OSA) may be at a higher risk for postoperative complications. During obstructive episodes, patients with OSA may show hypoxia, bradyarrhythmias or tachyarrhythmias, myocardial ischemia, and decreased cardiac output.[23] Postoperative pain management is therefore more complicated in the patient with OSA. Patients with OSA are at an increased risk for respiratory arrest, and the use of sedatives, such as benzodiazepines and opioids, may be especially dangerous. Avoiding respiratory depressants and optimizing the use of NSAIDs and epidural analgesia with a local anesthetic instead of opioids may attenuate the risk for respiratory depression and arrest.

Patients with diagnosed OSA who require postoperative opioid therapy should be admitted to the hospital overnight and continuously monitored by pulse oximetry.[23] This strategy is especially true of high-risk children after tonsillectomy and adenoidectomy, because the surgery involves the airway and the patients receive opioids for pain.[32] Moreover, children with sleep-disordered breathing and recurrent hypoxemia are more sensitive to the effects of opioids and require dose reductions.[33] Codeine is best avoided, because some children have increased conversion of codeine to morphine (extensive and ultrarapid metabolizer phenotypes), which can lead to an overdose.[34]

Acute on Chronic Pain

Patients with chronic pain conditions need to have a specific plan for the management of their postoperative pain, particularly patients already taking large doses of analgesics or patients with a history of analgesic abuse.[10] Postoperative pain management may be difficult in opioid-tolerant patients, because the standard assessment and therapy approaches are usually inadequate. Opioid-tolerant patients usually require higher doses of analgesic medications, but health care providers are often afraid to prescribe them as needed, because of concern for addiction or medication-related side effects and mistaking tolerance for addiction.[10] An APS, if available, should be consulted before surgery, and the patient's personal chronic pain physician should be contacted for perioperative recommendations. It is important to develop a treatment plan before surgery, and this plan should be discussed with the patient and the perioperative management teams. It is also important to recognize and address nonnociceptive sources of distress.[10] Patients on chronic pain medications should not have the medications weaned or held before surgery, unless they are using an NSAID or COX-2 inhibitor that needs to be held preoperatively. Patients should be told to take their usual morning does of pain medication, and all transdermal patches should remain on during the surgery. Even if they are already on high doses of pain medications, the chronic pain patient's postoperative analgesic needs should be expected to increase.[10]

High self-reported pain scores should also be expected, and therefore, treatment should be based on other assessments, such as ability to breathe deeply, cough, and ambulate, in conjunction with the patient's self-reported pain scores. The patient's required maintenance medications should continue, with additional medications added to treat the new surgical pain. Adjuvants such as NSAIDs and regional anesthesia techniques as well as a plan to transition the patient from IV to oral medications are all necessary. The oral medications should include a scheduled long-lasting controlled-release opioid as well as an as-needed immediate-release opioid for breakthrough pain. It is also important for the physician to recognize that the perioperative period is not the appropriate time to detoxify the patient.[23]

SUMMARY

Postoperative pain is an individual multifactorial experience influenced by patient culture, psychology, genetics, previous pain events, beliefs, mood, and ability to cope, as well as the type of procedure performed. Inadequate treatment of postoperative pain continues to occur, despite advances in analgesic techniques, placing patients at risk for CPSP and significant disability. Optimal pain results from proper management in the preoperative, intraoperative, and postoperative periods and requires appropriate education of physicians, nurses, other health care providers, and patients. An understanding of the pathophysiology of postoperative pain and the various options available for analgesia often results in a procedure-specific, multimodal approach, optimizing pain relief, decreasing adverse effects, and creating a better patient experience.

REFERENCES

1. Macintyre PE, Scott DA, Schug SA, et al. Acute pain management: scientific evidence [Systematic reviews and meta-analyses]. 3rd edition. 2010. Available

at: http://www.anzca.edu.au/resources/college-publications/pdfs/Acute%20Pain%20Management/books-and-publications/acutepain.pdf. Accessed June 25, 2014.
2. Butterworth J, Mackey D, Wasnick J. Morgan and Mikhail's clinical anesthesiology. New York (NY): Lange/McGraw-Hill; 2013.
3. Prospect: procedure specific postoperative pain management [Systematic reviews and meta-analyses]. Available at: http://www.postoppain.org/frameset.htm. Accessed June 12, 2014.
4. Kehlet H. Updated pain guidelines. What is new? Anesthesiology 2012;117:1397–8.
5. White PF, Kehlet H. Improving postoperative pain management: what are the unresolved issues? Anesthesiology 2010;112:220–5.
6. Khan R, Kamran A, Blakeway E, et al. Catastrophizing: a predictive factor for postoperative pain. Am J Surg 2011;201(1):122–31.
7. Grosu I, de Kock M. New concepts in acute pain management: strategies to prevent chronic postsurgical pain, opioid-induced hyperalgesia, and outcome measures. Anesthesiol Clin 2011;29(2):311–27.
8. Kodali BS, Oberoi J. Management of postoperative pain [Systematic reviews and meta-analyses]. In: Rosenquist EW, Doucette K, editors. UpToDate. Waltham (MA): UpToDate; 2014.
9. American Society of Anesthesiologists Task Force on Acute Pain Management. Practice guidelines for acute pain management in the perioperative setting: an updated report by the American Society of Anesthesiologists Task Force on Acute Pain Management. Anesthesiology 2012;116:248–73.
10. Fisher S, Bader A, Sweitzer B. Preoperative evaluation. In: Miller R, Eriksson L, Fleisher L, et al, editors. Miller: Miller's anesthesia. 7th edition. Philadelphia: Churchill Livingston; 2010. p. 1001–66.
11. Carr D, Bradshaw Y. Time to flip the pain curriculum? Anesthesiology 2014;120:12–4.
12. Kamibayashi T, Maze M. Clinical uses of alpha2-adrenergic agonists. Anesthesiology 2000;93:1345–9.
13. Choi PT, Bhandari M, Scott J, et al. Epidural analgesia for pain relief following hip or knee replacement [Systematic reviews and meta-analyses]. Cochrane Database Syst Rev 2003;(3):CD003071.
14. Findlay J. Transversus abdominus plane (TAP) blocks–a review. Surgeon 2012;10(6):361–7.
15. Singh M, Chin K, Chan V. Case report: ultrasound-guided transversus abdominus plane (TAP) block: a useful adjunct in management of postoperative respiratory failure. J Clin Anesth 2011;23(4):303–6.
16. Chan EY, Fransen M, Parker DA, et al. Femoral nerve blocks for acute postoperative pain after knee replacement surgery [Systematic reviews and meta-analyses]. Cochrane Database Syst Rev 2014;(5):CD009941. http://dx.doi.org/10.1002/14651858.CD009941.pub2.
17. Kehlet H, Liu SS. Continuous local anesthetic wound infusion to improve postoperative outcome: back to the periphery? Anesthesiology 2007;107:369–71.
18. Berde C, Strichartz G. Local anesthetics. In: Miller R, Eriksson L, Fleisher L, et al, editors. Miller: Miller's anesthesia. 7th edition. Philadelphia: Churchill Livingston; 2010. p. 2757–82.
19. Ventham NT, O'Neill S, Johns N, et al. Evaluation of novel local anesthetic wound infiltration techniques for postoperative pain following colorectal resection surgery: a meta-analysis [Systematic reviews and meta-analyses]. Dis Colon Rectum 2014;57(2):237–50.

20. Dasta J, Ramamoorthy S, Patou G, et al. Bupivacaine liposome injectable suspension compared with bupivacaine HCl for the reduction of opioid burden in the postsurgical setting. Curr Med Res Opin 2012;28(10):1609–15.
21. Gandhi G, Baratta JL, Heitz JW, et al. Acute pain management in the postanesthesia care unit. Anesthesiol Clin 2012;30(3):1–15.
22. US Food and Drug Administration. Fentanyl transdermal system (marketed as duragesic and generics) healthcare professional sheet. 2005. Available at: http://www.fda.gov/Drugs/DrugSafety/PostmarketDrugSafetyInformationforPatientsandProviders/ucm125840.htm. Accessed June 12, 2014.
23. Hurley R, Wu C. Acute postoperative pain. In: Miller R, Eriksson L, Fleisher L, et al, editors. Miller: Miller's anesthesia. 7th edition. Philadelphia: Churchill Livingston; 2010. p. 2757–82.
24. Melson T, Boyer DL, Minkowitz H, et al. Sufentanil nanotab PCA system: phase 3 active-comparator data versus iv PCA morphine for post-operative pain. Reg Anesth Pain Med 2013 [abstract: A009]. Available at: http://www.asra.com/display_spring_2013.php?id=9. Accessed June 26, 2014.
25. Elvir-Lazo O, White P. Postoperative pain management after ambulatory surgery: role of multimodal analgesia. Anesthesiol Clin 2010;28(2):217–24.
26. Elia N, Lysakowski C, Tramer MR. Does multimodal analgesia with acetaminophen, nonsteroidal antiinflammatory drugs, or selective cyclooxygenase-2 inhibitors and patient-controlled analgesia morphine offer advantages over morphine alone? Meta-analyses of randomized trials [Systematic reviews and meta-analyses]. Anesthesiology 2005;103(6):1296–304.
27. Remy C, Marret E, Bonnet F. Effects of acetaminophen on morphine side-effects and consumption after major surgery: meta-analysis of randomized controlled trials [Systematic reviews and meta-analyses]. Br J Anaesth 2005;94(4):505–13.
28. Melemeni A, Staikou C, Fassoulaki A. Review article: gabapentin for acute and chronic post-surgical pain. Signa Vitae 2007;2(1):S42–51.
29. Ventham NT, Hughes M, O'Neill S, et al. Systematic review and meta-analysis of continuous local anaesthetic wound infiltration versus epidural analgesia for postoperative pain following abdominal surgery [Systematic reviews and meta-analyses]. Br J Surg 2013;100(10):1280–9.
30. Gebhardt R, Mehran RJ, Soliz J, et al. Epidural versus On-Q local anesthetic-infiltrating catheter for post-thoracotomy pain control. J Cardiothorac Vasc Anesth 2013;27:1–8.
31. Karthikesalinigam A, Walsh SR, Marker SR, et al. Continuous wound infusion of local anesthetic agents following colorectal surgery: systematic review and meta-analysis [Systematic reviews and meta-analyses]. World J Gastroenterol 2008;14(34):5301–5.
32. Cote CJ, Posner KL, Domino KB. Death or neurologic injury after tonsillectomy in children with a focus on obstructive sleep apnea: Houston, we have a problem! Anesth Analg 2014;118:1276–83.
33. Brown KA, Laferrière A, Lakheeram I, et al. Recurrent hypoxemia in children is associated with increased analgesic sensitivity to opiates. Anesthesiology 2006;105:665–9.
34. US Food and Drug Administration drug safety communication: codeine use in certain children after tonsillectomy and/or adenoidectomy may lead to rare, but life-threatening adverse events or death. Available at: http://www.fda.gov/drugs/drugsafety/ucm313631.htm. Accessed July 3, 2014.

Endpoints of Resuscitation

Ramon F. Cestero, MD*, Daniel L. Dent, MD

KEYWORDS

• Shock • Resuscitation • Hypoperfusion • Oxygen demand

KEY POINTS

- The state of shock, regardless of cause, essentially consists of oxygen supply not meeting tissue metabolic demands.
- Shock can progress along a continuum of compensatory processes, starting with catecholamine-based vasoconstriction, progressing to tachycardia and moderate hypotension, and terminating with loss of vascular autoregulation, cellular hypoxia, and severe metabolic acidosis.
- Various endpoints of resuscitation are in clinical use and can be broadly divided into 2 groups: hemodynamic markers, which provide global information regarding hemodynamic status, and perfusion endpoints, which can be useful indicators of oxygenation at the cellular level.
- Despite the availability of multiple endpoints of resuscitation in clinical use, there is no one single data point or laboratory value that can be used to identify the patient who has been completely resuscitated from the shock state, as each value or technique has its own benefits and limitations.
- At this point, global markers of oxygenation and perfusion, such as central venous oxygen saturation, base deficit, and lactate, are practical and easily available indices that are useful as supplements to experienced clinical assessments during resuscitation.

INTRODUCTION

Definition of Shock

Shock is broadly defined as the abnormal physiologic state in which inadequate tissue oxygenation does not meet metabolic demands. As early as 1872, shock was described by Gross[1] as a "manifestation of the crude unhinging of the machinery of life" as well as "a peripheral circulatory failure, resulting from a discrepancy in the size of the vascular bed and the volume of the intravascular fluid" by Blalock in 1937.[2]

In an attempt to better define the shock state, the 2006 International Consensus Conference on hemodynamic monitoring in shock defined it as a "failure to deliver

Disclosures: None.

Division of Trauma and Emergency Surgery, Department of Surgery, UT Health Science Center San Antonio, 7703 Floyd Curl Drive, Mail Code 7740, San Antonio, TX 78229-3900, USA
* Corresponding author.
E-mail address: cestero@uthscsa.edu

Surg Clin N Am 95 (2015) 319–336
http://dx.doi.org/10.1016/j.suc.2014.10.004 surgical.theclinics.com
0039-6109/15/$ – see front matter

and/or utilize adequate amounts of oxygen."[3] Using degrees of derangements in physiologic parameters such as heart rate, blood pressure, and urine output to classify hypovolemic shock into 4 stages, the American College of Surgeons Advanced Trauma Life Support manual broadly defines shock as "an abnormality of the circulatory system that results in inadequate organ perfusion and tissue oxygenation.[4]

Although multiple causes of shock exist, including hypovolemic/traumatic, cardiogenic, septic, and neurogenic, all shock states have the common abnormality of oxygen supply not meeting tissue metabolic demands.

Compensated and Uncompensated Shock

The body's response to shock involves several stages of compensation. These compensatory stages proceed sequentially, starting with a phase of catecholamine-mediated vasoconstriction during which blood is diverted toward the heart and brain and away from other organs and tissues. The combination of catecholamines and fluid shifts from extracellular regions to the intravascular compartment helps to maintain blood pressure during these early stages of shock. Although patients may have lost up to 15% of blood volume in the setting of bleeding, they may still exhibit a normal pulse, blood pressure, and other physiologic parameters because of these compensatory mechanisms.

As shock progresses, the patient will then enter a state of partial compensation exhibited by mild to moderate hypotension, tachycardia, and a decreased pulse pressure. As the metabolic needs of tissues are not met, an imbalance between oxygen delivery (DO_2) and oxygen utilization occurs, resulting in oxygen debt. Because of this lack of oxygen, tissues activate anaerobic metabolism to produce energy, and anaerobic byproducts such as lactate are released. Ultimately, this is followed by a state of decompensation, or uncompensated shock, in which autoregulation of vascular beds fails, blood flow becomes pressure dependent, and cellular hypoxia leads to significant metabolic acidosis.

Resuscitation

Resuscitation from shock involves the restoration of normal physiology, particularly at the cellular level. Despite the achievement of normal physiologic values, persistent hypoxemia, lactic acidosis, and anaerobic metabolism may still exist. Physiologic parameters, which are typically used to monitor hemodynamic and oxygenation status, such as heart rate, blood pressure, urine output, and blood gases, can be normal in the setting of tissue hypoxia and cannot be used to rule out imbalances between oxygen supply and demand.[5] Dysoxia and capillary flow abnormalities may well be present despite normalization of these traditional markers. Physiologic markers, or endpoints of resuscitation, have therefore been sought to better guide resuscitative efforts in the setting of shock.

Endpoints of Resuscitation

Various endpoints have been identified to better guide resuscitation in the setting of shock. These endpoints can be broadly divided into 2 groups based on the information they provide. Hemodynamic markers, such as arterial blood pressure, central venous pressure (CVP), mixed and central venous oxygen saturation (SvO_2), arterial pulse waveform analysis, and values obtained from echocardiography, can provide global information regarding hemodynamic status. Perfusion endpoints including lactate, base deficit (BD), near-infrared spectroscopy (NIRS), and gastric or sublingual tonometry can be useful indicators of oxygenation at the cellular level (**Table 1**).

HEMODYNAMIC MARKERS/TARGETS

Mean Arterial Pressure

Restitution of a normal blood pressure in the management of a patient in shock is intuitive, because most clinicians are accustomed to using blood pressure as a marker of cardiovascular status. The mean arterial pressure (MAP), determined by the formula: (MAP = diastolic pressure + 1/3 [systolic pressure − diastolic pressure]), is commonly used as a blood pressure endpoint during resuscitation, despite no universally accepted MAP goal exists.

In the acutely bleeding patient in hypovolemic shock, establishing a target blood pressure can be difficult, because restoration of a normal blood pressure in the setting of uncontrolled arterial bleeding has been shown to increase both blood loss and mortality.[6] In addition, fluids administered before surgical control of bleeding sites can disrupt an effective thrombus, leading to a fatal secondary hemorrhage.[7]

To address whether there is a benefit to delaying resuscitation (and therefore normalization of blood pressure) until the time of operative intervention in trauma patients, Bickell and colleagues[8] studied 598 adults with penetrating torso injuries who presented with a blood pressure of 90 or less and compared immediate resuscitation in the field to delayed resuscitation after patients reached the operating room. Interestingly, those who did not receive resuscitation until operative intervention (hypotensive resuscitation) had a higher survival rate (70% vs 62%), fewer complications (23% vs 30%), and a shorter length of stay (11 vs 14 days). Although this was a landmark trial supporting delayed, or hypotensive, resuscitation, subsequent studies have been inconsistent in the results, and not all have shown an improvement in outcomes when hypotensive resuscitation is instituted.[9] Despite some controversy in the civilian community, the US Military currently recommends permissive hypotension in the management of combat casualties without central nervous system injury, because hypotension in patients with neurologic injuries is associated with adverse outcomes.[10]

In the setting of sepsis, resuscitation using mean arterial blood pressure endpoints has been used since the landmark 2001 trial by Rivers and colleagues,[11] which reported substantial benefits of early goal-directed therapy. In that trial, they demonstrated a significant mortality decrease (16.5%) in septic patients treated with an algorithm including MAP, CVP, and mixed venous oxygen saturation (SvO_2). However, on post hoc analysis, Donnino and colleagues[12] reported that, despite normalization of MAP, a significant number of patients still exhibited signs of global hypoxia as evidenced by lactic acidosis, defined as cryptic septic shock. Despite the controversies surrounding this study, the 2012 Surviving Sepsis Guidelines recommend a goal MAP of 65 or more during the first 6 hours of resuscitation in septic shock.[13]

Central Venous Pressure

CVP is a common measurement of preload in critically ill patients. Preload, defined as the load present before contraction of the ventricle has started, is an important determinant of cardiac output (CO).[14] CVP measurements are therefore frequently used in the management of fluid resuscitation and titration. In fact, the 2012 Surviving Sepsis Campaign guidelines recommend a CVP of 8 to 12 mm Hg as a "recommended physiologic target for resuscitation" during the first 6 hours of resuscitation in septic shock.[13]

Despite this strong recommendation of CVP use to guide resuscitation in septic patients, the reliability of CVP measurements as an indicator of fluid status is

Table 1
Benefits and limitations of hemodynamic markers and perfusion markers

Technique	Variable Measured	Benefits	Limitations
Hemodynamic markers			
MAP	Arterial blood pressure	Universally available and interpretable	Lack of universal MAP goals to guide therapy
		Hypotensive MAP goals may improve outcomes	Normalization of blood pressure may increase bleeding
			Tissue hypoxia may exist despite normal MAP
CVP	Venous blood pressure	Common measurement in critically ill	Static value, poor relationship between CVP and overall volume
			Central venous access required
$ScvO_2$	Oxygen extraction (pulmonary artery)	Marker of total body DO_2/consumption	Pulmonary artery catheter required, global measurement
			May be more useful as predictor of survival
			Does not provide information on tissue perfusion
SvO_2	Oxygen extraction (central line)	PA catheter not required	Central venous access required
		Regional marker of oxygenation	Does not provide information on tissue microcirculation
Arterial pulse waveform analysis	SVV	Accurate in determination of fluid responsiveness	Special equipment required
		Arterial line typically present in critically ill patients	Data support use only in mechanically ventilated patients
			Inaccurate in arrhythmias, vascular disease, aortic regurgitation

Echocardiography	Cardiac anatomy/function	Noninvasive mode available (transthoracic) Real-time data on volume and CO	Special equipment and training required Limited data on use as endpoint of resuscitation
Perfusion markers			
Lactate	Marker of anaerobic metabolism	Universally available Reliable estimate of anaerobic metabolism	Decreased clearance in hepatic or renal disease May be elevated in settings other than shock (seizures, drugs)
BD	Base required to normalize pH	Sensitive measure of hypoperfusion/acidosis	Inaccurate in hypothermia, hypocapnea, intravenous $NaHCO_3$ Limited specificity in renal failure, DKA, CO_2 retention Does not correlate well with lactate levels in operating room or ICU patients
NIRS	StO_2	Measures regional tissue oxygenation Noninvasive Provides continuous data	Inconclusive data regarding reliability Requires specialized equipment
Gastric tonometry	Gastric CO_2, intramucosal pH (pHi)	Minimally invasive Indicator of gastrointestinal ischemia	Limited availability May not improve outcomes, undefined clinical benefit Values affected by enteral feeding and technical limitations
Sublingual capnometry	Sublingual mucosal CO_2	Easy accessibility of sublingual mucosa Provides real-time information	Limited availability Limited data as endpoint of resuscitation

controversial. Multiple studies of various patient populations (trauma, sepsis, cardiovascular surgery, and other critical illnesses) have suggested that static pressure–derived values, such as CVP, do not accurately predict volume status.[15–18] Similarly, Marik and colleagues,[19] in a 2008 systematic review of 24 studies, found a "very poor relationship between CVP and blood volume" and recommended that "CVP should not be used to make clinical decisions regarding patient management." In addition, the 2006 International Consensus Conference on hemodynamics in shock recommended that "preload measurement alone not be used to predict fluid responsiveness," because "poor correlation between assessments of preload and predictions of fluid responsiveness has been widely reported."[3]

Overall, despite consensus recommendations of using CVP as a resuscitation target in the setting of septic shock, most data do not support the use of CVP as a global endpoint of resuscitation.

CENTRAL AND MIXED VENOUS OXYGEN SATURATION

The adequacy of tissue oxygenation is determined by a balance between DO_2 and oxygen consumption ($\dot{V}O_2$). This balance is reflected by the percentage of oxygen extracted from hemoglobin by the tissues, defined as either the SvO_2 or the $ScvO_2$, depending on where the venous sample is obtained.

Mixed Venous Oxygen Saturation

SvO_2 requires the placement of a pulmonary artery catheter, and the values obtained from the catheter tip represent total body oxygen extraction because it is a true mixed venous sample. Normal values typically range between 65% and 75%.[20] A decrease in SvO_2 to less than 65% represents a decrease in DO_2 (normally due to anemia or a low CO), and values near 50% are associated with inadequate tissue oxygenation.

In a general population of critically ill patients, Gattinoni and colleagues[21] resuscitated patients to a normal SvO_2, normal cardiac index (CI), or supranormal CI. No differences in mortality or multiorgan failure (MOF) were found. Durham and colleagues[22] found that resuscitating critically ill patients to specific oxygenation parameters did not improve rate of death or organ failure compared with conventional parameters. In trauma patients, Velmahos and colleagues[23] reported that optimization of DO_2 did not improve outcome, with 40% of patients achieving the desired parameters spontaneously versus 70% of the protocol patients. Although none of those who reached the desired oxygenation parameters died, 30% of those who did not achieve them died, suggesting that oxygenation parameters were more predictive of survival than useful as a goal of resuscitation.

Central Venous Oxygen Saturation

An alternate method of obtaining similar information is using a venous sample from a central line catheter ($ScvO_2$), which represents regional rather than global venous oxygen saturation and normally has a value near 70%. Although the use of $ScvO_2$ provides the practical benefit of eliminating the need for a pulmonary artery catheter, $ScvO_2$ values tend to be higher than SvO_2 by an average of $7 \pm 4\%$ in critically ill patients, with the largest discrepancies noted in sepsis, heart failure, and cardiogenic shock.[20,24] However, despite discrepancies in absolute values, trends in $ScvO_2$ generally correlate with changes in SvO_2.[24]

It is important to note, however, that the placement of the central line catheter tip plays an important role in the correlation of $ScvO_2$ to SvO_2. Kopterides and colleagues[25] found that as the central venous catheter tip was located closer to the right atrium, the discrepancy between $ScvO_2$ and SvO_2 decreased. When the tip was 15 cm away from the inlet of the right atrium, $ScvO_2$ overestimated SvO_2 by 8%. When the tip was advanced to the right atrium, $ScvO_2$ overestimated SvO_2 by only 1%.

Increasing evidence has supported the use of $ScvO_2$ as an indicator of shock,[26] and decreased values have been noted in both cardiogenic shock[27] and hypovolemic shock.[28] In septic shock, Rivers and colleagues[11] showed that using a goal $ScvO_2$ of greater than 70% as part of an "early goal-directed therapy" protocol improved survival by 16%,[11] and this has become a recommendation in the Surviving Sepsis Campaign guidelines.[13] Increased use of $ScvO_2$ values as an endpoint of resuscitation, particularly in septic shock, has gained favor despite controversies regarding the Rivers study.

In summary, SvO_2 and $ScvO_2$ represent oxygen balance in the tissues, and low values indicate tissue hypoxia and the need for continued resuscitation. Unfortunately, neither one indicates the cause of the hypoxia, because they are general markers. As such, they are not able to provide information regarding locoregional or microcirculatory perfusion, specifically in septic shock, whereby conditions such as perfusion heterogeneity may lead to a combination of highly saturated open capillaries along with closed capillaries with low saturation.[29,30] However, despite their limitations and until further data are available, normal SvO_2 and $ScvO_2$ parameters can be used as reasonable resuscitation goals.

ARTERIAL PULSE WAVEFORM ANALYSIS/PULSE CONTOUR ANALYSIS

Arterial pulse waveform analysis involves the determination of stroke volume (SV) by analyzing the pulse pressure waveform using the data obtained from an intra-arterial line. When arterial compliance and systemic vascular resistance are known, CO can be calculated because the pulse pressure is directly proportional to SV and inversely related to vascular compliance.

In addition to CO, the pulse pressure waveform also provides information on changes in the SV affected by positive pressure ventilation. Specifically, during the inspiratory phase of positive pressure ventilation, intrathoracic pressure increases and leads to an increase in right atrial pressure. In volume-depleted patients, right ventricular filling is decreased, and after a few cycles, results in a variation in left ventricular filling as blood is pumped through the lungs and back to the left side of the heart. In hypovolemic patients, this then leads to a variation in SV, termed stroke volume variation (SVV).[31]

Monitoring SVV has proved useful in accurately predicting patients who are fluid responsive.[32] In septic patients, Michard and colleagues[33] showed that systolic pressure variations of 13% or more in mechanically ventilated patients were highly sensitive and specific for fluid responsiveness. Zhang and colleagues,[34] in a recent meta-analysis of 568 patients from 23 studies, found that SVV is effective in predicting fluid responsiveness, with a sensitivity and specificity of 81% and 80%, respectively.

Several devices are available to evaluate the arterial pressure waveform. The Vigileo/FloTrac system (Edwards Lifesciences, Irvine, CA, USA) uses a proprietary software algorithm to determine CO by analyzing the arterial waveform, and it has the advantage of being able to be used with any arterial catheter in any location. Although software upgrades have improved the accuracy of the values obtained from this device,[35] some limitations exist when using the algorithm in critically ill patients.[36] The LiDCO Plus system (LiDCO, Cambridge, UK) also uses pulse contour analysis to determine SV and CO, but to estimate SV, it uses a lithium-based dye dilution technique, which has been shown to be as reliable as other thermodilution methods.[37] The PiCCO monitor (Pulsion, Munich, Germany) combines waveform analysis with thermodilution to determine CO as well as several additional hemodynamic parameters, including global end-diastolic volume measurements of all cardiac chambers and extravascular lung water measurements. However, cannulation of both a central arterial and a central venous vessel is required.[38]

Although each device has its advantages and disadvantages, a common limitation to using any arterial waveform system is decreased validity in the setting of cardiac arrhythmias, severe peripheral vascular disease, and aortic valve regurgitation. In addition, the necessity of mechanical ventilation with tidal volumes of 8 mL/kg or greater and a respiratory rate of less than 17 per minute further limit their use,[32] although in critically ill patients these requirements are typically fulfilled.

Unfortunately, data from multicenter randomized trials using these techniques are limited. Although several encouraging single-center small-scaled studies have shown improved outcome using arterial waveform analysis and goal-directed therapy,[39–41] limited multicenter data exist to support the clinical value of these devices with respect to patient outcomes.

ECHOCARDIOGRAPHY

As point-of-care ultrasound devices have become more commonplace, the use of echocardiography in critical care settings has increased. Bedside echocardiography can assist the clinician in assessing hemodynamically unstable patients, providing information on both cardiac anatomy and function. Transthoracic and transesophageal modalities are available, and both provide information on left ventricular and right ventricular function, ejection fraction, ventricular volume, and CO.[42]

Echocardiography has been used to assess patients with hemodynamic failure. Although originally used for evaluation of static parameters of cardiac preload such as volumes and estimated filling pressures, dynamic parameters were eventually found to be more useful. Echocardiography can measure left ventricular SV by multiplying the area under the curve of aortic flow (velocity time interval, or VTI) by the cross-sectional area of the aortic annulus,[43] and changes in VTI reflect changes in SV. In 38 mechanically ventilated patients, Monnet and colleagues[44] have shown that changes in VTI detected hypovolemia and predicted fluid responsiveness. Similarly, in mechanically ventilated patients in septic shock, Feissel and colleagues[45] reported that VTI changes can predict increases in CO after fluid infusion with a high sensitivity and specificity.

Echocardiography has also been used to evaluate the size of the inferior vena cava (IVC) to assess preload and volume responsiveness in critically ill patients, and IVC diameter change after a fluid challenge has been shown to be a potential determinant of fluid status. In 73 surgical patients who received a fluid bolus when their IVC was determined to be "FLAT" (<2 cm) by transthoracic echocardiogram (TTE), Ferrada and colleagues[46] found that all patients had an increase in their IVC diameter to "FAT" (>2 cm) and 97% of these patients had resolution of hypotension after this initial fluid bolus. In mechanically ventilated septic patients, both Barbier and colleagues[47] and Feissel and colleagues[48] showed that respiratory variations in IVC diameter can be used to predict fluid responsiveness.

A major limitation to the use of echocardiography in critical care regards the training necessary to acquire several of the dynamic parameters. Although only basic skills in critical care echocardiography are required to obtain IVC diameter values to identify preload-dependent patients, advanced TTE skill levels are necessary to appreciate the respiratory changes in SV determined by VTI. The International Expert Consensus Statement on Advanced Critical Care Echocardiography, recently published by Viellard-Baron and colleagues,[49] describes the current competencies and training standards recommended for critical care ultrasound, including requirements for national-level certification.

It appears that bedside echocardiography can be a useful adjunct in the evaluation of the patient in shock, providing information regarding volume status and fluid responsiveness. Although data regarding its use as an endpoint of resuscitation are lacking, its increasing use will likely lead to further studies as to its potential role in the management of the patient in shock.

PERFUSION MARKERS

Lactate

Lactate is created as a byproduct of glucose as it is metabolized during glycolysis. As glucose molecules are processed for energy in the cytoplasm, pyruvate is created, which can either be directly converted into lactate (producing two molecules of adenosine triphosphate [ATP]) or enter the mitochondria where it can generate 36 molecules of ATP as a result of oxygen-dependent reactions. In the setting of hypoxia or hypoperfusion where oxygen supplies are diminished, pyruvate does not enter the mitochondria, resulting in increased lactate production.[50]

Lactate concentration in the blood is a balance between lactate production and clearance. Most lactate clearance occurs in the liver, with a small amount removed by the kidneys.[51,52] In situations where liver and/or renal clearance is impaired, such as hepatic dysfunction or renal disease, lactate concentrations may be increased despite the absence of hypoperfusion.

The time to correction and normalization of elevated lactate concentrations is associated with mortality, because longer times result in poorer outcomes. In a study of 95 critically ill patients requiring hemodynamic monitoring, those who normalized lactate in less than 24 hours had the lowest mortality (3.9%) compared with those who were corrected in 24 to 48 hours (13.3%) and 48 to 96 hours (42.5%).[53] Patients who did not normalize their lactate during hospitalization experienced a rate of 100% mortality. On multivariate analysis, time to lactate clearance was shown to be an independent predictor of survival.

In another study evaluating both lactate and BD, these markers were shown to be associated with increased mortality. In this study of 137 patients, mortality was 10% when lactate was normalized within 2 hours, 24% if normalized after 48 hours, and 67% if lactate was not corrected.[54] The 2004 Eastern Association for Surgery of Trauma clinical practice guidelines state that standard hemodynamic parameters do not adequately quantify the degree of physiologic derangement in trauma patients and therefore initial BD, lactate level, or gastric pH can be used to stratify patients.[55]

More recently, attempts have been made to integrate lactate clearance as part of a goal-directed protocol-driven response to persistent elevation. In the randomized LACTATES trial, Jones and colleagues[56] compared early goal-directed therapy in septic patients using lactate clearance against a strategy using $ScvO_2$ as endpoints of resuscitation. Patients in the group resuscitated to a lactate clearance of 10% or higher had a rate of 6% lower in-hospital mortality than those resuscitated to a $ScvO_2 \geq 70\%$. In another study, Jansen and colleagues[57] randomized intensive care unit (ICU) patients to a group whose resuscitation was guided by lactate levels and another group that was not. Not only was mortality decreased in the lactate-guided group (33.9% vs 43.5%), but the lactate-guided patients had a shorter time in the ICU and were weaned faster from mechanical ventilation and inotropes.

Overall, lactate remains an easily measured laboratory value that can provide a reliable estimate of hypoperfusion or anaerobic metabolism. Despite data supporting its use as an endpoint of resuscitation, it does have some limitations, because it may be elevated due to causes other than hypoperfusion (seizures, drugs, liver failure) and its clearance may be impaired, resulting in persistently elevated values. In addition, lactate elevation may lack sensitivity, because it may be falsely normal in the settings of mesenteric ischemia[58] and sepsis.[59]

Base Deficit

BD is defined as the amount of base required to raise the serum pH of 1 L of whole blood to 7.40 at a temperature of 37°C and a P_{CO_2} of 40 mm Hg. It has been used as a marker of anaerobic metabolism and a surrogate marker for lactic acidosis. Normal values are between −3 and +3 mMol, with negative values representing metabolic acidosis.

Because of its rapid availability, multiple studies have been performed evaluating BD in the setting of shock. In trauma patients, it appears to be a sensitive measure of hypoperfusion. In a retrospective study of 3791 trauma patients, Rutherford and colleagues[60] reported that a BD of −15 mMol within 24 hours of injury was a significant marker of mortality in patients less than 55 years of age. In patients older than 55, a lower BD value of 8 mMol was found to be a significant predictor of mortality, suggesting that elderly patients may require a lower BD threshold. In a more recent study, Mutschler and colleagues[61] retrospectively classified more than 16,000 trauma patients into 4 groups based on worsening BD, from less than 2 mmol/dL (class I) to greater than 10 mMol/dL (class 4). BD class was linearly correlated to mortality, need for transfusion, and risk of coagulopathy. In addition, BD predicted hypovolemic shock better than the conventional Advanced Trauma Life Support classifications of shock, leading the authors to suggest that BD may be superior in early risk-stratification of severely injured patients.

BD has also been found to be predictive of complications. Davis and colleagues,[62] in a retrospective review of 2954 trauma patients, found that BD less than or equal to 6 correlated with the need for blood transfusion, increased hospital stays, and shock-related complications, including renal failure, acute respiratory distress syndrome, coagulopathy, and MOF. Similarly, in severely injured patients, Eberhard and colleagues[63] reported that the initial BD was significantly increased in patients who developed acute lung injury versus those who did not.

Despite data supporting the ability of BD to predict transfusion requirements, complications, and mortality, the use of BD as a marker of perfusion has significant limitations. The administration of sodium bicarbonate, hypothermia, and hypocapnea can all affect the BD. In trauma patients, alcohol intoxication can worsen BD values for similar degrees of injury severity and hemodynamics.[64] In addition to lactic acidosis, other causes of acidosis such as renal failure, diabetic ketoacidosis, and chronic CO_2 retention can also affect BD values, limiting the specificity of using the BD for resuscitation. Resuscitation with standard crystalloid solutions, such as normal saline or lactated Ringer, can also increase BD independent of injury severity.[65] BD also does not correlate well with lactate levels, in both the operating room[66] and the critically ill setting.[67] Because of these multiple limitations, BD is not recommended as a sole endpoint of resuscitation.

Near-Infrared Spectroscopy

Compared with other measurements of resuscitation that reflect total body perfusion and oxygenation, NIRS measures regional tissue oxygenation. NIRS uses fiber-optic light to determine the oxygen saturation of chromophomes noninvasively based on spectrophotometric principles. Tissue oxygen saturation (StO_2) is then derived by a complex mathematical algorithm, providing a measurement of both DO_2 and consumption in the selected tissues.[68] The current system available commercially uses the thenar eminence as the targeted tissue bed, and this area offers the advantages of relatively thin fat tissue over the muscle as well as limited edema formation, which provide the best setting for measuring StO_2. To enhance the value of NIRS, the StO_2 desaturation occlusion slope after vascular occlusion of the target tissue bed as well as the StO_2 reperfusion slope after release of occlusion has been studied.

Data using NIRS have been inconclusive in regards to its reliability as a sensitive indicator of oxygenation. Several studies have suggested that resting StO_2 values are insensitive indicators of tissue perfusion,[69–71] noting that both patients and control individuals had similar StO_2 levels despite evidence of impaired systemic oxygenation in the patient group. In a study using healthy volunteers, a 500-mL blood loss at blood donation did not result in changes in NIRS values despite causing an appreciable decrease in blood pressure.[72] However, in hemodynamically significant hypovolemia, StO_2 was found to be low.[73]

In the setting of hypovolemic shock, NIRS has been shown to identify the presence of hypoperfusion. Crookes and colleagues[74] studied 707 normal volunteers and 145 trauma patients who were stratified into 4 groups depending on severity of shock: no evidence of shock, mild shock, moderate shock, and severe shock. Although the StO_2 values were similar for the no-shock, mild-shock, and moderate-shock groups (87%, 83%, and 80%, respectively), StO_2 values were significantly decreased in the severe shock group (45%). Although NIRS values were not as useful in the setting of mild or moderate shock, the authors suggested that NIRS could be used to assess changes in tissue dysoxia. In a multicenter, prospective, observational study of trauma patients, Cohn and colleagues[75] studied the ability of StO_2 and BD obtained soon after patient arrival to predict MOF and death, using MOF as a surrogate for hypoperfusion. Both BD and StO_2 were equivalent in their ability to predict death and MOF, although StO_2 provided the added benefit of being continuous and noninvasive.

In sepsis, some studies report a difference in StO_2 between healthy subjects and patients in severe sepsis or septic shock,[69,71,76] although others do not.[77–79] However, at least according to data from one study using goal-directed therapy, persistently low StO_2 may be a marker of organ failure in sepsis. In a prospective observational study of critically ill patients with increased lactate levels (>3 mmol/L) who were observed during 8 hours of resuscitation, only half had low (<70%) StO_2 levels and StO_2 changes had no relationship with heart rate, MAP, or $ScvO_2$.[80] However, SOFA (sequential organ failure assessment) and APACHE (acute physiology and chronic health evaluation) scores were higher in those with decreased StO_2.

Despite encouraging results, data supporting NIRS as an endpoint of resuscitation remain inconclusive. It is still unclear if the small volume of distal muscle in the thenar region is an adequate indicator of organ perfusion or global oxygenation. Until further studies are conducted, the use of NIRS as a single resuscitative endpoint cannot be recommended at this time.

Gastric Tonometry

Gastric tonometry involves the measurement of CO_2 levels in the gastric wall to assess perfusion to the stomach and bowel. In hemodynamically compromised patients, blood flow is diverted from the gastrointestinal tract, resulting in an increase in P_{CO_2} in the wall of the stomach and a subsequent decrease in gastric mucosal pH (pHi). Through the use of a gastric tonometer, a specialized nasogastric tube with a silicone balloon filled with saline, samples can be obtained to measure CO_2 levels. Using the CO_2 results and the arterial bicarbonate level, pHi is calculated using a modified Henderson-Hasselbalch equation, providing a surrogate estimate of splanchnic ischemia.

Studies have shown that gastric tonometry is a sensitive predictor of outcomes in multiple settings, including trauma,[81] sepsis,[82] cardiac surgery,[83] and critically ill patients.[84] Although most studies have not shown an improvement in outcome using gastric tonometry, at least one study has shown that pHi-guided resuscitation may improve outcomes in critically ill patients.[84] However, in a prospective randomized trial of trauma patients comparing pHi-guided therapy and conventional shock management protocols, there was no difference in mortality, organ dysfunction, or length of stay.[85] In addition, Hameed and Cohn,[86] in a review of gastric tonometry, concluded that there was no evidence that pHi-guided resuscitation to a target pHi improved outcomes in critically ill patients or patients in septic shock.

Despite some initial enthusiasm and studies suggesting an undefined clinical benefit, several technical issues limited the use and widespread application of gastric tonometry. Perhaps most importantly, the calculation of pHi may be inherently flawed. In comparison to the CO_2 level that is directly measured, pHi is a derived value calculated using arterial bicarbonate values, which may not be equal to intramucosal gastric bicarbonate levels.[87] In addition, there are multiple confounders related to the low specificity associated with this technology, including enteral feeding, differences in arterial supply, buffering of gastric acid, and inappropriate measurement of gastric P_{CO_2}.

Sublingual Capnometry

As a result of the methodological limitations of gastric tonometry, attempts have been made to identify other areas of the gastrointestinal tract, which may serve as indicators of hypoperfusion. Using sublingual mucosal P_{CO_2} levels, sublingual capnometry has been shown to provide information regarding the adequacy of tissue perfusion in both hemorrhagic and septic shock.[88–91] In addition, it is able to differentiate between varying degrees of blood loss in trauma patients.[92]

Although the easy accessibility of the sublingual mucosa for P_{CO_2} sampling is attractive, there are limited data supporting the benefits of sublingual capnometry compared with conventional global assessments of hypoperfusion. In a prospective observational study of severely injured trauma patients, Baron and colleagues[93] found that although sublingual capnometry predicted survival, it had equivalent diagnostic ability to lactate and BD. Although the authors suggested that the ability to rapidly normalize sublingual P_{CO_2} may have played a role in survival, they recommended that sublingual capnometry may supplement standard measures of hemorrhagic shock.

SUMMARY

A significant number of clinical and laboratory markers is available to the clinician in regards to the evaluation and management of the patient in shock. Unfortunately, there is no one single data point or laboratory value that can be used to identify the patient who has been completely resuscitated from the shock state, because each value or technique has its own benefits and limitations. Resuscitation of patients in shock remains guided by a combination of multiple clinical tools, ranging from simple everyday data points such as physiologic values to methods and techniques that may require specialized equipment and/or extensive training. At this point, global markers of oxygenation and perfusion such as central venous oxygen saturation, BD, and lactate are practical and easily available indices that are useful as supplements to experienced clinical assessments during resuscitation. When a patient presents a mixed picture with some markers suggesting a shock state persists while others suggest resuscitation is complete, the clinician is encouraged to err on the side of continuing attempts to improve perfusion. As tools and techniques that assess the microcirculation are further studied and data become available, it is likely that we will eventually be able to consistently guide therapy to resolve hypoxia at the tissue level, and thereby improve patient outcomes in the setting of shock.

REFERENCES

1. Gross SD. A system of surgery: pathological, diagnostic, therapeutic and operative. 4th edition. Philadelphia: H. C. Lea; 1866.
2. Blalock A. Shock: further studies with particular reference to the effects of hemorrhage. 1934. Arch Surg 2010;145(4):393–4.
3. Antonelli M, Levy M, Andrews PJ, et al. Hemodynamic monitoring in shock and implications for management. International Consensus Conference, Paris, France, 27–28 April 2006. Intensive Care Med 2007;33(4):575–90.
4. American College of Surgeons, Committee on Trauma, ATLS. Advanced trauma life support for doctors. 8th edition. Chicago: American College of Surgeons; 2008. p. 366 xxxiii.
5. Shoemaker WC, Montgomery ES, Kaplan E, et al. Physiologic patterns in surviving and nonsurviving shock patients. Use of sequential cardiorespiratory variables in defining criteria for therapeutic goals and early warning of death. Arch Surg 1973;106(5):630–6.
6. Stern SA, Dronen SC, Wang X. Multiple resuscitation regimens in a near-fatal porcine aortic injury hemorrhage model. Acad Emerg Med 1995;2(2):89–97.
7. Shaftan GW, Chiu CJ, Dennis C, et al. Fundamentals of physiologic control of arterial hemorrhage. Surgery 1965;58(5):851–6.
8. Bickell WH, Wall MJ Jr, Pepe PE, et al. Immediate versus delayed fluid resuscitation for hypotensive patients with penetrating torso injuries. N Engl J Med 1994; 331(17):1105–9.
9. Dutton RP, Mackenzie CF, Scalea TM. Hypotensive resuscitation during active hemorrhage: impact on in-hospital mortality. J Trauma 2002;52(6):1141–6.
10. US Army, Institute of Surgical Research, Joint theater trauma system clinical practice guideline: damage control resuscitation at level IIb/III treatment facilities. 2013. Available at: http://www.usaisr.amedd.army.mil/assets/cpgs/Damage%20Control%20Resuscitation%20-%201%20Feb%202013.pdf.
11. Rivers E, Nguyen B, Havstad S, et al. Early goal-directed therapy in the treatment of severe sepsis and septic shock. N Engl J Med 2001;345(19):1368–77.
12. Donnino MW, Jørgensen NB, Jacobsen G, et al. Cryptic septic shock: a sub-analysis of early, goal-directed therapy. Chest 2003;124. 90S–90b.
13. Dellinger RP, Levy MM, Rhodes A, et al. Surviving Sepsis Campaign: international guidelines for management of severe sepsis and septic shock, 2012. Intensive Care Med 2013;39(2):165–228.

14. Opie LH. The heart: physiology, from cell to circulation. 3rd edition. Philadelphia: Lippincott-Raven; 1998. p. 637 xviii.
15. Osman D, Ridel C, Ray P, et al. Cardiac filling pressures are not appropriate to predict hemodynamic response to volume challenge. Crit Care Med 2007;35(1):64–8.
16. Michard F, Teboul JL. Predicting fluid responsiveness in ICU patients: a critical analysis of the evidence. Chest 2002;121(6):2000–8.
17. Kumar A, Anel R, Bunnell E, et al. Pulmonary artery occlusion pressure and central venous pressure fail to predict ventricular filling volume, cardiac performance, or the response to volume infusion in normal subjects. Crit Care Med 2004;32(3):691–9.
18. Bendjelid K, Romand JA. Fluid responsiveness in mechanically ventilated patients: a review of indices used in intensive care. Intensive Care Med 2003; 29(3):352–60.
19. Marik PE, Baram M, Vahid B. Does central venous pressure predict fluid responsiveness? A systematic review of the literature and the tale of seven mares. Chest 2008;134(1):172–8.
20. Maddirala S, Khan A. Optimizing hemodynamic support in septic shock using central and mixed venous oxygen saturation. Crit Care Clin 2010;26(2):323–33 [table of contents].
21. Gattinoni L, Brazzi L, Pelosi P, et al. A trial of goal-oriented hemodynamic therapy in critically ill patients. SvO2 Collaborative Group. N Engl J Med 1995;333(16):1025–32.
22. Durham RM, Neunaber K, Mazuski JE, et al. The use of oxygen consumption and delivery as endpoints for resuscitation in critically ill patients. J Trauma 1996; 41(1):32–9 [discussion: 39–40].
23. Velmahos GC, Demetriades D, Shoemaker WC, et al. Endpoints of resuscitation of critically injured patients: normal or supranormal? A prospective randomized trial. Ann Surg 2000;232(3):409–18.
24. Reinhart K, Kuhn HJ, Hartog C, et al. Continuous central venous and pulmonary artery oxygen saturation monitoring in the critically ill. Intensive Care Med 2004; 30(8):1572–8.
25. Kopterides P, Bonovas S, Mavrou I, et al. Venous oxygen saturation and lactate gradient from superior vena cava to pulmonary artery in patients with septic shock. Shock 2009;31(6):561–7.
26. Rivers EP, Ander DS, Powell D. Central venous oxygen saturation monitoring in the critically ill patient. Curr Opin Crit Care 2001;7(3):204–11.
27. Ander DS, Jaggi M, Rivers E, et al. Undetected cardiogenic shock in patients with congestive heart failure presenting to the emergency department. Am J Cardiol 1998;82(7):888–91.
28. Scalea TM, Holman M, Fuortes M, et al. Central venous blood oxygen saturation: an early, accurate measurement of volume during hemorrhage. J Trauma 1988; 28(6):725–32.
29. De Backer D, Ospina-Tascon G, Salgado D, et al. Monitoring the microcirculation in the critically ill patient: current methods and future approaches. Intensive Care Med 2010;36(11):1813–25.
30. Trzeciak S, Rivers EP. Clinical manifestations of disordered microcirculatory perfusion in severe sepsis. Crit Care 2005;9(Suppl 4):S20–6.
31. Pinsky MR. Hemodynamic evaluation and monitoring in the ICU. Chest 2007; 132(6):2020–9.
32. Marik PE, Cavallazzi R, Vasu T, et al. Dynamic changes in arterial waveform derived variables and fluid responsiveness in mechanically ventilated patients: a systematic review of the literature. Crit Care Med 2009;37(9):2642–7.

33. Michard F, Boussat S, Chemla D, et al. Relation between respiratory changes in arterial pulse pressure and fluid responsiveness in septic patients with acute circulatory failure. Am J Respir Crit Care Med 2000;162(1):134–8.
34. Zhang Z, Lu B, Sheng X, et al. Accuracy of stroke volume variation in predicting fluid responsiveness: a systematic review and meta-analysis. J Anesth 2011; 25(6):904–16.
35. Zimmermann A, Kufner C, Hofbauer S, et al. The accuracy of the Vigileo/FloTrac continuous cardiac output monitor. J Cardiothorac Vasc Anesth 2008;22(3): 388–93.
36. Tsai YF, Liu FC, Yu HP. FloTrac/Vigileo system monitoring in acute-care surgery: current and future trends. Expert Rev Med Devices 2013;10(6):717–28.
37. Sundar S, Panzica P. LiDCO systems. Int Anesthesiol Clin 2010;48(1):87–100.
38. Oren-Grinberg A. The PiCCO Monitor. Int Anesthesiol Clin 2010;48(1):57–85.
39. Benes J, Chytra I, Altmann P, et al. Intraoperative fluid optimization using stroke volume variation in high risk surgical patients: results of prospective randomized study. Crit Care 2010;14(3):R118.
40. Cecconi M, Fasano N, Langiano N, et al. Goal-directed haemodynamic therapy during elective total hip arthroplasty under regional anaesthesia. Crit Care 2011;15(3):R132.
41. Pearse R, Dawson D, Fawcett J, et al. Early goal-directed therapy after major surgery reduces complications and duration of hospital stay. A randomised, controlled trial [ISRCTN38797445]. Crit Care 2005;9(6):R687–93.
42. Manasia AR, Nagaraj HM, Kodali RB, et al. Feasibility and potential clinical utility of goal-directed transthoracic echocardiography performed by noncardiologist intensivists using a small hand-carried device (SonoHeart) in critically ill patients. J Cardiothorac Vasc Anesth 2005;19(2):155–9.
43. Huntsman LL, Stewart DK, Barnes SR, et al. Noninvasive Doppler determination of cardiac output in man. Clinical validation. Circulation 1983;67(3):593–602.
44. Monnet X, Rienzo M, Osman D, et al. Esophageal Doppler monitoring predicts fluid responsiveness in critically ill ventilated patients. Intensive Care Med 2005;31(9):1195–201.
45. Feissel M, Michard F, Mangin I, et al. Respiratory changes in aortic blood velocity as an indicator of fluid responsiveness in ventilated patients with septic shock. Chest 2001;119(3):867–73.
46. Ferrada P, Anand RJ, Whelan J, et al. Qualitative assessment of the inferior vena cava: useful tool for the evaluation of fluid status in critically ill patients. Am Surg 2012;78(4):468–70.
47. Barbier C, Loubieres Y, Schmit C, et al. Respiratory changes in inferior vena cava diameter are helpful in predicting fluid responsiveness in ventilated septic patients. Intensive Care Med 2004;30(9):1740–6.
48. Feissel M, Michard F, Faller JP, et al. The respiratory variation in inferior vena cava diameter as a guide to fluid therapy. Intensive Care Med 2004;30(9):1834–7.
49. Vieillard-Baron A, Mayo PH, Vignon P, et al. Expert Round Table on Echocardiography in ICU. International consensus statement on training standards for advanced critical care echocardiography. Intensive Care Med 2014;40(5): 654–66.
50. Levy B. Lactate and shock state: the metabolic view. Curr Opin Crit Care 2006; 12(4):315–21.
51. Consoli A, Nurjhan N, Reilly JJ Jr, et al. Contribution of liver and skeletal muscle to alanine and lactate metabolism in humans. Am J Physiol 1990;259(5 Pt 1): E677–84.

52. Connor H, Woods HF, Ledingham JG, et al. A model of L(+)-lactate metabolism in normal man. Ann Nutr Metab 1982;26(4):254–63.
53. McNelis J, Marini CP, Jurkiewicz A, et al. Prolonged lactate clearance is associated with increased mortality in the surgical intensive care unit. Am J Surg 2001; 182(5):481–5.
54. Husain FA, Martin MJ, Mullenix PS, et al. Serum lactate and base deficit as predictors of mortality and morbidity. Am J Surg 2003;185(5):485–91.
55. Tisherman SA, Barie P, Bokhari F, et al. Clinical practice guideline: endpoints of resuscitation. J Trauma 2004;57(4):898–912.
56. Jones AE, Shapiro NI, Trzeciak S, et al. Lactate clearance vs central venous oxygen saturation as goals of early sepsis therapy: a randomized clinical trial. JAMA 2010;303(8):739–46.
57. Jansen TC, van Bommel J, Schoonderbeek FJ, et al. Early lactate-guided therapy in intensive care unit patients: a multicenter, open-label, randomized controlled trial. Am J Respir Crit Care Med 2010;182(6):752–61.
58. Acosta S, Block T, Bjornsson S, et al. Diagnostic pitfalls at admission in patients with acute superior mesenteric artery occlusion. J Emerg Med 2012;42(6): 635–41.
59. Dugas AF, Mackenhauer J, Salciccioli JD, et al. Prevalence and characteristics of nonlactate and lactate expressors in septic shock. J Crit Care 2012;27(4): 344–50.
60. Rutherford EJ, Morris JA Jr, Reed GW, et al. Base deficit stratifies mortality and determines therapy. J Trauma 1992;33(3):417–23.
61. Mutschler M, Nienaber U, Brockamp T, et al. Renaissance of base deficit for the initial assessment of trauma patients: a base deficit-based classification for hypovolemic shock developed on data from 16,305 patients derived from the TraumaRegister DGU(R). Crit Care 2013;17(2):R42.
62. Davis JW, Parks SN, Kaups KL, et al. Admission base deficit predicts transfusion requirements and risk of complications. J Trauma 1996;41(5):769–74.
63. Eberhard LW, Morabito DJ, Matthay MA, et al. Initial severity of metabolic acidosis predicts the development of acute lung injury in severely traumatized patients. Crit Care Med 2000;28(1):125–31.
64. Dunham CM, Watson LA, Cooper C. Base deficit level indicating major injury is increased with ethanol. J Emerg Med 2000;18(2):165–71.
65. Brill SA, Stewart TR, Brundage SI, et al. Base deficit does not predict mortality when secondary to hyperchloremic acidosis. Shock 2002;17(6):459–62.
66. Chawla LS, Nader A, Nelson T, et al. Utilization of base deficit and reliability of base deficit as a surrogate for serum lactate in the peri-operative setting. BMC Anesthesiol 2010;10:16.
67. Chawla LS, Jagasia D, Abell LM, et al. Anion gap, anion gap corrected for albumin, and base deficit fail to accurately diagnose clinically significant hyperlactatemia in critically ill patients. J Intensive Care Med 2008;23(2):122–7.
68. Santora RJ, Moore FA. Monitoring trauma and intensive care unit resuscitation with tissue hemoglobin oxygen saturation. Crit Care 2009;13(Suppl 5):S10.
69. Creteur J, Carollo T, Soldati G, et al. The prognostic value of muscle StO2 in septic patients. Intensive Care Med 2007;33(9):1549–56.
70. Gomez H, Torres A, Polanco P, et al. Use of non-invasive NIRS during a vascular occlusion test to assess dynamic tissue O(2) saturation response. Intensive Care Med 2008;34(9):1600–7.
71. Skarda DE, Mulier KE, Myers DE, et al. Dynamic near-infrared spectroscopy measurements in patients with severe sepsis. Shock 2007;27(4):348–53.

72. Jeger V, Jakob SM, Fontana S, et al. 500 ml of blood loss does not decrease non-invasive tissue oxygen saturation (StO2) as measured by near infrared spectroscopy - A hypothesis generating pilot study in healthy adult women. J Trauma Manag Outcomes 2010;4:5.
73. Bartels SA, Bezemer R, de Vries FJ, et al. Multi-site and multi-depth near-infrared spectroscopy in a model of simulated (central) hypovolemia: lower body negative pressure. Intensive Care Med 2011;37(4):671–7.
74. Crookes BA, Cohn SM, Bloch S, et al. Can near-infrared spectroscopy identify the severity of shock in trauma patients? J Trauma 2005;58(4):806–13 [discussion: 813–6].
75. Cohn SM, Nathens AB, Moore FA, et al. Tissue oxygen saturation predicts the development of organ dysfunction during traumatic shock resuscitation. J Trauma 2007;62(1):44–54 [discussion: 54–5].
76. Payen D, Luengo C, Heyer L, et al. Is thenar tissue hemoglobin oxygen saturation in septic shock related to macrohemodynamic variables and outcome? Crit Care 2009;13(Suppl 5):S6.
77. Doerschug KC, Delsing AS, Schmidt GA, et al. Impairments in microvascular reactivity are related to organ failure in human sepsis. Am J Physiol Heart Circ Physiol 2007;293(2):H1065–71.
78. Nanas S, Gerovasili V, Renieris P, et al. Non-invasive assessment of the microcirculation in critically ill patients. Anaesth Intensive Care 2009;37(5):733–9.
79. Pareznik R, Knezevic R, Voga G, et al. Changes in muscle tissue oxygenation during stagnant ischemia in septic patients. Intensive Care Med 2006;32(1): 87–92.
80. Lima A, van Bommel J, Jansen TC, et al. Low tissue oxygen saturation at the end of early goal-directed therapy is associated with worse outcome in critically ill patients. Crit Care 2009;13(Suppl 5):S13.
81. Kirton OC, Windsor J, Wedderburn R, et al. Failure of splanchnic resuscitation in the acutely injured trauma patient correlates with multiple organ system failure and length of stay in the ICU. Chest 1998;113(4):1064–9.
82. Marik PE. Gastric intramucosal pH. A better predictor of multiorgan dysfunction syndrome and death than oxygen-derived variables in patients with sepsis. Chest 1993;104(1):225–9.
83. Mythen MG, Webb AR. Perioperative plasma volume expansion reduces the incidence of gut mucosal hypoperfusion during cardiac surgery. Arch Surg 1995; 130(4):423–9.
84. Gutierrez G, Palizas F, Doglio G, et al. Gastric intramucosal pH as a therapeutic index of tissue oxygenation in critically ill patients. Lancet 1992;339(8787): 195–9.
85. Miami Trauma Clinical Trials Group. Splanchnic hypoperfusion-directed therapies in trauma: a prospective, randomized trial. Am Surg 2005;71(3):252–60.
86. Hameed SM, Cohn SM. Gastric tonometry: the role of mucosal pH measurement in the management of trauma. Chest 2003;123(5 Suppl):475S–81S.
87. Creteur J. Gastric and sublingual capnometry. Curr Opin Crit Care 2006;12(3): 272–7.
88. Marik PE. Regional carbon dioxide monitoring to assess the adequacy of tissue perfusion. Curr Opin Crit Care 2005;11(3):245–51.
89. Marik PE. Sublingual capnometry: a non-invasive measure of microcirculatory dysfunction and tissue hypoxia. Physiol Meas 2006;27(7):R37–47.
90. Creteur J, De Backer D, Sakr Y, et al. Sublingual capnometry tracks microcirculatory changes in septic patients. Intensive Care Med 2006;32(4):516–23.

91. Weil MH, Nakagawa Y, Tang W, et al. Sublingual capnometry: a new noninvasive measurement for diagnosis and quantitation of severity of circulatory shock. Crit Care Med 1999;27(7):1225–9.
92. Baron BJ, Sinert R, Zehtabchi S, et al. Diagnostic utility of sublingual PCO2 for detecting hemorrhage in penetrating trauma patients. J Trauma 2004;57(1):69–74.
93. Baron BJ, Dutton RP, Zehtabchi S, et al. Sublingual capnometry for rapid determination of the severity of hemorrhagic shock. J Trauma 2007;62(1):120–4.

Optimal Glucose Management in the Perioperative Period

Charity H. Evans, MD, MHCM*, Jane Lee, MD, PhD,
Melissa K. Ruhlman, MD

KEYWORDS

- Blood glucose • Glucose management • Glycemic control • Hyperglycemia
- Hypoglycemia • Perioperative • Surgical • Tight glycemic control

KEY POINTS

- Hyperglycemia, defined as a level of blood glucose (BG) greater than 180 mg/dL, in the perioperative period is associated with poor clinical outcomes; treating hyperglycemia in critically ill patients can lead to decreased morbidity and mortality.
- The gold standard for BG measurement is a venous plasma sample evaluated through the clinical laboratory.
- Intensive insulin therapy, defined as a target treatment BG range of 80 to 110 mg/dL, significantly increases the incidence of hypoglycemia and has not been proven to be beneficial in surgical patients.
- When determining when to treat surgical patients for hyperglycemia and what target BG to achieve, the surgeon must take into account the patient's clinical status, because the evidence has shown optimal benefit at different levels.
- In critically ill and noncritically ill surgical patients, insulin therapy should be used with a goal BG of 140 to 180 mg/dL.

INTRODUCTION

Hyperglycemia is a common finding in patients undergoing surgery. Up to 40% of noncardiac surgery patients have a postoperative level of blood glucose (BG) greater than 140 mg/dL, with 25% of those patients having a level greater than 180 mg/dL.[1] Perioperative hyperglycemia has been associated with increased morbidity, decreased survival, and increased resource utilization.[2–4] For example, McConnell and researchers[5] found a mean 48-hour postoperative glucose greater than

Disclosure Statement: No actual or potential conflict of interest in relation to this review.
Department of Surgery, University of Nebraska Medical Center, 983280 Nebraska Medical Center, Omaha, NE 68198-3280, USA
* Corresponding author.
E-mail address: charity.evans@unmc.edu

Surg Clin N Am 95 (2015) 337–354
http://dx.doi.org/10.1016/j.suc.2014.11.003 surgical.theclinics.com
0039-6109/15/$ – see front matter Published by Elsevier Inc.

200 mg/dL in patients after colorectal surgery was associated with an increased incidence of surgical site infection. Similar associations have been found in patients following total joint arthroplasty, infra-inguinal vascular surgery, orthopedic spinal surgery, hepato-biliary-pancreatic surgery, and mastectomy.[6–10] As a treatable and therefore preventable complication, optimal perioperative glycemic control is quickly becoming standard of care.

Evidence suggesting hyperglycemia is a modifiable and independent predictor of adverse outcomes in surgical patients led to widespread implementation of intensive insulin therapy (IIT) with perioperative BG targets of 80 to 110 mg/dL. However, further investigation into the use of IIT failed to show a survival benefit, leading researchers to question what constitutes "normoglycemia" in the perioperative period. The purpose of this review is to summarize the pertinent research on perioperative glucose management, evaluate the pathophysiology of glucose control and glycemic disturbances, discuss the workup and assessment of preoperative patients, and analyze optimal management strategies.

NATURE OF THE PROBLEM

Hyperglycemia in the critically ill was once viewed as a normal adaptive response to the stress placed on the body by disease. Insulin resistance was thought to be causative factor, because it has been demonstrated in greater than 80% of all critically ill patients.[11] Additional research showed that hyperglycemia is the clinical endpoint of multiple physiologic processes, including increased cortisol, catecholamines, glucagon, growth hormone, gluconeogenesis, and glycogenolysis.[12] Once viewed as an adaptive response essential for survival, hyperglycemia was not routinely monitored or controlled in the perioperative patient.

In the late 1980s, researchers discovered improved cardiac function with glucose-insulin-potassium (GIK) infusion for 48 hours after coronary artery bypass grafting.[13] GIK was found to be safe and effective in the treatment of refractory left ventricular failure after grafting. Early studies involving GIK emphasized the importance of glucose and insulin in surgical patients, but offered little insight to glycemic control. The beneficial effect of GIK on cardiac function was likely due to the metabolic effects of insulin, including the ability to promote the use of glucose as a primary myocardial energy substrate. However, these effects were unrelated to glycemic control because BG was not corrected or controlled.

The adverse outcomes of individuals with diabetes were established in the early 1990s and were thought to be secondary to the direct effect of hyperglycemia on immune function, pathogen growth, and vascular permeability, and the indirect effect via the long-term consequences of hyperglycemia on the microvascular system.[14,15] In critically ill patients in the intensive care unit (ICU), levels of BG greater than 180 mg/dL are associated with impaired neutrophil function, increased infection risk, longer hospital stays, and increased mortality.[3] Further studies showed that IIT with intravenous (IV) insulin to a level of target glucose less than 150 mg/dL reduced the incidence of myocardial infarction (MI) and cerebrovascular accidents (CVA) in diabetics with known atherosclerosis. MI and CVA constituted most of the postoperative complications in diabetics. Therefore, researchers proposed that better glycemic control may improve other perioperative complications in patients with diabetes. Early studies focused on perioperative glycemic control and the risk of infectious complications after coronary artery bypass surgery. Researchers showed that postoperative hyperglycemia is an independent predictor of short-term infectious complications and recommended a glucose target level of less than 200 mg/dL to reduce the risk of infection.[16]

In 2001, Brownlee[17] demonstrated under experimental conditions that concentrations of glucose greater than 300 mg/dL were clearly deleterious, mediated by a hyperglycemia-induced process of overproduction of superoxide by the mitochondrial electron-transport chain. These studies were completed in animals, but provided the only scientific guidance for glycemic targets in humans. A landmark study published by van den Berghe and colleagues in 2001 then changed the long-held beliefs about stress hyperglycemia. In contrast to earlier beliefs that hyperglycemia was just a normal adaptive response to the stress placed on the body by disease, the Leuvin I researchers postulated that elevations in serum glucose contributed to the pathophysiology of critical illness. Leuvin I compared the conventional management in which BG was treated only when greater than 200 mg/dL to IIT regimen targeting a level of BG between 80 and 110 mg/dL. Van den Berghe and colleagues[18] demonstrated a 4% decrease in the mortality of surgical critical care patients randomized to the IIT group. This study included mostly surgical patients, of which 63% underwent a cardiac procedure.

The Leuven II study published in 2006 focused on nonsurgical patients. Similar to the Leuven I study, patients were randomly assigned to strict normalization of BG between 80 and 110 mg/dL with the use of insulin infusion or to conventional therapy, with insulin administered when level of BG exceeded 215 mg/dL, with the infusion tapered when the level decreased to less than 180 mg/dL. This study was unable to show the mortality benefit seen in the Leuven I study because IIT reduced levels of BG but did not significantly reduce mortality.[19] The external validity of the Leuven studies has been questioned and may explain why the results are considered inconclusive. Although inconclusive, the Leuven trials clearly showed that a level of BG higher than 180 mg/dL cannot be considered acceptable. Additional retrospective trials by Krinsley[20] and Finney and colleagues[21] in 2003 and 2004, respectively, found that when BG was controlled less than 150 mg/dL, patients had better outcomes than those with higher levels.

The external validity of the Leuven studies led researchers to question the evidence. In the late 2000s, several large single-center and multicenter prospective trials were completed to further evaluate target BG ranges. All studies to date titrated insulin therapy to maintain a level of BG between 80 and 110 mg/dL in the intervention group. Prior studies, including Leuven I and II, managed the control groups with insulin to a BG range of 180 to 200 mg/dL. In comparison, the NICE-SUGAR and GluControl trials used a control target value of 140 to 180 mg/dL. Review of pertinent trials of tight glucose control by IIT (**Table 1**) revealed no significant difference in primary outcome, specifically mortality, between the 2 groups, with the exception of the Leuven I and NICE-SUGAR studies, in opposite directions. A significant secondary outcome revealed in several studies is tight glucose control by IIT, associated with a 4-fold to 6-fold increase in the incidence of hypoglycemia.[22,23]

Guidelines for perioperative glycemic control are limited by the available evidence. However, when viewed as a whole, the evidence clearly shows that perioperative hyperglycemia is associated with worse outcomes. There is insufficient evidence to support tight glucose control to a target of 80 to 120 mg/dL over conventional glucose control to a target of less than 180 mg/dL in the perioperative period.

PATHOPHYSIOLOGY

Fasting plasma glucose (FPG) is tightly regulated in healthy nondiabetic individuals with levels between 60 and 90 mg/dL and rarely increases to greater than 140 mg/dL in the postprandial period. According to the current guidelines of the American College of

Table 1
Summary of pertinent prospective randomized controlled trials of tight glucose control by intensive insulin therapy

Publish Year	Papers	No of Subjects (Intervention and Control)	Subject Classification	Study Design	Intervention (BG Target, mg/dL)	Control (BG Target, mg/dL)	Primary Outcome Variable	Significant Secondary Outcomes
2001	Van den Berghe, et al. (Leuven I)	765/783	Surgical	Single center, single blind	80–110	180–200	ICU mortality (4% decrease)	Multiorgan failure (decreased)
2006	Van den Berghe, et al. (Leuven II)	595/605	Medical	Single center, single blind	80–110	180–200	ICU mortality (no significant change)	Acute kidney injury (decreased)
2008	Arabi	266/257	Medical (~80%) Surgical (~20%)	Single center, single blind	80–110	180–200	ICU mortality (no significant change, increased hypoglycemia)	Hypoglycemic episodes (increased)
2008	De La Rosa	254/250	Medical (~50%) Surgical (~50%)	Single center, single blind	80–110	180–200	28-d mortality (no significant change)	Hypoglycemic episodes (increased)
2009	Brunkhorst, et al. (VISEP)	247/289	Medical (46.9%) Surgical (52.9%)	Multicenter, single blind	80–110	180–200	28-d mortality (no significant change)	Hypoglycemic episodes (increased)
2009	Finfer, et al. (NICE-SUGAR)	3054/3050	Medical (~63%) Surgical (~37%)	Multicenter, single blind	80–110	140–180	90-d mortality (increased in intervention group)	Hypoglycemic episodes (increased)
2009	Preiser, et al. (GluControl)	542/536	Medical (~42%) Surgical (~58%)	Multicenter, single blind	80–110	140–180	ICU mortality (lack of benefit in intervention group)	Hypoglycemic episodes (increased)

Data from Refs.[18,19,22,23,64–66]

Endocrinology and the American Diabetes Association, individuals with FPG levels greater than 126 mg/dL or hemoglobin A1c greater than 5.7% have diabetes mellitus (DM).[24] The aforementioned studies identified these individuals as having increased incidence of operative complications, thus leading to the concept that tight glucose control during the perioperative period in both healthy and diabetic patients may lead to improved outcomes. However, it became evident that understanding the pathophysiology of the disease was required to develop a comprehensive perioperative glucose control model.

The principal organs involved in glucose control include the brain, pancreas, muscle, adipose tissue, liver, and kidneys.[25] The interactions between these organs have been elucidated as outlined in **Fig. 1**, but the understanding is far from complete. Insulin mediates glucose control by regulating the transport of glucose into cells either by facilitated diffusion or by active transport. Glucose transport is facilitated by specific glucose transporters, which include GLUT 1–12, H^+/myoinositol transporter, and sodium-dependent glucose cotransporter 1–6.[26] Activation of the insulin receptor is the rate-limiting step in moving glucose out of the serum into the cells to maintain FPG levels; therefore, both insulin level regulation and insulin receptor sensitivity are involved in maintaining glucose homeostasis.

Insulin is secreted from β-cells in the pancreatic islets of Langerhans, with a half-life of 4 to 6 minutes. Basal rate of 0.5 to 0.7 U/h is secreted constitutively and increases acutely with increased levels of glucose. Glucose levels are detected by pancreatic cells via binding of glucose with GLUT2.[27] The secretion of insulin is directly modulated by other hormones, including those from the pancreas (glucagon, somatostatin,

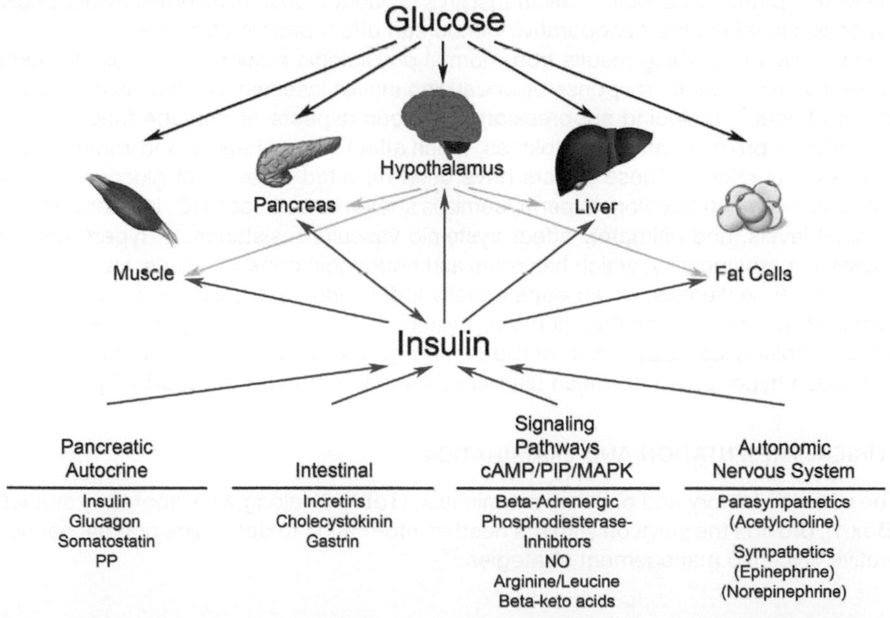

Fig. 1. Modulation of the secretion of insulin. Interactions between glucose, insulin, and multiple organ systems. Glucose had direct effects on various systems through glucose-specific receptors (*black arrows*). Multiple organ systems communicate with each other through their neural pathways (*gray arrows*). Insulin release is activated by both glucose and various other mechanisms as summarized in the figure (*red arrows*). cAMP, cyclic adenosine monophosphate; PIP, phosphatidylinositol phosphate; NO, nitric oxide; PP, pancreatic polypeptide.

and pancreatic polypeptide) and intestine (incretins), as depicted in **Fig. 1**.[28] Indirect modulation occurs through other hormones that promote islet cells neogenesis (cholecystokinin and gastrin) and growth factors (insulin-like growth factor-1 and insulin-like growth factor-2). Other factors that increase insulin release are those that activate cytosolic cyclin adenosine monophosphate, which results in increases in intracellular calcium levels, such as nitric oxide (NO), arginine, leucine, and β-keto acids. Increases in intracellular calcium can also affect parasympathetic signaling pathways, such as those activated by acetylcholine. Conversely, sympathetic pathways mediated by catecholamines decrease insulin levels.[29] The physiology of insulin regulation brings light to how operative stress and various agents used in the perioperative period can influence glucose levels.

Insulin affects glucose transport via binding of Insulin Receptor (IR) in organ systems involved in glucose regulation, and IRs present other organ systems through activation of downstream signaling pathways, which can be loosely categorized as proliferative (mitogenic) and metabolic. These pathways are not mutually exclusive and many times synergistic. IRs are present on cells involved in hemostasis and inflammation, which activate the proliferative pathways through mitogen-activated protein kinase (MAPK).[30] These pathways affect the immune system by suppressing proinflammatory transcription factors and endotoxin-mediated inflammatory mediators. Metabolic pathways are activated by phosphatidylinositol-3 kinase, which affects growth, adaptation to fasting and feeding, and response to stress.[31] In addition, PI3 kinase increases NO production,[32] which affects both platelets and endothelium and decreases expression of several factors that ultimately highlight insulin's antioxidant, antithrombotic, and antifibrinolytic properties, all of which are also affected through the MAPK pathway as well.[33] Given insulin's broad actions, it becomes evident how hyperinsulinemia in the perioperative period can affect patient outcomes.

Hyperglycemia, which results from normal physiologic response to stress through actions of sympathetic response or underlying insulin insensitively, has its own pathologic effects,[12] including suppression of various aspects of immune function and activation of proinflammatory cytokines, which affect wound healing and immunologic defensive function.[34] These effects have been reported in levels of glucose greater than 200 mg/dL. In addition, hyperglycemia is known to decrease NO, increase angiotensin II levels, and ultimately affect systemic vascular resistance.[35] Hyperglycemia causes hyperosmolality, which has renal and neurologic consequences. Hyperosmolality can cause dieresis, which leads to dehydration and electrolyte and acid-base imbalances as well as central nervous system dysfunction.[36] Rapid correction of hyperosmolality can cause cerebral edema. **Fig. 2** depicts how perioperative injury can cause hyperglycemia, which ultimately leads to mortality and morbidity.

CLINICAL PRESENTATION AND EXAMINATION

The patient's history and physical examination (**Table 2**), along with laboratory studies (**Box 1**), provide the surgeon with the needed information to determine optimal perioperative glycemic management strategies.[24]

DIAGNOSTIC PROCEDURES

Determining the best modality for evaluating BG in the perioperative period requires knowledge of the advantages and disadvantages of each. A variety of options are available for testing including hemoglobin A1c, point-of-care (POC) testing, arterial, venous, capillary, and plasma blood sampling, and continuous glucose monitoring.

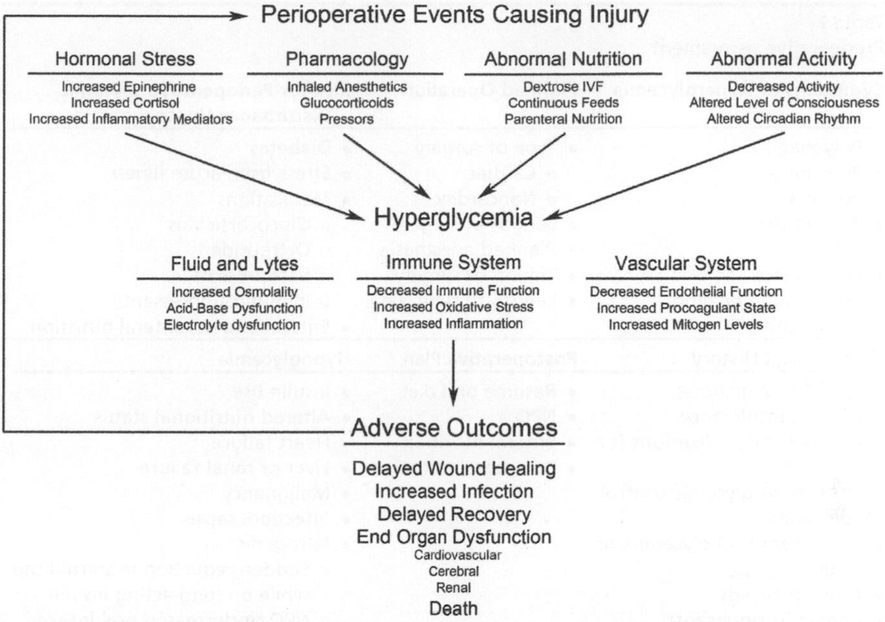

Fig. 2. Influence of perioperative events on hyperglycemia. Perioperative stress-related hyperglycemia may start a downward spiral resulting in significant morbidity and mortality. Perioperative stressors cause hyperglycemia, which activates mechanisms that result in adverse outcomes. Often these adverse outcomes worsen the same perioperative stressors or activate other perioperative stressors, which compounds itself, resulting in further injury and, if not controlled, eventually resulting in death. IVF, intravenous fluid.

The terms blood glucose and plasma glucose, although at times used interchangeably, can have significant variability. Plasma glucose is typically 10% to 15% higher than whole BG due to higher water concentration in plasma (93%) compared with erythrocytes (73%). Plasma glucose is a more physiologic measurement because whole BG can vary significantly with the hematocrit.[37,38] The American Diabetes Association and World Health Organization recommend the use of venous plasma glucose for measuring and reporting BG. Capillary glucose is the most imprecise measurement of BG, mostly because of the type and accuracy of devices used for measuring. The difference between venous and capillary glucose is typically small in fasting patients without major physiologic derangements. The difference in glucose values between these 2 measurements has been shown to be up to 8% higher in capillary blood after meals or glucose load. Capillary glucose also tends to underestimate whole BG in situations with poor peripheral perfusion or increased tissue extraction of glucose.[37,38] Classically, in the operating room, whole BG evaluation is obtained in conjunction with an arterial blood gas. Arterial BG is accepted to be more accurate than capillary glucose but has been shown in some cases to provide higher glucose values than either venous or capillary samples.[37]

POC devices are readily available and quick and require a minimal sample size. POC devices typically measure whole BG but most self-correct internally and report results as plasma glucose.[37] Although these devices are useful, the rapid physiologic changes that occur in the operating room and in the postoperative patient may lead to significantly less accurate results. Factors such as hemoglobin, temperature changes, fluid shifts, and hypotension can all affect the accuracy of the rapid-acting

Table 2
Preoperative assessment

Symptoms of Hyperglycemia	Planned Operation	Risk for Perioperative Glycemic Disturbance Hyperglycemia

• Polyphagia
• Polydipsia
• Polyuria
• Blurred vision
• Fatigue
• Weight loss
• Poor wound healing
• Dry mouth
	• Type of surgery
	  ○ Cardiac
	  ○ Noncardiac
	• Length of surgery
	• Planned anesthesia
	• Timing of surgery
	• Length of time NPO
		• Diabetes
		• Stress from acute illness
		• Medications
		  ○ Glucocorticoids
		  ○ Octreotide
		  ○ Vasopressors
		  ○ Immunosuppressants
		• Enteral and parenteral nutrition

Past Medical History	**Postoperative Plan**	**Hypoglycemia**

• Type 1 or 2 diabetes
• Glucose intolerance
• Previous hospitalizations for diabetes
• Outpatient glycemic control
Medications
• Outpatient oral glycemics or insulin
• Glucocorticoids
• Immunosuppressants
	• Resume oral diet
	• NPO
	• Enteral nutrition
	• Parenteral nutrition
		• Insulin use
		• Altered nutritional status
		• Heart failure
		• Liver or renal failure
		• Malignancy
		• Infection, sepsis
		• Iatrogenic
		  ○ Sudden reduction in steroid use while on long-acting insulin
		  ○ NPO or decreased oral intake
		  ○ Inappropriate timing of insulin administration
		  ○ Decreased dextrose administration
		• Interruptions in enteral or parenteral nutrition

POC machines. It appears that these inaccuracies are more pronounced in the hypoglycemic range, with up to 20% variation in either direction, and in the anemic patient, with inaccuracies up to 30%. These wide variations can lead to alterations in clinical decision-making and potentially cause adverse outcomes in patient care. Clinical laboratory measurements using arterial or venous samples are much more accurate than POC meters and should be used whenever possible.[37,39] Hemoglobin A1c, or glycated hemoglobin, is a marker of long-term glucose control. A preoperative hemoglobin A1c less than 7% confers good long-term glucose control and has been associated with decreased risk of infectious complications.[40]

Continuous glucose monitoring devices can be used to obtain real-time BG analysis and allow for closer monitoring and for prevention of the deleterious effects associated with hypoglycemia. These devices can be quite accurate but require frequent calibration. This type of device might prove beneficial in a diabetic patient undergoing a long, complicated, or high-risk procedure in which frequent and accurate glucose monitoring is required.[40]

As an alternative to blood sampling, subcutaneous sensors for continuous monitoring are available and have been found to correlate with BG values. These devices may not have the needed accuracy for routine use in an acute care setting such as with surgical patients. Ellmerer and researchers[41] found good correlation of blood and subcutaneous glucose measurements in ICU postcardiac surgery patients using a subcutaneous sensor.These devices require frequent calibrations with the patient's blood, which may limit the benefit of the device.[40]

Box 1
Preoperative laboratory studies

Patient with known diabetes

- Hemoglobin A1C (HgA1C)
- Fasting level of BG

Patient without diabetes

- Based on risk factors
- Hemoglobin A1C (HgA1C)
- Fasting level of BG *IF*
  - Adults with BP greater than 135/80 mm Hg
  - Adults with body mass index greater than or equal to 25 kg/m^2 *AND*
    - Physical inactivity
    - First-degree relative with diabetes
    - High-risk ethnicity
    - History of gestational diabetes or delivery of baby greater than 9 lbs (4.1 kg)
    - Hypertension
    - HDL less than 35 mg/dL or triglycerides greater than 250 mg/dL
    - History of polycystic ovarian syndrome
    - History of cardiovascular disease
    - History of impaired glucose tolerance or impaired fasting glucose

MANAGEMENT

Insulin is used in the management of perioperative hyperglycemia. Insulin requirements are determined by the balance between endogenous insulin secretion and insulin resistance. Exogenous insulin comes in several forms, typically classified as short and fast-acting, or long and slow-acting, based on the time to onset, peak activity, and duration of action of each. The time to onset, peak activity, and duration of action can only be approximated, because the degree of absorption of any dose can vary as much as 25% to 50%, leading to fluctuation in glucose control.[42,43] **Fig. 3** displays the properties of different types of insulin. The intermediate to long-acting preparations are used as a basal supplement, suppressing hepatic glucose production and maintaining normal levels of BG in the fasting state. Short-acting bolus doses of insulin are used to cover extra insulin requirements. In critically ill patients, the short-acting insulins allow the patient to reach goal BG ranges in the shortest duration of time and allows for rapid changes in doses given its short half-life.

Exogenous insulin can be delivered as a bolus, premeal or prandial, correctional, basal, or basal-bolus dose. The decision of the type of insulin dose to administer is based on the patient's basal insulin requirements, degree of hyperglycemia, level of perioperative stress, and clinical status. A description of each is provided in **Table 3**.

Exogenous insulin can be administered subcutaneously or intravenously, each with its own advantages and disadvantages (**Table 4**).

Although most surgeons agree that glycemic control is required in the perioperative period, the optimal BG range remains controversial. Review of the evidence provides surgeons with recommendations based on the clinical status of the patient, as

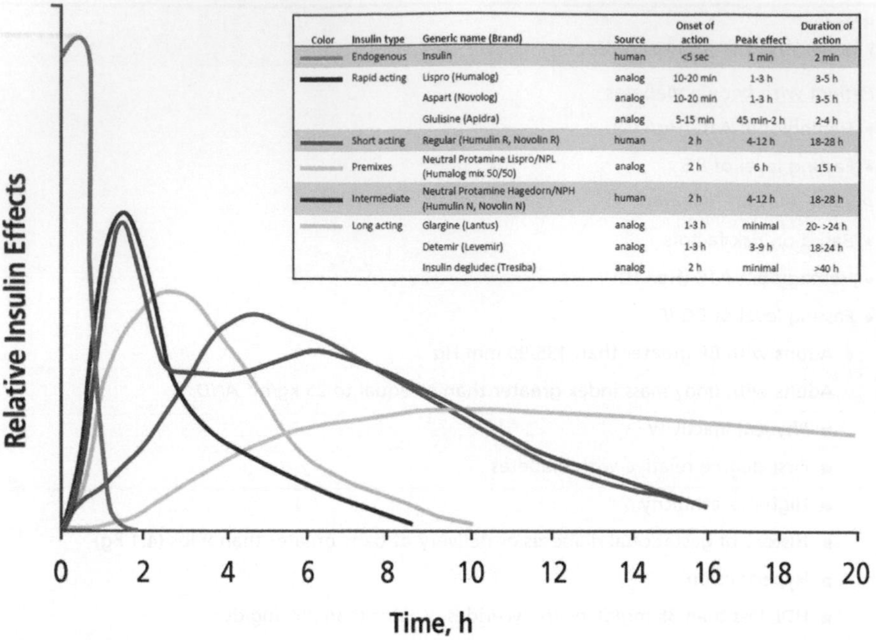

Color	Insulin type	Generic name (Brand)	Source	Onset of action	Peak effect	Duration of action
	Endogenous	Insulin	human	<5 sec	1 min	2 min
	Rapid acting	Lispro (Humalog)	analog	10-20 min	1-3 h	3-5 h
		Aspart (Novolog)	analog	10-20 min	1-3 h	3-5 h
		Glulisine (Apidra)	analog	5-15 min	45 min-2 h	2-4 h
	Short acting	Regular (Humulin R, Novolin R)	human	2 h	4-12 h	18-28 h
	Premixes	Neutral Protamine Lispro/NPL (Humalog mix 50/50)	analog	2 h	6 h	15 h
	Intermediate	Neutral Protamine Hagedorn/NPH (Humulin N, Novolin N)	human	2 h	4-12 h	18-28 h
	Long acting	Glargine (Lantus)	analog	1-3 h	minimal	20- >24 h
		Detemir (Levemir)	analog	1-3 h	3-9 h	18-24 h
		Insulin degludec (Tresiba)	analog	2 h	minimal	>40 h

Fig. 3. Insulin action guideline. There are several categories of insulin that vary in time of onset and duration. Shorter-acting insulin is used in acute insulin control, such as after meals. Intermediate-acting and long-acting insulin is used to provide baseline insulin levels. Intermediate dosing is dosed several times during the day, whereas long-acting insulin is dosed once daily. Combination insulin is used for immediate action as well as providing baseline levels of insulin.

summarized in **Fig. 4** and **Box 2**. The proposed insulin infusion protocol presented in **Fig. 4** is a modified version of the protocol recommended by Goldberg and colleagues.[44]

Once the perioperative patient on IV insulin is more stable, the prehospital insulin regimen can be resumed, assuming that it was optimal in achieving glycemic targets. Because of the short half-life of IV regular insulin, the first dose of subcutaneous (SQ) insulin must be given before discontinuation of the IV insulin infusion. If intermediate-acting or long-acting insulin is used, it should be given 2 to 3 hours before stopping the infusion, whereas short-acting or rapid-acting insulin should be given 1 to 2 hours before discontinuation.

SPECIAL POPULATIONS

The concept of perioperative glycemic control was born in the research of special populations, including patients undergoing cardiovascular surgery, pediatric population, trauma patients, patients with traumatic brain injury (TBI), and patients on steroids. The evidence and recommendations vary from the management of the critically ill and noncritically ill patients, and therefore, warrant special attention.

Cardiovascular

The very concept of intense glucose control in the critically ill was first studied in cardiac patients.[18] Since this landmark article by Van den Berghe about the benefit of IIT,[45] the debate has centered on who may benefit from glucose control and to

Table 3
Types of insulin doses

Bolus	Basal
• Commonly used for noncritical patients with or without DM • Short-acting (regular) or rapid-acting (lispro, aspart, or glulisine) insulin • Typically provided as a premeal bolus to cover the extra requirements after food is absorbed • Does not provide patient with basal level of insulin • Or as a "sliding scale" titrated to level of BG • Little data to support its benefit and some evidence of potential harm when the "sliding scale" is applied in a rote fashion (Queale)	• Intermediate- to long-acting preparations (neutral protamine hagedron; neutral protamine lispro, detemir, or glargine) • Typically administered once or twice daily to provide basal insulin levels to suppress hepatic glucose production and maintain near normoglycemia in the fasting state • Provides patient with basal level of insulin • Basal insulin levels can also be achieved by continuous infusion of a short-acting or rapid-acting insulin via an insulin pump, used almost exclusively in type 1 diabetes
Correctional	**Basal-bolus**
• Additional doses of short-acting or rapid-acting insulin • Given premeal to patients on basal-bolus regimens to correct premeal hyperglycemia • Dose of correction insulin should be based on patient characteristics such as previous level of glucose control, prior insulin requirements, and, if possible, the carbohydrate content of meals	• Combination of short-acting and long-acting insulins, given separately (not premixed) • Increasing use for inpatient hyperglycemia in the noncritically ill patient (Umpierrez)

Data from Queale WS, Seidler AJ, Brancati FL. Glycemic control and sliding scale insulin use in medical inpatients with diabetes mellitus. Arch Intern Med 1997;157(5):545–52; and Umpierrez GE, Smiley D, Hermayer K, et al. Randomized study comparing a Basal-bolus with a basal plus correction insulin regimen for the hospital management of medical and surgical patients with type 2 diabetes: basal plus trial. Diabetes Care 2013;36(8):2169–74.

Table 4
Comparison of subcutaneous and intravenous delivery of insulin

SQ Delivery of Insulin	IV Delivery of Insulin
• Most noncritically ill patients with or without DM can be treated with SQ insulin • Little data showing that IV insulin is superior to SQ insulin in the noncritically ill patient • Injection sites include upper arms, abdominal wall, upper legs, and buttocks • Injection sites should be rotated • Insulin is absorbed more rapidly when injected into the abdomen than the arms or legs • The variability in absorption is increased and net absorption is reduced with increasing size of the subcutaneous depot	• Any patient with BG >180 mg/dL should be managed with IV insulin • Patients with type 1 DM, especially those undergoing a long surgery, also should be treated with IV insulin • Changes of IV dose have a more immediate effect compared with SQ therapy • Little data showing that IV insulin is superior to SQ insulin in the noncritically ill patient • The best IV insulin protocols take into account not only the prevailing BG but also its rate of change and the current insulin requirements

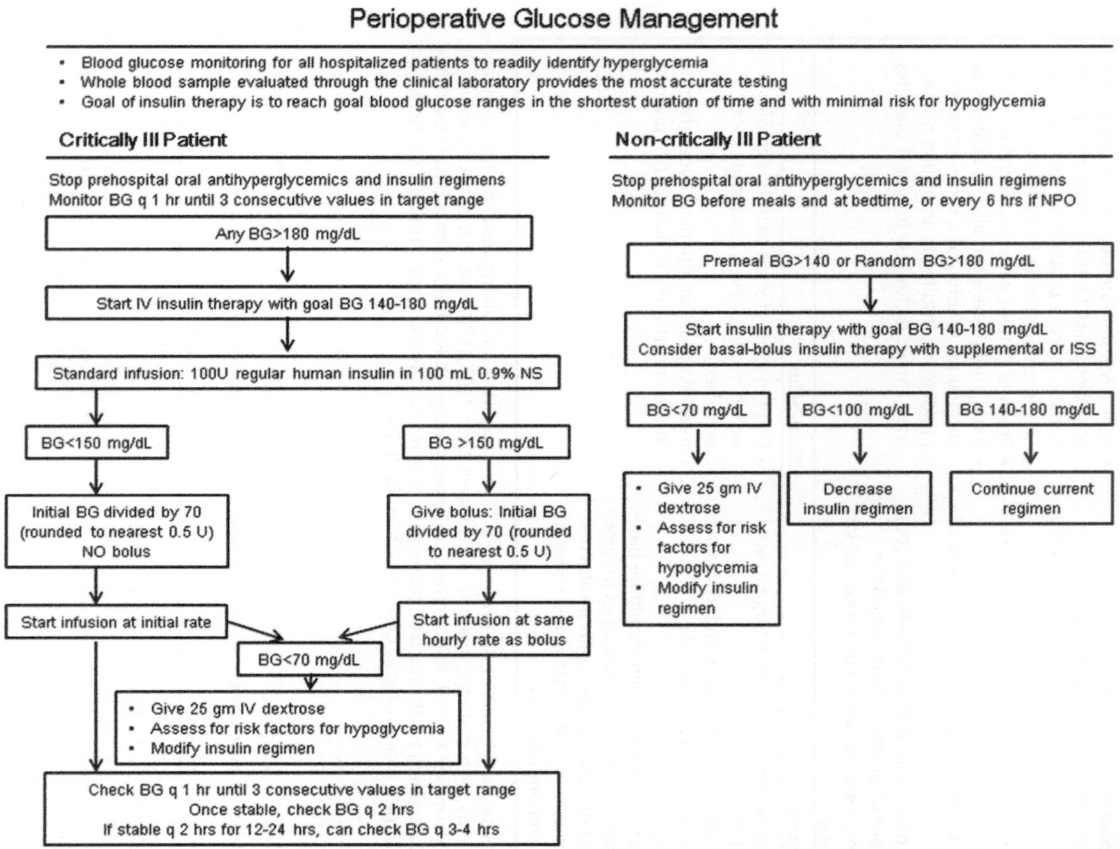

Fig. 4. Recommendations for perioperative glucose management. ISS, insulin sliding scale; NS, normal saline; NPO, nothing by mouth. (*Adapted from* Goldberg PA, Siegel MD, Sherwin RS, et al. Implementation of a safe and effective insulin-infusion protocol in a medical intensive care unit. Diabetes Care 2004;27:461–7.)

Box 2
Indications for intravenous insulin therapy

- Type 1 diabetics who are instructed as nothing by mouth (NPO), perioperative, or in labor and delivery
- Any ICU patient with BG greater than 180 mg/dL
- Poorly controlled hyperglycemia despite subcutaneous insulin therapy
- Patients with known diabetes status postcardiac surgery
- Patients with acute coronary syndrome or acute MI with BG greater than 180 mg/dL
- Patients with diabetic ketoacidosis or hyperosmolar hyperglycemic syndromes

what degree of glucose control is required for the benefits to outweigh the risks of hypoglycemia, also an independent risk factor for poor outcomes.[46] Hyperglycemia is postulated to be cardiotoxic because of its direct effects on the myocardium membranes and mitochondria,[47] and its indirect effects via activation of proinflammatory mediators.[48] Contrary to the seminal article on this topic, studies in both neonatal and adult cardiac surgery patients revealed that IIT contributes to severe hypoglycemia, and moderately intense glucose control has demonstrated no difference in outcome compared with IIT. Currently, the Society of Thoracic Surgeons advocate a target range of 120 to 180 mg/dL for patients undergoing cardiac bypass surgery.[49]

Pediatric

Neonates, infants, and young children less than 8 years of age have a higher incidence of hypoglycemia because of poor glycogen stores in their liver and their intrinsic higher metabolism. In pediatric trauma patients, early administration of glucose-containing solutions in the form of D5 or D10 is recommended after initial resuscitation.[50] However, it is also known that hyperglycemia is associated with poor neurologic outcomes in the pediatric traumatic head-injury patients. In addition, in infants on pressor support with necrotizing enterocolitis, hyperglycemia is associated with longer lengths of stay and increased rates of death.[51] The studies that showed improved outcomes of IIT in cardiac surgery patients spurred investigations in glucose control in neonatal and infant cardiac surgery patients, which showed similar findings.[52] Researchers then focused on perioperative glucose control in the pediatric population. Several studies showed the danger of hypoglycemia in normal healthy infants and children is rare and dextrose-containing fluids should be avoided perioperatively.[53] However, neonates and patients on parenteral or continuous enteral feeds should not be categorized as normal, and administration of dextrose solution would be appropriate. D5 solutions should be avoided, but 1% to 2% dextrose solutions in normal saline or lactated Ringer is recommended at an infusion rate of 120 to 300 mg/kg/h to maintain adequate levels of glucose and to avoid lipid metabolism.[54]

Trauma

Hyperglycemia is a normal metabolic response to stress and trauma due to activation of the sympathetic nervous system. Studies showed that hyperglycemia in trauma patients is more strongly associated with poor outcomes than sick patients in the ICU.[55,56] Despite these associations, trauma patients account for only a small percentage of patients addressed in studies of critically ill patients and IIT.[57] Theoretically, critically ill trauma patients can be treated as ICU patients; yet hyperglycemia in the noncritically ill trauma patient is largely uninvestigated at this time. At the authors' institution, glucose monitoring is initiated on admission of all trauma patients regardless of diabetes or level of care status and is discontinued if levels of glucose remain within institutionally acceptable levels for 48 hours. This practice is based on the empiric knowledge of the literature and has yet to be shown to decrease mortality or morbidity in all trauma patients.

Neurologically Critical Ill Patients

The brain is one of few organ systems that exclusively use glucose as an energy source. Hypoglycemia is detrimental to critically ill neurologic patients, including those who suffered TBIs. Furthermore, in congruency with the studies of critical ill patients, hyperglycemia defined as greater than 200 mg/dL has also been linked to higher mortality and worse outcomes in these patients.[58,59] Similarly, tight glucose control had been shown to not improve neurologic outcome while increasing the risk of hypoglycemia. In fact, a large body of evidence is available that shows that tight glucose control causes reduced cerebral extracellular glucose and increased incidence of brain energy crisis.[60] A microdialysis study of severe brain injury cohort demonstrated that systemic levels of glucose closely reflects to levels in the cerebrospinal fluid and, furthermore, hypoglycemia in the brain was detected even in systemic levels of glucose in the intermediate range.[61] Given that the traumatized brain has several metabolic changes including dysfunction of glucose transport mechanism, probable increased metabolic needs, and mitochondrial dysfunction, hypoglycemia defined as less than 80 mg/dL has been associated with brain energy crisis and poor outcomes, leading to the assumption that glucose control range in TBI is somewhere between 80 and 200 mg/dL. Further studies on the subject will eventually elucidate BG goals in TBI.[58]

Steroids

Steroids are used perioperatively as a prophylaxis for nausea, stress steroids for patients with adrenal insufficiency, and an induction agent before organ transplantation. Steroids are released when the sympathetic nervous system is activated to mobilize energy reserves during stressful states. Incidentally, steroid boluses and drips are used as an adjunct to pressors during septic shock.[62] However, steroids can also induce hyperglycemia and insulin intolerance. Intraoperatively, steroid use has not been shown to significantly affect levels of BG and outcomes.[63] Hence, denying steroids for indicated perioperative uses for fear of hyperglycemia appears to be unsubstantiated that this time.

SUMMARY

Hyperglycemia, defined as any level of BG greater than 140 mg/dL in the hospital setting, is a common finding in surgical patients during the perioperative period. Factors contributing to poor glycemic control include counterregulatory hormones, insulin resistance, decreased glucose uptake, immune suppression, activation of proinflammatory cytokines, use of dextrose-containing IV fluids and enteral and parenteral nutrition. Hyperglycemia in the perioperative period is associated with increased morbidity, decreased survival, and increased resource utilization. Optimal glucose management in the perioperative period contributes to reduced morbidity and mortality. To readily identify hyperglycemia, BG monitoring should be instituted for all hospitalized patients. The gold standard for BG measurement is a venous plasma sample evaluated through the clinical laboratory. When determining when to treat surgical patients for hyperglycemia and what target BG to achieve, the surgeon must take into account the patient's clinical status, because the evidence has shown optimal benefit at different levels. IIT, defined as target treatment BG in the range of 80 to 110 mg/dL, significantly increases the incidence of hypoglycemia and has not been proven to be beneficial in surgical patients. In critically ill and noncritically ill surgical patients, insulin therapy should be used with a goal BG of 140 to 180 mg/dL. The avoidance of hypoglycemia, specifically in TBI and pediatrics, has been shown to be as significant as treating hyperglycemia. Therefore, treatment protocols must allow a margin of error when targeting the optimal BG range.

REFERENCES

1. Frisch A, Chandra P, Smiley D, et al. Prevalence and clinical outcome of hyperglycemia in the perioperative period in noncardiac surgery. Diabetes Care 2011;33:1783–8.
2. Yang W, Dall TM, Halder P, et al. Economic costs of diabetes in the U.S. in 2012. Diabetes Care 2013;36(4):1033–46.
3. Moghissi ES, Korytkowski MT, DiNardo M, et al. American Association of Clinical Endocrinologists and American Diabetes Association consensus statement on inpatient glycemic control. Diabetes Care 2009;32(6):1119–31.
4. Umpierrez GE, Isaacs SD, Bazargan N, et al. Hyperglycemia: an independent marker of in-hospital mortality in patients with undiagnosed diabetes. J Clin Endocrinol Metab 2002;87(3):978–82.
5. McConnell YJ, Johnson PM, Porter GA. Surgical site infections following colorectal surgery in patients with diabetes: association with postoperative hyperglycemia. J Gastrointest Surg 2009;3:508–15.
6. Marchant HM Jr, Viens NA, Cook C, et al. The impact of glycemic control and diabetes mellitus on perioperative outcomes after total joint arthroplasty. J Bone Joint Surg Am 2009;91(7):1621–9.
7. Malmstedt J, Wahlberg E, Jorneskog G, et al. Influence of perioperative blood glucose levels on outcome after infrainguinal bypass surgery in patients with diabetes. Br J Surg 2006;93(11):1360–7.
8. Olsen MA, Nepple JJ, Riew KD, et al. Risk factors for surgical site infection following orthopaedic spinal operations. J Bone Joint Surg Am 2008;90(1):62–9.
9. Ambiru S, Kato A, Kimura F, et al. Poor postoperative blood glucose control increases surgical site infections after surgery for hepato-biliary-pancreatic cancer: a prospective study in a high-volume institution in Japan. J Hosp Infect 2008; 68(3):230–3.
10. Vilar-Compte D, Alvarez de Iturbe I, Martin-Onraet A, et al. Hyperglycemia as a risk factor for surgical site infections in patients undergoing mastectomy. Am J Infect Control 2008;36(3):192–8.
11. Saberi F, Heyland D, Lam M, et al. Prevalence, incidence, and clinical resolution of insulin resistance in critically ill patients: an observational study. JPEN J Parenter Enteral Nutr 2008;32:227–35.
12. McCowen KC, Malhotra A, Bistrian BR. Stress-induced hyperglycemia. Crit Care Clin 2001;17(1):107–24.
13. Gradinac S, Coleman GM, Taegtmeyer H, et al. Improved cardiac function with glucose-insulin-potassium after aortocoronary bypass grafting. Ann Thorac Surg 1989;48(4):484–9.
14. Pozzilli P, Leslie R. Infections and diabetes: mechanism and prospects for prevention. Diabet Med 1994;11:935–41.

15. Currie B, Casey J. Host defense and infections in diabetes mellitus. In: Porte D Jr, Sherwin R, editors. Ellenburg and Rifkin's diabetes mellitus. 5th edition. Stamford (CT): Appleton and Lange; 1997. p. 861–74.
16. Golden SH, Peart-Vigilance C, Kao WH, et al. Perioperative glycemic control and the risk of infectious complications in a cohort of adults with diabetes. Diabetes Care 1999;22(9):1408–14.
17. Brownlee M. Biochemistry and molecular cell biology of diabetic complications. Nature 2001;414:813–20.
18. Van de Berghe G, Wouters P, Weekers F, et al. Intensive insulin therapy in critically ill patients. N Engl J Med 2001;345(19):1359–67.
19. Van den Berghe G, Wilmer A, Hermans G, et al. Intensive insulin therapy in the medical ICU. N Engl J Med 2006;354(5):449–61.
20. Krinsley JS. Effect of an intensive glucose management protocol on the mortality of critically ill adult patients. Mayo Clin Proc 2004;79(8):992–1000.
21. Finney SJ, Zekveld C, Elia A, et al. Glucose control and mortality in critically ill patients. JAMA 2003;290(15):2041–7.
22. Finfer S, Chittock DR, Su SY, et al, NICE-SUGAR Study Investigators. Intensive versus conventional glucose control in critically ill patients. N Engl J Med 2009; 360(13):1283–97.
23. Preiser JC, Devos P, Ruiz-Santana S, et al. A prospective randomized muli-centre controlled trial on tight glucose control by intensive insulin therapy in adult intensive care units: the Glucontrol study. Intensive Care Med 2009;35(10):1738–48.
24. Garber AJ, Abrahamson MJ, Barzilay JI, et al, American Association of Clinical Endocrinologists. AACE comprehensive diabetes management algorithm 2013. Endocr Pract 2013;19(2):327–36.
25. Herman M, Kahn B. Glucose transport and sensing in the maintenance of glucose homeostasis and metabolic harmony. J Clin Invest 2006;116(7):1767–75.
26. Zhao FQ, Keating A. Functional properties and genomics of glucose transporters. Curr Genomics 2007;8(2):113–28.
27. Thorens B. GLUT2 in pancreatic and extra-pancreatic gluco-detection. Mol Membr Biol 2001;18(4):265–73.
28. Rorsman P, Braun M. Regulation of insulin secretion in human pancreatic islets. Annu Rev Physiol 2012;75:155–79.
29. Thorens B. Brain glucose sensing and neural regulation of insulin and glucagon secretion. Diabetes Obes Metab 2011;13:82–8.
30. Chang L, Chiang S, Saltiel A. Insulin signaling and the regulation of glucose transport. Mol Med 2004;10(7–12):65–71.
31. Herlaar E, Brown Z. p38 MAPK signalling cascades in inflammatory disease. Trends Mol Med 1999;5(10):439–47.
32. Morello F, Perino A, Hirsch E. Phosphoinositide 3-kinase signaling in the vascular system. Cardiovasc Res 2009;82(2):261–71.
33. Kim J, Montagnani M, Koh KK, et al. Reciprocal relationships between insulin resistance and endothelial dysfunction: molecular and pathophysiological mechanisms. Circulation 2006;113(15):1888–904.
34. Alexandraki K, Piperi C, Kalofoutis C, et al. Inflammatory process in type 2 diabetes. Ann N Y Acad Sci 2006;1084(1):89–117.
35. Hamed S, Brenner B, Roguin A. Nitric oxide: a key factor behind the dysfunctionality of endothelial progenitor cells in diabetes mellitus type-2. Cardiovasc Res 2011;91(1):9–15.
36. Steenkamp DW, Alexanian SM, McDonnell ME. Adult hyperglycemic crisis: a review and perspective. Curr Diab Rep 2013;13(1):130–7.

37. Pitkin AD, Rice MJ. Challenges to glycemic measurement in the perioperative and critically ill patient. J Diabetes Sci Technol 2009;3(6):1270–81.
38. Carstensen B, Lindstrom J, Sundvall J, et al. Measurement of blood glucose: comparison between different types of specimens. Ann Clin Biochem 2008;45:140–8.
39. Mraovic B, Schwenk ES, Epstein RH. Intraoperative accuracy of a point-of-care glucose meter compared with simultaneous central laboratory measurements. J Diabetes Sci Technol 2012;6(3):541–6.
40. Raju TA, Torjman MC, Goldberg ME. Perioperative blood glucose monitoring in the general surgical population. J Diabetes Sci Technol 2009;3(6):1282–7.
41. Ellmerer M, Haluzik M, Blaha J, et al. Clinical evaluation of alternative-site glucose measurements in patients after major cardiac surgery. Diabetes Care 2006;29(6): 1275–81.
42. Binder C, Lauritzen T, Faber O, et al. Insulin pharmacokinetics. Diabetes Care 1984;7:188.
43. Sindelka G, Heinemann L, Berger M, et al. Effect of insulin concentration, subcutaneous fat thickness and skin temperature on subcutaneous insulin absorption in healthy subjects. Diabetologia 1994;37:377.
44. Goldberg PA, Siegel MD, Sherwin RS, et al. Implementation of a safe and effective insulin-infusion protocol in a medical intensive care unit. Diabetes Care 2004; 27:461–7.
45. Van den Berghe G. Intensive insulin therapy to maintain normoglycemia after cardiac surgery. Proc Intensive Care Cardiovasc Anesth 2011;3(2):97–101.
46. D'Ancona G, Bertuzzi F, Sacchi L, et al. Iatrogenic hypoglycemia secondary to tight glucose control is an independent determinant for mortality and cardiac morbidity. Eur J Cardiothorac Surg 2011;40(2):360–6.
47. Cai L, Li W, Wang G, et al. Hyperglycemia-induced apoptosis in mouse myocardium: mitochondrial cytochrome c–mediated caspase-3 activation pathway. Diabetes 2002;51(6):1938–48.
48. Ansley DM, Wang B. Oxidative stress and myocardial injury in the diabetic heart. J Pathol 2013;229(2):232–41.
49. Leibowitz G, Raizman E, Brezis M, et al. Effects of moderate intensity glycemic control after cardiac surgery. Ann Thorac Surg 2010;90(6):1825–32.
50. Spinella P, Martin J, Azarow KS. Pediatric trauma. In: Savitsky E, Eastridge B, editors. Combat casualty care: lessons learned from OEF and OIF. Fort Detrick (MD): Office of the Surgeon General & Borden Institute; 2012. p. 533–91.
51. Wintergerst KA, Buckingham B, Gandrud L, et al. Association of hypoglycemia, hyperglycemia, and glucose variability with morbidity and death in the pediatric intensive care unit. Pediatrics 2006;118(1):173–9.
52. Polito A, Thiagarajan RR, Laussen PC, et al. Association between intraoperative and early postoperative glucose levels and adverse outcomes after complex congenital heart surgery. Circulation 2008;118(22):2235–42.
53. Murat I, Dubois M. Perioperative fluid therapy in pediatrics. Pediatr Anesth 2008; 18:363–70.
54. Culpepper TL. AANA Journal course: update for nurse anesthetists–intraoperative fluid management for the pediatric surgical patient. AANA J 2000;68(6):531–8.
55. Kerby JD, Griffin RL, MacLennan P, et al. Stress-induced hyperglycemia, not diabetic hyperglycemia, is associated with higher mortality in trauma. Ann Surg 2012;253(3):446–52.
56. Vogelzang M, Nijboer JM, van der Horst IC, et al. Hyperglycemia has a stronger relation with outcome in trauma patients than in other critically ill patients. J Trauma 2006;80(4):873–9.

57. Matsushima K, Khan M, Frankel H. Trauma-related critical care. Scand J Surg 2014;103(2):138–42.
58. Griesdale DE, Tremblay M, McEwen J, et al. Glucose control and mortality in patients with severe traumatic brain injury. Neurocrit Care 2009;11(3):311–6.
59. Jeremitsky E, Omert L, Dunham M, et al. The impact of hyperglycemia on patients with severe brain injury. J Trauma Acute Care Surg 2005;58(1):47–50.
60. Vespa P, McArthur DL, Stein N, et al. Tight glycemic control increases metabolic distress in traumatic brain injury: a randomized controlled within-subjects trial. Crit Care Med 2012;40(6):1923–9.
61. Oddo M, Schmidt JM, Carrera E, et al. Impact of tight glycemic control on cerebral glucose metabolism after severe brain injury: a microdialysis study. Crit Care Med 2008;36(12):3233–8.
62. Loisa P, Parviainen I, Tenhunen J, et al. Effect of mode of hydrocortisone administration on glycemic control in patient with septic shock: a prospective randomized trial. Crit Care 2007;11(1):R21.
63. Abdelmalak BB, Bonilla AM, Yang D, et al. The hyperglycemic response to major noncardiac surgery and the added effect of steroid administration in patients with and without diabetes. Anesth Analg 2013;116(5):1116–22.
64. Arabi YM, Dabbagh OC, Tamim HM, et al. Intensive versus conventional insulin therapy: a randomized controlled trial in medical and surgical critically ill patients. Crit Care Med 2008;36:190–7.
65. De La Rosa GD, Donado JH, Restrepo AH, et al. Strict glycaemic control in patients hospitalised in a mixed medical and surgical intensive care unit: a randomised clinical trial. Crit Care 2008;12:R120.
66. Brunkhorst FM, Engel C, Bloos F, et al. Intensive insulin therapy and pentastarch resuscitation in severe sepsis. N Engl J Med 2008;358:125–39.

Essentials of Sepsis Management

John M. Green, MD

KEYWORDS

• Sepsis • Sepsis syndrome • Surgical infection • Septic shock
• Goal-directed therapy

KEY POINTS

- Successful treatment of perioperative sepsis relies on the early recognition, diagnosis, and aggressive treatment of the underlying infection; delay in resuscitation, source control, or antimicrobial therapy can lead to increased morbidity and mortality.
- When sepsis is suspected, appropriate cultures should be obtained immediately so that antimicrobial therapy is not delayed; initiation of diagnostic tests, resuscitative measures, and therapeutic interventions should otherwise occur concomitantly to ensure the best outcome.
- Early, aggressive, invasive monitoring is appropriate to ensure adequate resuscitation and to observe the response to therapy.
- Any patient suspected of having sepsis should be in a location where adequate resources can be provided.

INTRODUCTION

Sepsis is among the most common conditions encountered in critical care, and septic shock is one of the leading causes of morbidity and mortality in the intensive care unit (ICU). Indeed, sepsis is among the 10 most common causes of death in the United States.[1] Martin and colleagues[2] showed that surgical patients account for nearly one-third of sepsis cases in the United States. Despite advanced knowledge in the field, sepsis remains a common threat to life in the perioperative period. Survival relies on early recognition and timely targeted correction of the syndrome's root cause as well as ongoing organ support. The objective of this article is to review strategies for detection and timely management of sepsis in the perioperative surgical patient. A comprehensive review of the molecular and cellular mechanisms of organ dysfunction and sepsis management is beyond the scope of this article. The information presented herein is divided into sections devoted to definitions and diagnosis, source

The author has nothing to disclose.
Department of Surgery, Carolinas Medical Center, 1000 Blythe Boulevard, Suite 601, Charlotte, NC 28203, USA
E-mail address: john.m.green@carolinashealthcare.org

Surg Clin N Am 95 (2015) 355–365
http://dx.doi.org/10.1016/j.suc.2014.10.006 surgical.theclinics.com
0039-6109/15/$ – see front matter

control, fluid therapy, antibiotic therapy, and organ support for clarity of discussion, but the practitioner should understand that these approaches occur simultaneously at the bedside, and each action is related to, and should act in concert with, the others.

DEFINITION AND DIAGNOSIS

The most important aspect of intervention in sepsis is early recognition of the signs and symptoms of the condition. Reducing time to diagnosis and initiation of therapy for severe sepsis is considered a critical component of mortality reduction.[3] The Society of Critical Care Medicine and the American College of Chest Physicians proposed standard definitions of this illness spectrum in a consensus published in 1992. The systemic inflammatory response syndrome describes an immune response consisting of 2 or more of the following:

- Temperature greater than 38°C or less than 35°C
- Heart rate greater than 90 beats per minute
- Respiratory rate higher than 20 breaths per minute or a $Paco_2$ below 32 mm Hg
- Leukocytosis of 12,000/mm^3 or less than 4000/mm^3

This inflammatory reaction in the presence of infection is known as sepsis. Complications of organ failure and hypotension constitute severe sepsis. Finally, septic shock is defined by severe sepsis accompanied by hypoperfusion and organ failure refractory to fluid resuscitation.[4]

As with all clinical maladies, a focused history and physical examination can provide vital information about potential risk factors for infection and the most likely site of origin. Several clinical clues may support the clinician's suspicion of infection. For example, unexplained tachycardia is frequently the first indicator of inadequate organ perfusion or a hyperdynamic state of inflammation and should be thoroughly investigated in a perioperative patient. Septic patients, unlike those in cardiac failure or hemorrhagic shock, frequently have warm skin on examination because their peripheral vasculature is not constricted. Acute glucose elevation can be a predictor of infection and should raise the provider's suspicion when present.[5] Inadequate urine output, while useful in monitoring volume and perfusion status, is a late finding in sepsis and septic shock.

Sepsis in the surgical patient is likely an underappreciated cause of morbidity and mortality in the perioperative period. In the postoperative period beyond 24 hours, sepsis is by far the most common cause of shock. Sources include surgical site infections, catheter-related bloodstream infections (CRBSI), pneumonia, and urinary tract infections. Moore and colleagues[6] found that the abdomen was the most common site of infection in their general surgery ICU population, accounting for 63% of cases, followed by the lungs (17%), wound/soft tissue (10%), urinary tract (7%), and all other sites (4%). In fact, the authors demonstrated that the incidence of sepsis and septic shock exceeded those of pulmonary embolism and myocardial infarction by 10-fold. Gram-negative species were the most prevalent culprits, particularly in abdominal sources of sepsis.[6] An understanding of the patient's recent clinical trajectory is invaluable, particularly in the perioperative period. Host defense mechanisms can be compromised by many factors, including surgery, implanted devices, or previous antibiotic use. Knowledge of the patient's surgical history can give clues to mental status changes, increased minute ventilation, decreased urine output, glucose intolerance, thrombocytopenia, or gastrointestinal failure.

Appropriate cultures should be obtained before initiating antimicrobial therapy, provided the antimicrobials are not delayed. These cultures should include one set of blood cultures drawn from any indwelling device, and a separate set drawn peripherally. If the site of origin is not clear, prompt imaging studies should be performed, as required, to investigate suspected sources of infection, and any potential source should be sampled.

Any patient suspected of being in septic shock should be immediately moved to the ICU and administered antibiotics within 1 hour. Septic shock, a result of infection and the attendant inflammatory response, is composed of metabolic derangements attributable to inadequate perfusion, resulting in the buildup of lactic acid and the disruption of normal cellular function. However, the other significant challenge of the shock syndrome consists of the organism's neuroendocrine responses aimed at restoring adequate perfusion. One of these responses, glucose dysregulation, is a common clue to the presence of an infectious source. One prospective study of 2200 trauma patients admitted to the ICU revealed a 91% positive predictive value of acute glucose elevation in the diagnosis of infection.[5] This stress-induced hyperglycemia is generally seen as a transient plasma glucose level greater than 200 mg/dL and is thought to occur following increases in cortisol, glucagon, and epinephrine. Acute glucose elevation should stimulate clinicians to search for a new source of infection.

When septic shock is diagnosed, fluid bolus should be given, unless there is indisputable evidence of acute left heart failure. Electrocardiogram tracing should be obtained immediately to determine the likelihood of cardiac dysfunction. Arterial blood gas should be measured, as pH will drop below neutral due to anaerobic metabolism and lactic acid accumulation, if a shock state exists.

After the syndrome is recognized and resuscitation is begun, a review of the patient's medical history is paramount to determine causation. Surgical sites must be quickly examined for erythema, drainage, bullous changes, or other signs of infection. Surgeons and those caring for surgical patients should have specific knowledge of any operative procedure a patient has undergone, because this will surely help them focus on possible causes for sepsis and septic shock. If sepsis occurs in the first 24 hours after surgery, surgical site infection should be entertained. A streptococcal wound infection can quickly progress to myofascial necrosis. If this is present, radical debridement in the operating room is mandatory, supported by antibiotic therapy.

SOURCE CONTROL

A specific, treatable source of sepsis should always be aggressively sought and addressed as rapidly as possible. Specifically, abscess drainage, wound exploration, debridement of necrotic tissue, removal of infected implanted device, or surgical control of infectious source should occur simultaneously with resuscitation and antibiotic administration. An identified source should always be sampled and cultured for targeted therapy. A rare exception for surgical intervention exists with pancreatic necrosis, in which delayed surgical intervention has been shown to produce better outcomes.[7] Without adequate source control, resuscitative efforts will not be successful. Definitive operation in the case of abdominal sepsis is not as important as limiting the ongoing physiologic insult. A damage-control approach is appropriate for septic shock from abdominal sources using the same principles as the damage-control approach to trauma care.[8]

FLUID THERAPY AND HEMODYNAMIC SUPPORT

The ultimate goal of any hemodynamic intervention is the improvement of tissue perfusion and oxygenation. Subtle changes in a patient's condition are valuable signs in early recognition of hypoxemia or acidosis. Adequate fluid resuscitation should ideally be achieved before the use of vasopressors, although these are sometimes necessary earlier in severe cases. Initial fluid resuscitation should consist of crystalloid resuscitation of 30 mL/kg per ideal body weight. Patients with evidence of tissue hypoperfusion after initial fluid challenge, or those with persistent blood lactate concentration of 4 mmol/L or less, should receive ongoing, protocolized resuscitation. Evidence of hypoperfusion can appear in many ways, and treatment requires the physician to be at the bedside observing the effects of current therapy. Patients with early sepsis, whose vital signs may still fall within an expected range, might display metabolic derangements, such as confusion, a change in their state of wakefulness, or decreased urine output. If raising the blood pressure with volume or vasopressors mitigates these derangements, then central nervous system responsiveness or urine volume can be a good indicator of the adequacy of tissue perfusion.[9]

The Surviving Sepsis Campaign (SSC) suggests goals of this resuscitation are central venous pressure of 8 to 12 mm Hg, mean arterial pressure (MAP) of 65 mm Hg or more, urine output of 0.5 mL/kg/h or more, mixed venous oxygen saturation of at least 65%, or superior vena cava oxygen saturation of 70% (grade 1C recommendation).[10] A randomized controlled trial targeting these goals in the initial 6-hour period demonstrated a 15.9% reduction in 28-day mortality. This strategy was termed *early goal-directed therapy*.[11] Although the SSC demonstrated that adherence to fluid resuscitation targets was low, the goals remain a strong recommendation endorsed by the SSC.[12] Further study has determined goal-directed therapy is both clinically sound and economically beneficial.[13]

No clear benefit has been shown from the use of colloid solution over crystalloid in resuscitation for sepsis. A low-level recommendation comes from the SSC for the consideration of albumin in severe sepsis and septic shock.[10] The SAFE trial showed albumin to be as safe and effective as normal saline.[14] In a meta-analysis of 17 randomized trials, albumin administration showed small and variable benefit across different protocols. Although its use remains controversial, it can be considered in severe sepsis and septic shock in patients who have received large-volume crystalloid resuscitation.

Commonly, patients in septic shock decompensate to a point whereby their endogenous mechanisms can no longer maintain adequate oxygen delivery. In refractory shock, vasopressors are desirable aids to help compensate for distributive shock. If vasopressors are needed to reach the target of MAP of 65 or greater, norepinephrine is the first choice with strong α-1 and β-1 characteristics, and epinephrine may be added. Vasopressin (0.03 U/min) may be combined with norepinephrine but should not be used as the initial medication.[10,15] Clinicians must be aware, however, that these vasopressors are associated with serious adverse events, including dysrhythmias, chest pain, myocardial infarction, limb ischemia, mesenteric ischemia, and stroke. Patients who have such adverse events may also have significantly increased mortality.[16]

Phenylephrine is not recommended for use in septic shock unless norepinephrine is associated with severe dysrhythmia or as salvage therapy when other vasopressors have failed to achieve the target MAP.[17] Low-dose dopamine is not recommended for the purpose of maintaining renal function.[18] In the setting of myocardial dysfunction or ongoing hypoperfusion, despite intravascular volume replacement and adequate MAP, dobutamine should be considered at a rate up to 20 μm/kg/min.

Measurement of blood flow and intravascular volume status at the bedside can be assisted with multiple available technologies.[19] The use of these tools requires knowledge of their methods and limitations, however, so the data they generate can be correctly interpreted. The efficacy of these monitoring technologies requires further study before these tools are deemed standard of care in sepsis management. An arterial catheter for monitoring and continuous analysis should be placed in any patient requiring vasopressors and aggressive blood pressure management. Pulmonary artery catheters, while used much less frequently than in past decades, may still be considered in shock management. A large meta-analysis of randomized controlled trials concluded that use of a pulmonary artery catheter did not increase overall mortality or days in the hospital, nor did it confer any other benefit.[20] Use of these technologies is based on clinician judgment and experience in interpreting data. Ultimately, the goal remains the same: to restore circulation to a normal state and reverse hypoperfusion while inflicting no further harm on the patient.

If hemodynamic targets can be met and perfusion restored with volume and vasopressors, additional corticosteroids provide no real benefit.[10] However, there may be a role for hydrocortisone supplementation in refractory hypotension, dosed at 200 mg per day. The CORTICUS trial, a large European multicenter trial, failed to show benefit from steroid therapy in patients with septic shock, although it included patients whether or not they were responsive to vasopressors.[21] Several other randomized trials have shown significant shock reversal with steroid therapy.[22–25] Random cortisol levels and adrenocorticotropic hormone stimulation testing have not been demonstrated to be useful or predictive of patients who will benefit from steroid supplementation.[21,22]

ANTIMICROBIAL THERAPY

The timely administration of appropriate antimicrobials is critically important to reduce morbidity and mortality from sepsis.[26–29] The choice of agents is based on multiple factors, including patient history, details and timing of surgical procedures, previous antibiotic exposure, and hospital antimicrobial susceptibility patterns. Cultures of blood, urine, pulmonary secretions, wound drainage, or other potential infectious sites should be performed *before* initiation of antibiotics. Broad-spectrum antimicrobial therapy should begin within 1 hour of recognizing the presence of severe sepsis or septic shock.[10]

The initiation of broad-spectrum antibiotics, meant to cover a host of possible culprit organisms, should be able to contain the most common infectious agents in a given hospital or ICU and be effective at limiting superinfection and resistant organisms. The prevalence of methicillin-resistant *Staphylococcus aureus* should be considered, and initial antimicrobial therapy should include agents active against this strain. In addition, antifungal therapy should be considered if candidemia is a likely pathogen. Recent Infectious Diseases Society of America guidelines recommend antifungal therapy in immunosuppressed or neutropenic patients, those who have received prior antibiotic therapy, or those who have fungal colonization.[30] Combination therapy including an extended-spectrum β-lactam and an aminoglycoside or fluoroquinolone should be used if complicated or multidrug-resistant infections such as *Acinetobacter* and *Pseudomonas* species are suspected.[10] Combination therapy for suspected or known *Pseudomonas aeruginosa* or other multidrug-resistant gram-negative pathogens increases the likelihood that at least one agent will be effective.[31]

Daily assessments of the antibiotic regimen should examine clinical progress of the patient, culture data to guide de-escalation of the broad-spectrum regimen and target specific culprit organisms as soon as they are known, and compliance with antibiotic stewardship guidelines to ensure appropriate combinations and length of therapy. Such stewardship programs are in place to prevent resistance, reduce toxicity, and reduce costs.[10] Once the causative pathogen is identified, the most appropriate and cost-effective regimen should be implemented. This practice reduces the likelihood of superinfection with opportunistic organisms such as *Candida* species, *Clostridium difficile*, or vancomycin-resistant *Enterococcus* species, which can all be sources of septic shock and subsequent mortality. Once started, antimicrobial therapy should generally not exceed 7 to 10 days. Certainly, variables exist that necessitate longer therapy including certain patient factors relating to response and immune susceptibility, undrained foci of infection, and some fungal infections.

A common challenge in critical care is determining when to stop antibiotics. Occasionally, patients appear septic, and broad-spectrum antibiotics are initiated, but culture data never identify causative pathogens. Clinicians are then presented with the conundrum of continuing antibiotics in a patient who might be clinically improving, although there is no specific infection identified, or stopping the regimen to prevent opportunistic infection, resistance, and wasted resources. Multidrug resistance increases the cost of antimicrobial treatment by as much as 50%.[32] The use of biomarkers such as C-reactive protein and procalcitonin to differentiate between infection and inflammation without an infectious source remains undefined.[33] Procalcitonin levels might aid in the decision to discontinue antibiotics in this scenario, although available evidence remains conflicting.[33–35] Clinicians should recognize that even though bacterial and fungal sources are likely, blood cultures may be negative in as many as half the cases of severe sepsis if empiric therapy is administered.[10] The decision to continue, narrow, or stop antimicrobial therapy is made on clinician judgment with available information. Antimicrobial agents should not be used in states of severe inflammation determined to be of noninfectious cause.

Clinicians should also consider sepsis of viral origin, and antivirals should be initiated similar to antimicrobials. Viruses such as influenza, cytomegalovirus, and other herpes viruses can all induce septic shock and should be considered in cases with no clear bacterial infection. The role of some viruses in sepsis remains unclear, and active viremia may act as a marker of disease severity rather than an actual agent of organ injury and death in septic patients.[36]

ORGAN SUPPORT AND MONITORING

A comprehensive discussion of the mechanism and therapies for shock is beyond the scope of this review, but the practitioner's understanding of the essentials of managing septic shock is critical to patient survival. Knowledge of the shock syndrome has increased dramatically over the past several decades, and all advances point to the goal of prompt restoration of oxygen delivery. Invasive devices such as arterial blood pressure monitors, central venous catheters, and urinary catheters are helpful to guide therapy, although their placement should not detract from focusing on ongoing resuscitation of the patient.

Tachypnea is common in the septic patient, as is mental status deterioration. Intubation and mechanical ventilation might be warranted, depending on clinical findings. Resuscitation should be ongoing while intubation is performed. Ventilation strategies should be based on lung-protective strategies that have been supported by clinical trials and widely accepted. The precise choice of ventilator mode and tidal volume varies according to degree of respiratory distress and hypoxemia, sedation required, volume status, and other factors that make ventilator support in the septic patient a dynamic and individualized process. Positive end-expiratory pressure, recruitment maneuvers for hypoxemia due to acute respiratory distress syndrome (ARDS), and prone positioning in sepsis-induced ARDS with Pao_2/Fio_2 ratio less than or equal to

100 are all available adjunctive tools to improve oxygenation in the septic patient. Rescue therapies such as high-frequency oscillatory ventilation, airway pressure release ventilation, and extracorporeal membrane oxygenation require experienced personnel with significant expertise.[37]

Although the optimum hemoglobin concentration in sepsis is not defined, red blood cell transfusion is an important tool in organ support. The American College of Critical Care Medicine Taskforce of the Society of Critical Care Medicine and the Canadian Critical Care Trials Group endorse evidence-based transfusion for hemoglobin concentration less than 7 g/dL.[38,39] In patients with ongoing myocardial ischemia, hemorrhage, ischemic coronary disease, or other comorbidities, this transfusion trigger may be altered based on clinician judgment.

Immediately available indicators of global tissue perfusion include arterial pH and lactic acid. These indicators of the metabolic state are important, and mortality is as high as 46.1% in patients with both hypotension and lactate greater than 4.[12] Once resuscitation has restored adequate oxygen delivery, lactate should be metabolized and pH should return to normal. Persistent acidosis indicates inadequate source control such as ongoing bleeding or tissue necrosis. Lactic acid can be used as a marker of hypoperfusion and the depth of the shock state.

NUTRITION AND GLUCOSE CONTROL

Nutrition management in critically ill patients is an important and frequently overlooked aspect of care. Nutrition strategies that take into account information specific to the patient's perioperative condition, first-hand knowledge of the patient's operative history, and available nutritional access and support options should be in place. It is preferable that patients be fed enterally, which can be accomplished orally or via gastric or enteric feeding tube. If enteral feeding is not possible, total parenteral nutrition can be instituted per hospital protocols. Nutrition is frequently withheld in the perioperative period because of ileus and intestinal surgery, among other reasons. No direct evidence defines benefit or harm of parenteral nutrition in the first 48 hours in sepsis.[10] An adjunct to nutritional regimens is stress-ulcer prophylaxis. Patients with severe sepsis or septic shock who have bleeding risk factors should be placed on H2-blocker or proton pump inhibitor. Patients who are not coagulopathic, do not require mechanical ventilation for at least 48 hours, and are normotensive do not require stress-ulcer prophylaxis.[10] In addition, those receiving enteral nutrition do not need prophylaxis, and some evidence suggests that ulcer prophylaxis in this group might increase the risk of pneumonia and death.[40]

Glucose regulation can be a challenge in the perioperative period when nutrition is variable, and an infection state complicates this further. The largest study to date addressing glucose control in ICU patients is the NICE-SUGAR trial, which used a glucose level of 180 mg/dL as the upper limit of control. Multiple consensus statements for glycemic control in hospitalized patients have emerged, generally targeting levels between 140 and 180 g/dL.[41–43] Goals should be within this range, and efforts should be made to avoid wide swings in glucose levels. Of note, clinicians should adjust insulin regimens when nutrition is withheld or discontinued, because this is a common risk factor for hypoglycemia and there are large variations in glucose levels.

SPECIFIC PERIOPERATIVE ISSUES

Surgeons and those caring for surgical patients such as rapid response teams or critical care support teams should be aware of hospital protocols for resuscitation of acutely ill patients. Patients in the perioperative period frequently require pain control, and many agents can suppress respiratory drive if not closely monitored. Drug interactions can cause delirium, hypoxemia, tachycardia, and other signs similar to early sepsis that must be detected and treated appropriately to rescue patients from potential decline.

Septic patients are at increased risk for deep venous thrombosis. Patients with sepsis need daily venous thromboembolism prophylaxis, usually with daily low-molecular-weight heparin unless there is a contraindication to heparin use. Consequences of pulmonary embolism, particularly if a septic patient is already hemodynamically compromised, can be fatal.

NOSOCOMIAL SEPSIS PREVENTION

Prevention of secondary sepsis remains an important goal in surgical critical care. The nosocomial contributors of in-hospital sepsis are widely known but still poorly controlled. Rigorous infection control practices, as recommended by the SSC, should be enforced in any health care environment.[44] Multiple well-designed studies have demonstrated efficacy of focused interventions to reduce nosocomial infections.[45,46] Many health care facilities have specific policies to reduce nosocomial infection, which should be strictly followed by all who enter patient care areas, including family members and visitors, although they are frequently not required to do so.

Ninety percent of nosocomial sepsis cases are associated with central lines,[47] and research in this area is accordingly active due to both the clinical implications and the fact that Medicare and private insurers are discontinuing reimbursement for treatment of CRBSI and hospitals are being forced to assume these costs.

Strategies for preventing CRBSIs include proper hand hygiene for providers, the use of sterile barrier precautions for placement of central venous catheters, including skin antiseptic preparation, early removal of catheters as soon as they are no longer required, and routine replacement of connector tubing.[45,48] Antibiotic-impregnated catheters have also been used as a CRBSI-prevention strategy, with multiple studies supporting their effectiveness in reducing CRBSI incidence and cost. The Institute for Healthcare Improvement has advocated for a central-line infection prevention bundle comprising 5 elements: optimal hand hygiene, maximal sterile barrier precautions for catheter insertion, optimal catheter site selection, chlorhexidine skin antisepsis, and the daily evaluation of central line necessity.[49]

SUMMARY

This review outlines essentials of sepsis management in the surgical patient across the spectrum of care. Early recognition, aggressive fluid resuscitation, source control, and antibiotic therapy result in the best possible survival for patients suffering from sepsis. The Surviving Sepsis Guidelines should be reviewed and understood by any clinician caring for perioperative patients. Sepsis bundles, or protocols to enact evidence-based best practice, should be structured so that they can be implemented in a timely fashion to improve care delivery.

REFERENCES

1. Mokdad AH, Marks JS, Stroup DF, et al. Actual causes of death in the United States, 2000. JAMA 2004;291(10):1238–45.
2. Martin GS, Mannino DM, Eaton S, et al. The epidemiology of sepsis in the United States from 1979 through 2000. N Engl J Med 2003;348(16):1546–54.

3. Jones AE, Shapiro NI, Trzeciak S, et al. Lactate clearance vs central venous oxygen saturation as goals of early sepsis therapy: a randomized clinical trial. JAMA 2010;303(8):739–46.
4. Bone RC, Balk RA, Cerra FB, et al. Definitions for sepsis and organ failure and guidelines for the use of innovative therapies in sepsis. The ACCP/SCCM Consensus Conference Committee. American College of Chest Physicians/ Society of Critical Care Medicine. 1992. Chest 2009;136(5 Suppl):e28.
5. Bochicchio GV, Bochicchio KM, Joshi M, et al. Acute glucose elevation is highly predictive of infection and outcome in critically injured trauma patients. Ann Surg 2010;252(4):597–602.
6. Moore LJ, McKinley BA, Turner KL, et al. The epidemiology of sepsis in general surgery patients. J Trauma 2011;70(3):672–80.
7. Mier J, Leon EL, Castillo A, et al. Early versus late necrosectomy in severe necrotizing pancreatitis. Am J Surg 1997;173(2):71–5.
8. Waibel BH, Rotondo MF. Damage control for intra-abdominal sepsis. Surg Clin North Am 2012;92(2):243–57, viii.
9. Magder SA. The highs and lows of blood pressure: toward meaningful clinical targets in patients with shock. Crit Care Med 2014;42(5):1241–51.
10. Dellinger RP, Levy MM, Rhodes A, et al. Surviving sepsis campaign: international guidelines for management of severe sepsis and septic shock: 2012. Crit Care Med 2013;41(2):580–637.
11. Rivers E, Nguyen B, Havstad S, et al. Early goal-directed therapy in the treatment of severe sepsis and septic shock. N Engl J Med 2001;345(19):1368–77.
12. Levy MM, Dellinger RP, Townsend SR, et al. The Surviving Sepsis Campaign: results of an international guideline-based performance improvement program targeting severe sepsis. Crit Care Med 2010;38(2):367–74.
13. Ebm C, Cecconi M, Sutton L, et al. A cost-effectiveness analysis of postoperative goal-directed therapy for high-risk surgical patients. Crit Care Med 2014;42(5): 1194–203.
14. Finfer S, Bellomo R, Boyce N, et al. A comparison of albumin and saline for fluid resuscitation in the intensive care unit. N Engl J Med 2004;350(22):2247–56.
15. Russell JA, Walley KR, Singer J, et al. Vasopressin versus norepinephrine infusion in patients with septic shock. N Engl J Med 2008;358(9):877–87.
16. Anantasit N, Boyd JH, Walley KR, et al. Serious adverse events associated with vasopressin and norepinephrine infusion in septic shock. Crit Care Med 2014; 42(8):1812–20.
17. Morelli A, Ertmer C, Rehberg S, et al. Phenylephrine versus norepinephrine for initial hemodynamic support of patients with septic shock: a randomized, controlled trial. Crit Care 2008;12(6):R143.
18. Kellum JA, M Decker J. Use of dopamine in acute renal failure: a meta-analysis. Crit Care Med 2001;29(8):1526–31.
19. Pinsky MR, Payen D. Functional hemodynamic monitoring. Crit Care 2005;9(6): 566–72.
20. Shah MR, Hasselblad V, Stevenson LW, et al. Impact of the pulmonary artery catheter in critically ill patients: meta-analysis of randomized clinical trials. JAMA 2005;294(13):1664–70.
21. Sprung CL, Annane D, Keh D, et al. Hydrocortisone therapy for patients with septic shock. N Engl J Med 2008;358(2):111–24.
22. Annane D, Sebille V, Charpentier C, et al. Effect of treatment with low doses of hydrocortisone and fludrocortisone on mortality in patients with septic shock. JAMA 2002;288(7):862–71.

23. Briegel J, Forst H, Haller M, et al. Stress doses of hydrocortisone reverse hyperdynamic septic shock: a prospective, randomized, double-blind, single-center study. Crit Care Med 1999;27(4):723–32.
24. Annane D, Bellissant E, Bollaert PE, et al. Corticosteroids in the treatment of severe sepsis and septic shock in adults: a systematic review. JAMA 2009; 301(22):2362–75.
25. Sligl WI, Milner DA Jr, Sundar S, et al. Safety and efficacy of corticosteroids for the treatment of septic shock: a systematic review and meta-analysis. Clin Infect Dis 2009;49(1):93–101.
26. Kumar A, Roberts D, Wood KE, et al. Duration of hypotension before initiation of effective antimicrobial therapy is the critical determinant of survival in human septic shock. Crit Care Med 2006;34(6):1589–96.
27. Ibrahim EH, Sherman G, Ward S, et al. The influence of inadequate antimicrobial treatment of bloodstream infections on patient outcomes in the ICU setting. Chest 2000;118(1):146–55.
28. Barie PS, Hydo LJ, Shou J, et al. Influence of antibiotic therapy on mortality of critical surgical illness caused or complicated by infection. Surg Infect (Larchmt) 2005;6(1):41–54.
29. Leibovici L, Shraga I, Drucker M, et al. The benefit of appropriate empirical antibiotic treatment in patients with bloodstream infection. J Intern Med 1998; 244(5):379–86.
30. Pappas PG, Kauffman CA, Andes D, et al. Clinical practice guidelines for the management of candidiasis: 2009 update by the Infectious Diseases Society of America. Clin Infect Dis 2009;48(5):503–35.
31. Garnacho-Montero J, Sa-Borges M, Sole-Violan J, et al. Optimal management therapy for Pseudomonas aeruginosa ventilator-associated pneumonia: an observational, multicenter study comparing monotherapy with combination antibiotic therapy. Crit Care Med 2007;35(8):1888–95.
32. Vandijck DM, Depaemelaere M, Labeau SO, et al. Daily cost of antimicrobial therapy in patients with Intensive Care Unit-acquired, laboratory-confirmed bloodstream infection. Int J Antimicrob Agents 2008;31(2):161–5.
33. Tang BM, Eslick GD, Craig JC, et al. Accuracy of procalcitonin for sepsis diagnosis in critically ill patients: systematic review and meta-analysis. Lancet Infect Dis 2007;7(3):210–7.
34. Heyland DK, Johnson AP, Reynolds SC, et al. Procalcitonin for reduced antibiotic exposure in the critical care setting: a systematic review and an economic evaluation. Crit Care Med 2011;39(7):1792–9.
35. Jensen JU, Hein L, Lundgren B, et al. Procalcitonin-guided interventions against infections to increase early appropriate antibiotics and improve survival in the intensive care unit: a randomized trial. Crit Care Med 2011;39(9):2048–58.
36. Hotchkiss RS, Opal S. Immunotherapy for sepsis–a new approach against an ancient foe. N Engl J Med 2010;363(1):87–9.
37. Pipeling MR, Fan E. Therapies for refractory hypoxemia in acute respiratory distress syndrome. JAMA 2010;304(22):2521–7.
38. Napolitano LM, Kurek S, Luchette FA, et al. Clinical practice guideline: red blood cell transfusion in adult trauma and critical care. Crit Care Med 2009;37(12): 3124–57.
39. Hebert PC, Wells G, Blajchman MA, et al. A multicenter, randomized, controlled clinical trial of transfusion requirements in critical care. Transfusion Requirements in Critical Care Investigators, Canadian Critical Care Trials Group. N Engl J Med 1999;340(6):409–17.

40. Marik PE, Vasu T, Hirani A, et al. Stress ulcer prophylaxis in the new millennium: a systematic review and meta-analysis. Crit Care Med 2010;38(11):2222–8.
41. Qaseem A, Humphrey LL, Chou R, et al. Use of intensive insulin therapy for the management of glycemic control in hospitalized patients: a clinical practice guideline from the American College of Physicians. Ann Intern Med 2011; 154(4):260–7.
42. Jacobi J, Bircher N, Krinsley J, et al. Guidelines for the use of an insulin infusion for the management of hyperglycemia in critically ill patients. Crit Care Med 2012; 40(12):3251–76.
43. Moghissi ES, Korytkowski MT, DiNardo M, et al. American Association of Clinical Endocrinologists and American Diabetes Association consensus statement on inpatient glycemic control. Diabetes Care 2009;32(6):1119–31.
44. Aitken LM, Williams G, Harvey M, et al. Nursing considerations to complement the Surviving Sepsis Campaign guidelines. Crit Care Med 2011;39(7):1800–18.
45. Coopersmith CM, Zack JE, Ward MR, et al. The impact of bedside behavior on catheter-related bacteremia in the intensive care unit. Arch Surg 2004;139(2): 131–6.
46. Pronovost P, Needham D, Berenholtz S, et al. An intervention to decrease catheter-related bloodstream infections in the ICU. N Engl J Med 2006;355(26): 2725–32.
47. Chalupka AN, Talmor D. The economics of sepsis. Crit Care Clin 2012;28(1): 57–76, vi.
48. Edgeworth J. Intravascular catheter infections. J Hosp Infect 2009;73(4):323–30.
49. Berwick DM, Calkins DR, McCannon CJ, et al. The 100,000 lives campaign: setting a goal and a deadline for improving health care quality. JAMA 2006; 295(3):324–7.

Transfusion and Management of Surgical Patients with Hematologic Disorders

Wade G. Douglas, MD[a,*], Ekong Uffort, MD[b], David Denning, MD[b]

KEYWORDS

• Transfusion • Massive transfusion protocols • Transfusion-related lung injury
• Transfusion-related outcomes

KEY POINTS

- In the hemodynamically stable patient, restricted use of packed red blood cells appears to be at least equal to liberal use of packed red blood cells.
- The use of fresh frozen plasma and platelets along with packed red blood cells in the massively transfused patient appears to be of benefit.
- Transfusion-related lung injury is one of the leading causes of mortality in the transfused patient.
- Meta-analysis suggests that transfused patients with colorectal cancer have worse outcomes when compared with nontransfused patients.

Surgeons frequently encounter patients with hematologic disorders in the perioperative period. A fundamental understanding of the cause and the management of these clinical derangements is required. Most of these derangements occur as a result of abnormal production, dysfunction, or rapid loss.

This section explores the recent literature and how it has transformed how blood is used in the surgical patient, how blood transfusions impact other patient outcomes, and the current treatment schemes of the massively transfused patient.

LIBERAL VERSUS CONSERVATIVE TRANSFUSION

Recently, there has been a paradigm shift in packed red blood cell (PRBC) utilization. The studies that compare liberal versus restrictive transfusion policy and how these they impact patient outcomes are examined.

[a] Department of Clinical Sciences, Florida State University College of Medicine, 1401 Centerville Road, Suite 107, Tallahassee, FL 32308, USA; [b] Department of Surgery, Marshall University Joan C. Edwards School of Medicine, 1600 Medical Center Drive, Huntington, WV 25701, USA
* Corresponding author.
E-mail address: wade.douglas@med.fsu.edu

Surg Clin N Am 95 (2015) 367–377
http://dx.doi.org/10.1016/j.suc.2014.11.004 surgical.theclinics.com
0039-6109/15/$ – see front matter

Since the development of blood banks through the significant contributions of Dr Charles Drew around the beginning of World War II, the medical community has had many paradigm shifts on the appropriate clinical triggers for transfusion. In the acutely injured bleeding patient, the benefits outweigh the risks associated with blood transfusion. In all other surgical patients, the current paradigm would suggest that conservative clinical triggers provide the benefit and mitigate the risk. For many years, most clinicians used the 10/30 rule as a clinical trigger for transfusion of PRBCs. Because of concerns over transmission of blood-borne diseases and costs associated with a liberal transfusion rate, a re-examination of that clinical trigger began in the 1980s and continues to date. The 1988 National Institutes of Health Consensus Conference concluded that no one criterion should be used as an indication for transfusion and that multiple patient factors should be considered.[1] Since that time, many associations have published many guidelines in an attempt to determine the elusive trigger.[2–5] The indications and thresholds for PRBCs transfusion in adults are discussed in this section.

The support for a liberal transfusion protocol was developed primarily through observational studies that identified an association between anemia and poor outcomes.

- In a 1958 study of patients who declined blood transfusions for religious reasons, the mortality increased as the preoperative hemoglobin (Hgb) decreased.[6]
- That study had a mortality of 61.5% in the patients with an Hgb of less than 6.
- Patients with an Hgb of greater than10 had a 7.1% mortality.[7]
- These observational studies help formulate the 10/30 rule.

Also, studies suggested that there were groups of anemic patients that were at high risk for poor outcomes. Geriatric patients and patients with coronary artery disease are the groups that were determined to be most at risk when anemic in the perioperative period. When a patient is anemic, there are physiologic changes that occur to compensate for the anemia and hemodilution. Many articles describe the association of hemodilution and normalization of tissue oxygen delivery through increasing cardiac output.[7,8] However, in patients who cannot increase stroke volume because of coronary artery disease and/or decreased physiologic reserve, compensating during periods of anemia becomes the challenge.

- Multiple studies did not demonstrate worse outcomes with hemodilution; the animal studies illustrated that the hemodilution was mitigated by increased stoke volume and cardiac output in the animals with normal physiology. Patients who cannot increase their stroke volume or cardiac output have worse outcomes when they are anemic.[9]

The geriatric patient is a patient that surgeons care for frequently in the United States. Because anemia is quite prevalent in this population, many of these patients present anemic with a need for surgical intervention.

- Based on the World Health Organization definition of anemia, which is an Hgb less than13, 10% of patients 65 to 84 and 25% of patients 85 and older are anemic.
- Perioperative anemia constitutes a bad prognosis and increased mortality in elderly patients.[10]
- Symptomatic anemia and severe anemia should always be treated in the elderly.
- One observational study revealed a benefit for liberal transfusion rate in the elderly population.[11]

- A recent clinical trial, Functional Outcomes in Cardiovascular Patients Undergoing Surgical Hip Fracture, found the following characteristics[12]:
  - Average age of 78
  - Cardiac disease or coronary artery disease in 63% of the patients
  - No differences in functional outcome or mortality when restrictive versus liberal transfusion triggers were used
    - Higher myocardial infarction rate in the restrictive group, but not statistically significant.

The current literature does not support a liberal transfusion policy for the noncardiac and nongeriatric patient population. The recent prospective clinical trials and meta-analysis point toward a restrictive transfusion policy that has equal or better clinical outcomes when compared with a liberal policy.

- The transfusion requirements in critical care trial[13] did not find a benefit in keeping Hgb between 10 and 12 when compared with keeping Hgb between 7 and 9.
  - Liberal cohort trended toward worse mortality.
  - Ages 55 and younger had statistically worse outcomes when liberally transfused.
    - Mortality
    - Myocardial infarction
    - Congestive heart failure
- None of the current clinical trials reported statistically significantly higher mortality, and cardiac morbidity, infections, and length of hospital stay were associated with a lower use of red blood cell (RBC) transfusion.[14]
- In-hospital mortality and infections are associated with a liberal use of RBCs.[14]

Clinical Recommendations Made by the American Association of Blood Banks Clinical Transfusion Committee

In hospitalized, hemodynamically stable patients, at what Hgb concentration should a decision to transfuse be considered?

- The American Association of Blood Banks (AABB) recommends adhering to a restrictive transfusion strategy.[15]
- In adults and pediatric intensive care unit (ICU) patients, transfusion should be considered at Hgb concentrations of 7 g/dL or less.
- In postoperative surgical patients, transfusion should be considered at an Hgb concentration of 8 g/dL or less or for symptoms (chest pain, orthostatic hypotension or tachycardia unresponsive to fluid resuscitation, or congestive heart failure).
- Quality of evidence: high
- Strength of recommendation: strong

In hospitalized, hemodynamically stable patients with pre-existing cardiovascular disease, at what Hgb concentration should a decision to transfuse RBCs be considered?

- The AABB suggests adhering to a restrictive transfusion strategy.
- Transfusions should be considered at an Hgb concentration of 8 g/dL or less or for symptoms (chest pain, orthostatic hypotension or tachycardia unresponsive to fluid resuscitation, or congestive heart failure).
- Quality of evidence: moderate
- Strength of recommendation: weak

In hospitalized, hemodynamically stable patients with acute coronary syndrome, at what Hgb concentration should an RBC transfusion be considered?

- The AABB cannot recommend for or against a liberal or restrictive RBC transfusion threshold.
- Quality of evidence: very low
- Strength of recommendation: uncertain.

In hospitalized hemodynamically stable patients, should transfusion be guided by symptoms rather than Hgb concentrations?

- The AABB suggests that transfusion decisions be influenced by symptoms as well as Hgb concentrations.
- Quality of evidence: low
- Strength of recommendation: weak.

MASSIVE TRANSFUSION

An additional hematologic disorder encountered in the perioperative period is coagulopathy, typically seen in the critically ill patient; however, with timely recognition and proper treatment, good outcomes are attainable. Coagulopathies usually are a result of underlying clinical conditions, such as hepatic insufficiency, medication use such as Coumadin, injuries associated with hemorrhagic shock, or massive tissue destruction. This section examines how trauma-related coagulopathy has guided the scientific efforts and development of current treatment protocols of the massively transfused patient.

The definition of massive transfusion is to replace a person's blood volume within a 24-hour period; this is roughly equivalent to transfusing 10 units of PRBCs in an adult. The coagulopathy associated with massive transfusions is a result of dilutional and consumptive processes. Traumatic injuries that usually require massive transfusions cause the consumptive thrombocytopenias and coagulopathies. Furthermore, the dilutional effect of transfusing multiple units of PRBCs combined with infusing large volumes of crystalloid has led to the development of irreversible coagulopathies. Management of these critically ill patients requires close clinical observation and frequent laboratory evaluations. Surgeons should avoid hypothermia, hypovolemia, and acid/base imbalances and correct all coagulation and electrolyte abnormalities. Because of the frequency that irreversible coagulopathy is associated with massive transfusions, it is recommended that fresh frozen plasma (FFP) and platelets be transfused along with the PRBCs. However, there has been some debate over the optimal transfusion ratio of blood products.

Coagulopathy complicates the care of the critically injured patient; the liberal transfusion of FFP and PRBCs can be equally detrimental to this patient population. Transfusion of PRBCs to restore oxygen delivery and FFP to correct the associated coagulopathy has produced higher rates of multiorgan failure (MOF).

- A 2010 study identified that the absolute amount of FFP and the increased ratios of FFP and PRBCs increased the rate of MOF in the critically injured patient.[16]
- Another study looked at the non-massively transfused patient and found that the FFP transfusion was associated with increased complications[17]:
  - Acute respiratory distress syndrome
  - MOF
  - Pneumonia

- Long-term functional outcomes appear to be compromised when patients receive massive transfusion protocol (MTP).[18]
- Another study did identify an overuse of MTPs in the nontrauma patient but did not identify a higher rate of adverse outcomes.[19]

Acute traumatic coagulopathy (ATC) is the driving force behind the development of MTP, but the mechanisms and physiologic process that influence ATC are not completely understood. In the critically injured patient, presenting ATC is considered treatable, but there are risks associated with overuse of MTP. Currently, thromboelastography (TEG) is reported as a possible laboratory test that can help identify and guide the resuscitation.

- Initially, it was considered that iatrogenic causes (dilution, hypothermia, and acidosis) contributed to the development of ATC.
- There are endogenous processes that occur before and independent of the iatrogenic processes.
- The prospective, observational, multicenter major trauma transfusion (PROMMTT) study did identify ATC in the prehospital setting in 42.7% of the patients.[20] The major contributors to the endogenous factors were as follows:
  - Coagulation factor depletion as a result of tissue injury
  - Coagulation factor dysfunction associated with shock
- Early platelet dysfunction has been found to contribute to ATC. A recent study identified that trauma patients presented with normal platelet counts but profound platelet dysfunction.[21]
- This dysfunction was associated with the following:
  - Injury severity
  - Blood transfusion
  - Shock or base deficit of greater than or equal to 8.
- Although prothrombin time/partial thromboplastin time (PT/PTT), international normalized ratio (INR), and platelet levels are considered standard laboratory values to identify ATC, these tests were not developed to evaluate the acutely or critically injured patient. Also, they are not typically helpful during the hemostatic resuscitation.
- PT/INR and PTT fail to quantify clotting beyond the initiation phase. TEG and rapid TEG allow for the evaluation of how all of components are functioning as a unit.[22]
- Multiple studies confirmed that early use of TEG technology, FFP, and platelet transfusion in the massively transfused patient decreases mortality and treats ATC.[22–24]

Currently, there are multiple observational studies that suggest that MTP decreases mortality in the critically injured patient. A better understanding of the mechanisms and timing of ATC, along with studies that confirm that the early use of platelets and FFP decrease mortality, suggests that efforts are moving in the right direction. However, there are studies identifying the in-hospital and long-term risks associated with these protocols. The hope was that the recent clinical trials would alleviate the controversy. The data from the PROMMTT suggest that transfusion ratio greater than 1:2 for plasma:RBC and platelet:RBC within 6 hours of hospitalization improves outcomes.[25,26] The pragmatic randomized optimal platelets and plasma ratios trial is ongoing, and it is hoped it will provide some additional useful data on the topic.

Clinical Recommendations and Key Points

- PRBC transfusion is indicated for patients in hemorrhagic shock.[20]

- International and national trends are to move toward a formula-driven MTP incorporating point-of-care testing (TEG) to guide the ongoing transfusions.
- MTP with RBC:plasma:platelets ratios of 1:1:1 appears to improve survival in the critically injured patient, but additional data are needed.

TRANSFUSION-RELATED OUTCOMES

Many side effects to transfusion have been reported in the literature. Despite appearing in the literature, often the incidence and many of the mechanisms that promote these poor outcomes are not completely known. Transfusions are associated with the transmission of blood-borne pathogens, higher mortality, longer hospital stays, transfusion-related acute lung injury (TRALI), and poor outcomes in patients with cancer. Although some of these poor outcome measures have been discussed earlier, the mechanisms and risk factors associated with some of the transfusion-related poor outcomes that are pertinent to surgical patients are explored.

Transfusion-related Acute Lung Injury

TRALI is a clinical syndrome that presents as acute hypoxemia and noncardiogenic pulmonary edema during or after blood transfusion. TRALI is a leading cause of mortality in the transfused patient. Historically, this was underreported and underdiagnosed; however, work groups have brought needed attention to TRALI over the past decade.

- All transfused blood components (PLT, RBC, and FFP) have a risk of inducing TRALI.
- The true incidence of TRALI is unknown.
- A 2011 study of consecutive cardiac patients identified a possible incidence of 2.4% in transfused patients.[27]
  - An amount of 0.61% of blood products was transfused.
  - Only 1 patient was reported to the blood bank.
- The pathophysiology of TRALI is increased pulmonary microvascular permeability along with increased protein in the edema fluid.
- Two unique but not mutually exclusive mechanisms have been proposed as the cause of TRALI.
  - Transfused leukocyte antibodies reported a higher incidence with blood transfused from multiparous women and a higher percentage of lymphocyte and granulocyte antibodies in the transfused blood.[28]
  - The 2-hit theory is that a stressor (surgery, trauma, or sepsis) sequesters neutrophils in the lung. The second hit occurs with the transfusion of biologically active substances such as lipids or cytokines.[28]
- In confirmed cases of TRALI that were studied in a prospective manner, the TRALI patients had longer hospital and ICU stays, more days on the ventilator, and higher mortality.[29]

Cancer Outcomes and Transfusions

Surgery is the cornerstone of any multidisciplinary treatment plan for most solid organ malignancies. To improve outcomes, investigators constantly examine variables that will improve morbidity and mortality associated with treatment plans. Over the past 2 decades, the impact of surgical blood loss on outcomes in patients with cancer has been examined. Because many of these patients present with anemia, the surgical blood loss compounds this problem and usually results in a high transfusion rate in the perioperative period. Recently, the impact of blood transfusions on cancer-related outcomes has been debated in the literature and is examined in this section.

Perhaps the most intuitive clinical outcome of presenting anemia in the surgical oncology patient is the subsequent perioperative blood transfusion. Despite evidence that anemia is associated with poor patient outcomes, correction of this anemia has not improved these outcomes.

- A small, randomized study could show no benefit of a liberal transfusion policy (Hgb >10) compared with a restrictive transfusion policy (Hgb 8.5–10) in patients with resected lung cancer.[30]

It is estimated that the prevalence of anemia in the surgical oncology patient population is 25% to 75%, depending on the disease site.[31] Gastric cancer has one of the highest incidences of associated perioperative anemia. Most patients with gastric cancer require a total or subtotal gastrectomy and some form of lymph node dissection, and many have undergone some form of neoadjuvant therapy. The combination of presenting anemia and radical surgery usually results in the use of perioperative blood transfusion to correct the anemia.

- A retrospective study of 856 patients who had an R0 resection found that transfusion was an independent predictor of poor survival across all stages of disease.[32]
- The need for transfusion was significantly related to the T stage, preoperative albumin, Hgb, and operative time.[33]
- Also, this study found that blood transfusions were related to decreased patient survival, but the authors thought that the survival relationship was confounding and not prognostic.[33]

Another gastrointestinal tract malignancy associated with perioperative anemia and a high incidence of perioperative blood transfusion is colorectal cancer. There are some similarities between gastric and colorectal cancer, but colorectal cancer has a higher incidence and an opportunity to control the confounding variables. This section explores how blood transfusion impacts colorectal cancer–related treatment outcomes.

- Retrospective studies identified a negative relationship between perioperative blood transfusion and survival of the patient with colorectal cancer.[34]
- The authors thought that this relationship was confounded by many variables as stated above. Small prospective trials attempted to control for some of these variables.
- One proposed variable investigated the banking process of the allogeneic blood; this study randomized patients to receive leukocyte-reduced blood (LR), buffy coat depleted blood (BCD), or no blood transfusion (NT).[35]
  - Initial results found that blood transfusion regardless of how it was processed had a detrimental effect on overall survival.
  - However, the 15-year follow-up results found that 43% of the NT, 27% of the LR, and 28% of the BCD patients were alive at 15 years.
- Some authors thought the cause of the worse outcome could be explained by the difference between allogeneic and autologous blood transfusion. A randomized trial of 475 patients with a 30-month follow-up found that the transfused patients, regardless of whether it was allogeneic or autologous, did worse.
  - Worse local recurrence rate
  - Worse disease-free interval.
- The 20-year follow-up of that study found that there was no survival benefit to blood transfusion regardless of whether it was autologous or allogeneic.[36]

- With the conflicting results of the small trials, meta-analyses were performed to try to answer the question.
- Large meta-analyses found that transfused patients had worse clinical outcomes when compared with nontransfused patients.[37]
  - All-cause mortality, cancer-related mortality, recurrence or metastatic-related death, postoperative infections, and length of hospital stay.
  - This study had no patient-related or stage-related data.
- Cochrane analysis and meta-analysis found that perioperative blood transfusion increased the recurrence rate in patients with curable colorectal cancer. The heterogeneity detected in the study prevents the authors from assessing a causal relationship.[38]

Most of the data support the notion that perioperative blood transfusions negatively impact outcomes related to the patient with cancer. Because many of these patients present with anemia, consideration should be given to the development of an anemia management plan. This plan should focus on the correction of preoperative anemia with bank blood alternatives, minimization of perioperative blood loss, and the use of restrictive transfusion triggers.

PERIOPERATIVE MANAGEMENT OF SPECIFIC HEMATOLOGICAL DISORDERS

Von Willebrand Disease

Von Willebrand disease is the most common inherited abnormality affecting platelet function. It is caused by a deficiency or dysfunction of von Willebrand factors (vWF) that are essential to a platelet's adhesion. Common symptoms reported with this disorder are related to the skin and mucous membrane and include mucosal bleeding, gastrointestinal bleeding, menorrhagia, epistaxis, and easy bruising; however, because vWF is also a carrier protein for factor VIII (FVIII), these patients may also have prolonged active partial thromboplastin time (aPTT).

Preoperative evaluation should therefore include measurement of FVIII activity, vWF activity, and ristocetin cofactor activity laboratory tests to appropriately assign severity of the disease. Type 1 vWD or mild disease represents a partial quantitative deficiency in vWF; type 2 disease is dysfunctional vWF/qualitative deficiency, and type 3 or severe vWD is a complete deficiency of vWF.

Recommendations

Although the effectiveness of desmopressin (DDAVP) depends on the disease type, all surgical patients with vWD require preoperative desmopressin at 30 μg/kg intravenously over a period of 30 minutes or vWF/FVIII concentrate for surgical prophylaxis and a consultation by a hematologist. FVIII and vWF levels usually increase 30 to 60 minutes after administration of desmopressin and stay at that level for 8 to 10 hours. Desmopressin can be repeated in 12 to 24 hours for up to 36 hours if the patient has postoperative bleeding. The vWF/FVIII concentrate is indicated for patients who do not respond to desmopressin with concentrate dosing at 25 to 50 IU/kg depending on the FVIII activity and monitored every 12 hours for the first 24 hours and then every 24 hours, avoiding supratherapeutic levels.

Hemophilia A/B

Congenital FVIII deficiency (hemophilia A) and factor IX deficiency (hemophilia B) are coagulopathies that require perioperative management in surgical patients because they are associated with an increased risk of excessive bleeding with surgery. These patients usually have a prolonged aPTT and a normal PT.

Hemophilia A is an X-linked recessive disorder caused by a mutation of the FVIII gene. Its severity is proportional to FVIII level and activity. Severe hemophilia A has FVIII levels less than 1% of normal and so is usually diagnosed in childhood and is usually known by the patient before any surgery hence the importance of an excellent history. Patients with factor levels between 6% and 30% of normal are considered mildly affected and may go undiagnosed, because they do not spontaneously bleed into vital organs.

Hemophilia B is also an X-linked recessive disorder caused by a mutation in factor IX gene leading to factor IX deficiency.

Recommendations

Plasma-derived or recombinant FVIII or factor IX concentrate should be given as surgical prophylaxis before any surgical intervention and continued for 10 to 14 days following the procedure. The initial dose can be 50 to 60 U/kg (for hemophilia A) or 100 U/kg (for hemophilia B) depending on the factor activity level and can be repeated with doses of 25 to 30 U/kg every 8 to 12 hours for hemophilia A or 30 to 50 U/kg every 12 to 24 hours for hemophilia B if the respective factor levels drop to less than 80%. A consultation with a hematologist is recommended; the dosage required is to reach 80% to 100% of normal factor activity.

Idiopathic Thrombocytopenic Purpura

Idiopathic thrombocytopenic purpura (ITP) disorder is also known as primary immune thrombocytopenic purpura, and it involves antibodies against platelet antigen formed and leading to destruction of the platelets, hence thrombocytopenia. The immune-complex-coated platelets are destroyed and eliminated by the spleen. The patient presents with thrombocytopenia not related to drugs or other causes, and it is a diagnosis of exclusion. ITP can present as an acute form or a chronic form. Clinical features of ITP are different in adults and children, occurring acutely in children after a viral infection but self-limiting. In adults, it can be an acute onset but usually with no preceding infection and then proceeds to a chronic form with a high production rate of platelet in the bone marrow in an effort to maintain a low to near-normal platelet count. Presentation is highly variable, ranging from asymptomatic to mild symptoms of easy bruising and gastrointestinal bleeding, to severe symptoms such as intracranial bleeding.

Recommendations

If the surgical patient with ITP presents with bleeding, ITP should be treated as a medical emergency with high-dose corticosteroids for the first 3 days. The patient should also receive intravenous immunoglobulin and platelet transfusion every 8 to 12 hours. There are some adults who do not respond to corticosteroids and develop chronic ITP. Splenectomy is often recommended, but the patient will require pneumococcal, meningococcal, and haemophilus influenza vaccines before surgery.

REFERENCES

1. Consensus conference. Perioperative red blood cell transfusion. JAMA 1988; 260(18):2700–3.
2. Ferraris VA, Brown JR, Despotis GJ, et al. Update to the Society of Thoracic Surgeons and the Society of Cardiovascular Anesthesiologists blood conservation clinical practice guidelines. Ann Thorac Surg 2011;91(3):944–82.
3. Qaseem A, Humphrey LL, Fitterman N, et al, Clinical Guidelines Committee of the American College of Physicians. Treatment of anemia in patients with heart

disease: a clinical practice guideline from the American College of Physicians. Ann Intern Med 2013;159(11):770–9.
4. Hillis LD, Smith PK, Anderson JL, et al. 2011 ACCF/AHA guideline for coronary artery bypass graft surgery. A report of the American College of Cardiology Foundation/American Heart Association Task Force on practice guidelines. Developed in collaboration with the American Association for Thoracic Surgery, Society of Cardiovascular Anesthesiologists, and Society of Thoracic Surgeons. J Am Coll Cardiol 2011;58(24):e123–210.
5. Napolitano LM, Kurek S, Luchette FA, et al, American College of Critical Care Medicine of the Society of Critical Care, Eastern Association for the Surgery of Trauma Practice Management Workgroup. Clinical practice guideline: red blood cell transfusion in adult trauma and critical care. Crit Care Med 2009;37(12): 3124–57.
6. Carson JL, Duff A, Poses RM, et al. Effect of anemia and cardiovascular disease on surgical mortality and morbidity. Lancet 1988;1:727–9.
7. Carson JL, Reynolds RC. Transfusion policies in anemia; in search of the transfusion threshold. Hematology 2005;10(Suppl 1):86–8.
8. Crosby ET. Perioperative heamotherapy: I. Indications for blood component transfusion. Can J Anaesth 1992;39(7):695–707.
9. Geha AS, Baue AE. Graded coronary stenosis and coronary flow during acute normovolemic anemia. World J Surg 1978;2:645–52.
10. Beyer I, Compte N, Busuioc A, et al. Anemia and transfusions in geriatric patients: a time for evaluation. Hematology 2010;15(2):116–21.
11. Wu WC, Smith TS, Henderson WG, et al. Operative blood loss, blood transfusion and 30-day mortality in older patients after non-cardiac surgery. Ann Surg 2010; 252(1):11–7.
12. Carson JL, Terrin ML, Noveck H, et al. Liberal or restrictive transfusion in high-risk patients after hip surgery (FOCUS). N Engl J Med 2011;365(26):2453–62.
13. Hebert PC, Wells G, Laijchmann M, et al. A multicenter, randomized, controlled clinical trial of transfusion requirements in critical care. N Engl J Med 1999;340: 409–17.
14. Carson JL, Carless PA, Herbert PC. Transfusion thresholds and other strategies for guiding allogeneic red blood cell transfusion [review]. Cochrane Database Syst Rev 2012;(4):CD002042.
15. Carson JL, Grossman BJ, Klienman S, et al. Red blood cell transfusion: a clinical practice guideline from the AABB. Ann Intern Med 2012;157(1):49–58.
16. Johnson JL, Moore EE, Kashuk JL, et al. Effect of blood products transfusion on the development of post injury multiple organ failure. Arch Surg 2010;145(10): 973–7.
17. Inaba K, Branco BC, Rhee P, et al. Impact of plasma transfusion in trauma patients who do not require massive transfusion. J Am Coll Surg 2010;210(6): 957–64.
18. Mitra B, Gabbe BJ, Kaukonen KM, et al. Long-term outcomes of patients receiving a massive transfusion after trauma. Shock 2014;42(4):307–12.
19. McDaniel LM, Neal MD, Sperry JL, et al. Use of a massive transfusion protocol in nontrauma patients: activate away. J Am Coll Surg 2013;216(6):1103–9.
20. Cohen MJ, Kutcher M, Redick B, et al. Clinical and mechanistic drivers of acute traumatic coagulopathy. J Trauma Acute Care Surg 2013;75(1 Suppl 1):40–7.
21. Wohlauer MV, Moore EE, Thomas S, et al. Early platelet dysfunction: an unrecognized role in the acute coagulopathy of trauma. J Am Coll Surg 2012;214(5): 739–46.

22. Gonzalez E, Moore EE, Moore HB, et al. Trauma-induced coagulopathy: an institution's 35 year perspective on practice and research. Scand J Surg 2014;103: 89–103.
23. Branco BC, Inaba K, Ives c, et al. Thromboelastagram evaluation of the impact of hypercoagulability in trauma patients. Shock 2014;41(3):200–7.
24. McDaniel LM, Etchill EW, Raval JS, et al. State of the art: massive transfusion. Transfus Med 2014;24:138–44.
25. Del Junco DJ, Holcomb JB, Fox EF, et al. Resuscitate early with plasma and platelets balanced blood products gradually: findings from PROMMTT study. J Trauma Acute Care Surg 2013;75(1 Suppl 1):24–30.
26. Holcomb JB, del Junco DJ, Fox EF, et al. The prospective, observational, multicenter, major trauma transfusion (PROMMTT) study. JAMA Surg 2013;148(2): 127–36.
27. Vlaar AP, Hostra JJ, Determann RM, et al. The incidence, risk factors and outcome of transfusion-related acute lung injury in a cohort of cardiac surgery patients: a prospective nested case-control study. Blood 2011;117(16):1–13.
28. Toy P, Popovsky MA, Abraham E, et al. Transfusion-related acute lung injury: definition and review. Crit Care Med 2005;33(4):721–6.
29. Looney MR, Roubinian N, Gajic O, et al. Prospective study on the clinical course and outcomes in transfusion-related acute lung injury. Crit Care Med 2014;42(7): 1676–87.
30. Dougenis D, Patrinou V, Filos KS, et al. Blood use in lung resection for carcinoma; perioperative elective anemia does not compromise the early outcome. Eur J Cardiothorac Surg 2001;20:372–7.
31. Shander A, Knight K, Thurer R, et al. Prevalence and outcomes of anemia in surgery: a systematic review of the literature. Am J Med 2004;116(Suppl 7A):58–69.
32. Ojima T, Iwahashi M, Nakamori M, et al. Association of allogeneic blood transfusion and long-term survival of patients with gastric cancer after curative gastrectomy. J Gastrointest Surg 2009;13:1821–30.
33. Rausei S, Ruspi L, Galli F, et al. Peri-operative blood transfusion in gastric cancer surgery: prognostic or confounding factor? Int J Surg 2013;11:S100–3.
34. Busch OR, Hop WC, Marquet RL, et al. The effect of blood transfusion on survival after surgery for colorectal cancer. Eur J Cancer 1995;31A(7):1226–8.
35. Mortensen FV, Jensen LS, Sorensen HT, et al. Cause-specific mortality associated with leukoreduced, buffy coat-depleted, or no blood transfusion after elective surgery for colorectal cancer: a posttrial 15-year follow-up study. Transfusion 2011;51:259–63.
36. Harlaar JJ, Gosselink MP, Hop WC, et al. Blood transfusions and prognosis in colorectal cancer. Long-term results of a randomized controlled trial. Ann Surg 2012;252(5):681–7.
37. Acheson AG, Brookes MJ, Spahn D. Effects of allogeneic red blood cell transfusions on clinical outcomes in patients undergoing colorectal cancer surgery: a systematic review and meta-analysis. Ann Surg 2012;256(2):235–44.
38. Amato A, Pescatori M. Perioperative blood transfusion and recurrence of colorectal cancer. The Cochrane Collaboration 2011. 1–77.

Perioperative Management of Obese Patients

Kenji L. Leonard, MD[a], Stephen W. Davies, MD[b], Brett H. Waibel, MD[a,*]

KEYWORDS

• Obesity • Perioperative management • Surgery • Metabolic syndrome
• Bariatric surgery • Morbid obesity • Preoperative care • Postoperative care

KEY POINTS

- There is an increase in the prevalence of obesity within the United States, with an estimated 30% of the population considered obese; given the increase in prevalence, practicing surgeons will encounter more and more of this complex population.
- Obese patients are at increased risk for morbidity and mortality secondary to associated comorbidities and benefits from optimization of these morbidities before elective surgery.
- The perioperative management of obese patients is complex and requires the coordinated care of surgeons, anesthesiologists, nurses, and other hospital staff.
- There is still considerable controversy and variability in certain aspects of management of obese patients; this article reviews the literature ranging from expert opinion to guidelines set forth by regulatory organizations to provide up-to-date management recommendations.

INTRODUCTION

The prevalence of obesity in the United States has grown significantly within the past 2 decades, with current figures estimating that one-third of adults in the United States are obese[1,2]; a statistic that has quadrupled since the 1980s.[3] Paralleling the increased prevalence of obesity is the number of bariatric surgical procedures, which have increased from 8597 in 1993 to 220,000 in 2004.[4,5] The World Health Organization and US Centers for Disease Control and Prevention define obesity as body mass index (BMI) greater than or equal to 30.[2,6] Obese patients usually have other conditions associated with obesity, such as hypertension, type II diabetes mellitus, dyslipidemia, and cardiovascular disease.[7,8] The constellation of these comorbidities has been defined as metabolic syndrome, which has been shown in the literature to

Conflicts of interest: The authors have no conflicts of interest to report.

[a] Division of Trauma and Acute Care Surgery, Department of Surgery, The Brody School of Medicine, East Carolina University, 600 Moye Boulevard, Greenville, NC 27834, USA; [b] Department of Surgery, University of Virginia, School of Medicine, PO Box 800136, Charlottesville, VA 22908, USA
* Corresponding author.
E-mail address: brett.waibel@vidanthealth.com

Surg Clin N Am 95 (2015) 379–390
http://dx.doi.org/10.1016/j.suc.2014.10.008 surgical.theclinics.com
0039-6109/15/$ – see front matter

have increased morbidity and mortality.[9–11] Surgeons are likely to encounter this challenging population during the course of their practice and need to be adept at the often complex management of these patients.

ANESTHESIA, PARALYTICS, AND ANALGESIA

Obesity causes variation in drug pharmacokinetic profiles, which makes drug dosing complicated, because most data are from nonobese patients. The greater fat mass, extracellular volume, and lean body weight in obese patients all affect drug pharmacokinetics.[7] In addition, the volume of distribution of lipophilic drugs is substantially greater than in normal-weight individuals, whereas hydrophilic drugs do not vary as much.[12] The decision to use ideal body weight (IBW) or total body weight to calculate drug dosages is not always clear. For example, paralytics are dosed based on IBW and most analgesics are based on lean body weight.[7,12] **Table 1** shows common medications and how dosage should be based.

Given the larger dosages required with the increased distribution volume and the risk of prolonged effects after discontinuation, lipophilic drugs, such as barbiturates, benzodiazepines, and volatile inhalation agents, should be used with caution or minimally in obese patients.[3,10,12–16] Maintenance of anesthesia can safely be performed either by intravenous (IV) anesthesia or inhalation anesthesia. The ideal inhalational anesthetic has a short onset and short, reliable recovery profile. Desflurane is the inhalational agent of choice in obese patients, but sevoflurane can also be used, because it has similar results to desflurane.[3,12,17–20]

With regard to paralytics, rocuronium, vecuronium, and cisatracurium have been studied and should be dosed based on IBW. Succinylcholine should be based on total body weight, because obese patients recover more rapidly secondary to increased pseudocholinesterase activity.[7,12] Sugammadex, a reversal agent for paralytics, has been used in the obese population with good results and should be dosed based

Table 1
Common medications and suggested dosages based on weight

Medication	Dosing Weight
Propofol	Lean body weight (induction) Total body weight (maintenance)
Etomidate	Lean body weight
Succinylcholine	Total body weight
Vecuronium	IBW
Rocuronium	IBW
Cisatracurium	IBW
Fentanyl	Lean body weight
Sufentanil	Total body weight
Remifentanil	IBW Lean body weight
Morphine (PCA)	Lean body weight
Neostigmine	Total body weight
Sugammadex	IBW + 40% or total body weight
Lidocaine (local)	Total body weight

Abbreviation: PCA, patient controlled analgesia.
Data from Refs.[7,17,22,25]

on total body weight.[7,12] It is essential that full reversal of the muscle relaxant be performed once the patient is to be extubated, because inadequacy in reversal can cause residual curarization and lead to clinically significant respiratory depression and need for emergent reintubation.[7]

Fentanyl and its analogues can be used, but remifentanil is the drug of choice because it does not accumulate in fat.[21] Given the risk of respiratory depression when using opiates, nonsteroidal antiinflammatory drugs such as ketorolac, acetaminophen, local anesthetic wound infiltration, cyclooxygenase-2 inhibitors, and regional nerve blocks have been described as analgesic adjuncts to decrease the use of IV opiates.[7,14,15,19,22] A problematic issue with regional or local nerve blocks is the potential difficulty in delineating anatomic landmarks.[7,12,13] Also mentioned is dexmedetomidine, a highly selective alpha-adrenergic agonist with sedative, amnestic, and analgesic properties without the respiratory depressive side effect.[7,13,22] Epidurals have also been described,[8–10,23] although respiratory depression, epidural hematomas, and increased risk of rhabdomyolysis can also occur with their use.[8,23,24] Adequate postoperative pain control is essential for these patients to help them gain early mobility, quicker return of gastrointestinal function, and good pulmonary function.[14] Patient controlled analgesia (PCA) using opiates can help with postoperative pain, although caution should is needed to ensure that a limited dosage without a basal rate is used to limit the risk of respiratory depression.[14,15,25] The recommended dosage of an opiate PCA should be based on lean body mass.[22,25]

PULMONARY SYSTEM

Obese patients are at increased risk of having airways that are difficult to manage, because bag mask valve ventilation and intubation can be challenging.[7] Although increased BMI does not predict difficulty with laryngoscopy or tracheal intubation, larger neck circumference (>40 cm) and higher Mallampati score (>3) were better predictors of a difficult intubation.[3,12,25,26] The probability of difficult intubation with a neck circumference of 40 cm was 5%, which increased to 35% with a 60-cm neck circumference.[15,19] Although most patients can successfully undergo tracheal intubation in a supine position, other adjuncts, such as awake intubation with a flexible fiberoptic scope, video-assisted laryngoscopy, and laryngeal mask airway (LMA), should be readily available.[7,12,14,27]

Given that the functional residual capacity (FRC) is reduced in obese patients, long periods of apnea are not tolerated and patients deoxygenate rapidly.[12,20,21,23,28,29] The use of preoxygenation using 100% fraction of inspired oxygen (FiO_2) for denitrogenation is thus recommended.[7,12–15,17,18,29,30] The use of continuous positive airway pressure (CPAP) at 10 cm H_2O is also suggested in the preintubation phase to reduce the formation of atelectasis.[7,13,15,17,27] A common intubation position for obese patients is the reverse Trendelenburg or head-up position of 25° to 40° with the use of shoulder towels. This position aids in improving oxygenation to prolong the time until desaturation, preventing aspiration, and offloading abdominal contents on the diaphragm, which increases FRC and reduces the formation of atelectasis.[14,15,19,20,25,27]

With the increase in BMI, obese patients present with a restrictive pattern with decreased forced expiratory volume, FRC, and expiratory reserve volume.[14,15,19,27] Lung volume and lung and chest wall compliance decrease as well. An increase in oxygen consumption, respiratory resistance, and work of breathing is seen in obese patients.[14,15,19,27] These changes lead to gas trapping with ventilation-perfusion mismatching, hypoxemia, and atelectasis, which becomes worse with anesthesia and paralysis. In addition, a higher prevalence of obstructive sleep apnea (OSA) is present, with rates of 30% to 93% in bariatric patients.[30] Moderate to severe OSA causes an increased in all-cause mortality and adverse outcomes. The American Association of Clinical Endocrinologists (AACE), The Obesity Society (TOS), and the American Society for Metabolic and Bariatric Surgery (ASMBS) advocate preoperative screening with polysomnography and preoperative CPAP in at-risk patients.[31] Preoperative CPAP has been shown to decrease severe hypoxemia, pulmonary vasoconstriction, hospital length of stay, and the incidence of postoperative complications.[13,15,28,30,32] Postoperative CPAP reduces the risk of pulmonary restrictive disease and acute respiratory distress syndrome.[7,15,16,19,29,30] McGlinch and colleagues[18] suggested the use of postoperative CPAP therapy until pulse oximetry is greater than 90% while sleeping and IV narcotics for pain management are no longer needed.

No strict guidelines as to ventilator strategies or modes for obese patients exist; however, recommendations within the anesthesiology literature include use of at least 10 cm H_2O of post–end expiratory pressure (PEEP) after a recruitment maneuver, tidal volumes of 6 to 12 mL/kg IBW, and use of lower Fio_2 (<0.8) to maintain physiologic oxygenation.[14,17,27] The respiratory rate should be adjusted to maintain normocapnia and offload carbon dioxide absorbed from pneumoperitoneum.[27,33] Kaw and colleagues[15] reported using high tidal volumes, PEEP, and vital capacity maneuvers to improve ventilation and oxygenation, whereas Cullen and Fergusen[7] reported no benefit in high tidal volumes in an attempt to maintain FRC.

Extubation should be performed once return of protective airway reflexes and muscle strength recovery has been assessed, the patient is fully awake and able to follow commands,[7,12,13] and in the reverse Trendelenburg position.[17,27,29] Once extubated, continuous pulse oximetry is used to detect subclinical periods of desaturation. Supplemental oxygen should be provided after major surgery, with some clinicians recommending treatment times of at least 24 to 48 hours.[7,15,16,18,22,30] Nasal CPAP has also been recommended postoperatively, in addition to supplemental oxygen.[12,13,17,20,27,30]

CARDIOVASCULAR SYSTEM

Obesity is an independent risk factor for coronary artery disease and therefore all obese patients should undergo a cardiac evaluation before an elective surgery, because they are at higher risk for essential hypertension, left ventricular hypertrophy, pulmonary hypertension, and congestive heart failure.[9,20,33,34] Work-up includes chest radiograph, 12-lead echocardiogram, and polysomnography in those patients with OSA or hypercapnia, because arrhythmias are commonly caused by hypoxia from OSA.[20,33] The AACE/TOS/ASMBS guidelines recommend echocardiography, spirometry, and arterial blood gases only if the patient has additional risk factors. Their guidelines recommend that "patients at risk for heart disease should undergo evaluation for perioperative beta-adrenergic blockade."[31] Apovian and colleagues[35] recommend "perioperative beta blockers in patients with stable or suspected coronary artery disease, unless contraindicated." However, some side effects of beta-blockade, such as impaired glucose tolerance, increased insulin resistance, and other metabolic abnormalities, can be harmful in severely obese patients or patients with metabolic syndrome.[7] Other medications, such as antihypertensives, should be continued preoperatively up to the operation.[3,12]

Routine intraoperative hemodynamic monitoring should be initiated using telemetry and blood pressure monitoring.[19] Given the increased size of extremities in some obese patients, ankle and wrist pressures are acceptable, if it is not possible to obtain routine arm noninvasive pressures. Blood pressure cuffs should be long enough to encircle at least 75% of the arm and the wide enough to encircle 40% of the arm.[3,9,33] Invasive arterial or pulmonary catheter monitoring may be needed in the superobese (>60 BMI), patients with severe cardiopulmonary disease, those with access difficulties, and patients with unreliable noninvasive cuff readings.[3,7,9,10,14,17–19] Intraoperative transesophageal echocardiography has been used, but no data exist to support everyday use.[20,33] The American College of Cardiology (ACC) and American Heart Association (AHA) task force 2007 guidelines recommend postoperative cardiac monitoring in patients with single or multiple risk factors for coronary artery disease who are undergoing noncardiac surgery,[36] as does the AACE/TOS/ASMBS guideline recommendation for at least the first 24 hours.[31]

GASTROINTESTINAL SYSTEM/NUTRITION

Although most elective cases do not require extensive work-up of gastrointestinal reflux disease (GERD), cholelithiasis, *Helicobacter pylori*, or fatty liver and nonalcoholic steatohepatitis, the AACE/TOS/ASMBS guidelines recommend work-up in symptomatic patients when preparing for weight loss surgery.[31] GERD should be treated preoperatively with proton pump inhibitors or histamine receptor blockers.[14,19]

Obese patients commonly (15%–25%) have type 2 diabetes.[28] Hyperglycemia can delay wound healing, increase infection rate, and cause significant postoperative morbidity. The AACE/TOS/ASMBS guidelines indorse preoperative glycemic control targets of hemoglobin A1c of 6.5% to 7% or less, fasting blood glucose level of less than or equal to 110 mg/dL, and a 2-hour postprandial blood glucose level of less than or equal to 140 mg/dL.[31] Less stringent targets can be applied to patients with extensive comorbid conditions, long-standing and hard-to-control diabetes despite intensive medical therapy, and those with advance microvascular and macrovascular disease per the AACE/TOS/ASMBS guidelines.[31] Before surgery, oral hypoglycemics should be withheld and blood glucose should be controlled with a sliding scale.[3,12] Intensive insulin therapy (target of 110 mg/dL) is recommended in the perioperative period because of a reduction in in-hospital death, length of stay, and improvement in clinical outcomes.[37]

Proper nutrition is paramount to decrease morbidity and mortality postoperatively. Surgical stress can cause protein malnutrition, ureagenesis, and accelerated protein breakdown secondary to increased insulin levels from stress blocking lipid use in obese patients.[7,38]

The AACE/TOS/ASMBS guidelines and Apovian and colleagues[35] suggest preoperative nutritional screening, because deficiencies of nutrients such as iron, thiamine, vitamin B_{12}, and vitamin D are common.[31]

The American Society for Parenteral and Enteral Nutrition (ASPEN) guidelines weakly recommend a high-protein, hypocaloric diet.[39] They define hypocaloric feeds as 50% to 70% of estimated energy needs or less than 14 kcal/kg actual body weight, and define high protein as 1.2 g/kg actual body weight or 2 to 2.5 g/kg IBW, with adjustment of goal protein intake determined by nitrogen balance studies. They strongly recommend all patients be screened for nutrition risk within 48 hours of admission and for critically ill, obese patients to have a nutrition assessment and support plan in placed within 48 hours of intensive care unit admission.[39] To determine energy requirement, indirect calorimetry should be used.[7] If unavailable, the ASPEN guidelines recommend the Penn State University 2010 predictive equation to determine energy requirements, with the modified Penn State equation being used in patients more than 60 years old.[39] Although the 2013 AHA/ACC/TOS guidelines also suggest a hypocaloric, high-protein diet, they also offer options for nutrition, such as the AHA Step 1 diet, a macronutrient targeted diet, and a Mediterranean-style diet.[40]

RENAL SYSTEM/FLUIDS

The comorbidities (cardiovascular disease, hypertension, diabetes) associated with obesity lead to an increase in chronic kidney disease (CKD).[41–44] Obesity-related glomerulopathy is the process resulting in proteinuria and renal dysfunction associated with structural changes, such as glomerulomegaly and focal segmental glomerular sclerosis.[41,43–46] Other hypothesized mechanisms by which obesity affects kidney function are inflammatory cytokines, oxidative stress, intraoperative and postoperative hemodynamics, and pharmacologic nephrotoxicity.[43,44,47] However, the exact pathophysiology of these mechanisms is unknown at this time.

The literature has shown an association with obesity and acute kidney injury (AKI) postoperatively and in the intensive care unit.[42,45–48] Glance and colleagues[11] reported a 2-fold to 3-fold increased risk of postoperative AKI in obese patients using the American College of Surgeons (ACS) National Surgical Quality Improvement Program database. Risk factors for postoperative AKI in bariatric patients include age greater than 50 years; BMI greater than 35; hyperlipidemia; hypertension; preoperative CKD; diabetes; male gender; long operative times; intraoperative hypotension; and preoperative use of statins, angiotensin-converting enzyme inhibitors (ACE-Is), and angiotensin II receptor blockers (ARBs).[24,42,45,46,48,49] AKI related to long operative time is usually secondary to rhabdomyolysis, with an overall incidence of 7% in bariatric patients.[50] Recommendations regarding the optimization or reduction of AKI postoperatively include avoiding preoperative exposure to nephrotoxic agents (eg, antibiotics, ARBs, ACE-Is), adequate fluid administration, avoiding intraoperative and postoperative hypotension, avoiding long operative times, and use of invasive hemodynamic monitoring to aid in intraoperative hemodynamic monitoring.

Fluid management in obese surgical patients can be difficult, because body fluid compartments are different compared with nonobese patients.[12,51,52] A urine output of approximately 1 mL/kg/h based on lean body mass is a good predictor of adequate fluid replacement in obese patients, with 4 to 5 L of crystalloid as an average for a 2-hour operation.[12] Recommendations regarding fluid management in obese patients are limited, because there are no large randomized controlled trials on morbidity and mortality in liberal versus restrictive fluid management in this population. Ingrande and Brodsky[51] advise that fluid be goal directed, using maximal stroke volume via transesophageal Doppler monitoring.

SURGICAL SITE INFECTIONS

Surgical site infections are increased in the obese population and the cause is likely multifactorial, including such factors as diabetic and obesity-related immune dysfunction, decreased perioperative tissue oxygenation and perfusion, and inadequate antimicrobial dosing.[7,9,14,18,19,53–57] In the 2013 Clinical Practice Guidelines for Antimicrobial Prophylaxis in Surgery developed by the American Society of Health-System Pharmacists, the Infectious Diseases Society of America (IDSA), the Surgical Infection Society, and the Society for Health care Epidemiology of America, the optimal timing of initial antibiotic dosing was recommended to be 60 minutes before incision, with 120 minutes for fluoroquinolones or vancomycin. In addition, 3 g of cefazolin were recommended in patients weighing more than 120 kg and 2 g if using cefoxitin or cefotaxime in obese patients. The systematic review by Fischer and colleagues[58] reported that cefazolin is appropriate for prophylaxis, although a specific dose was not reported. Furthermore, conclusive recommendations for weight-based dosing in obese patients are not currently possible, because there are insufficient data showing better efficacy than standard dosage regimens.[53] Given the increased body mass and volume of distribution, studies evaluating the pharmacokinetics in the obese population, such as the piperacillin/tazobactam pharmacokinetics study, are needed.[59] Al-Benna[14] recommended that any skin infection, such as *Candida albicans*, should be treated preoperatively.

MUSCULOSKELETAL DISORDERS

Obesity is a well-known risk factor for several types of musculoskeletal disorder, such as arthritis and gout,[60] that can affect mobility. Nevertheless, early postoperative mobilization is vital to decreasing pulmonary, skin, and thrombotic complications[7,9,12,17–19,34] and should occur as soon as possible, even if only to a chair.[19] To achieve early mobilization, multiple modalities and services are needed, including adjustment to hospital facilities. The ACS and the ASMBS joined their bariatric surgery accreditation programs to form a unified national standard, the Metabolic and Bariatric Surgery Accreditation and Quality Improvement Program, which released detailed standards and pathways for accreditation of metabolic and bariatric surgery centers in 2014, describing the physical and human resources needed to manage obese patients in an ACS-designated bariatric surgery center. Resources dealing specifically with mobility and musculoskeletal health, such as equipment and staff needed for transfer and patient movement, are detailed within this standard.[61] Further recommendations included adequate radiological facilities, medical imaging equipment, blood pressure cuffs, specialized wheelchairs, beds, enlarged doorways, expanded gowns, rooms, and bathrooms.[10,14,18,19,61] The recommendation has been made that toilet and shower seats be floor mounted rather than wall mounted to avoid injurious falls if the facility breaks away from the wall.[10,18,19,62]

Operative tables capable of holding more than 250 to 350 kg are needed.[9,10,14,17,34] Proper restraints should be used to avoid patients slipping off the table during position changes.[9,10,14] O'Leary and colleagues[19] suggest the use of an extra-large table strap placed at the hips and a footrest and placement of the feet in the dorsiflexed position if using reverse Trendelenburg. A bean bag may help in securing the patient.[10,14,19] Care in positioning and padding to avoid nerve injuries and rhabdomyolysis is important because of an increased prevalence of these problems in obese patients.[9,10,14,17,34] Common nerves injured by positioning and traction are the brachial plexus, sciatic, lateral femoral cutaneous, and ulnar nerve, with increased BMI and male gender being risk factors for these injuries.[9,18,34] If postoperative neuropathies are found, neurologic consultation and nerve conduction studies may be warranted if severe, but most resolve over time.[9]

In 2008, Medicare stopped reimbursement for management of stage III and IV pressure ulcers if they developed within the hospital stay.[63] Preoperative evaluation for pressure ulcers on obese patients is needed to provide adequate documentation and treatment at the time of admission. After surgery, skin care should be assessed at frequent intervals, and patients unable to mobilize themselves should be turned every 2 hours, even if on a special mattress such as an air or rotating mattress.[10,62] Inspection of skin should include lifting, cleaning, and drying skin folds, and attention should be paid to skin areas that are touching structures, such as the bed side, lines, drains, and tracheostomy or endotracheal tubing.[62]

DEEP VENOUS THROMBOSIS/THROMBOEMBOLISM

Likely secondary from decreased mobility, increased pressure on the venous system, and increased venous stasis, obesity is a risk factor for deep venous thrombosis (DVT) and pulmonary embolism (PE).[7,8,14,64,65] Other risk factors include obesity hypoventilation syndrome, pulmonary hypertension, immobility, hormonal therapy, expected long operative times or an open approach, and male gender.[66] Even with perioperative prophylaxis, the estimated incidences of DVT and PE in obese patients range from 0.2% to 2.4%,[12,14] therefore a combined protocol of pneumatic-compression lower extremity devices and anticoagulant chemoprophylaxis is needed to reduce the risk of DVT and PE.[12,18,28,31,66]

However, there are currently no universal dosing protocols, standard type of chemoprophylaxis used, or dosage duration. The American College of Chest Physicians has suggested higher dosages of low-molecular-weight heparin (LMWH) for obese patients.[67] The American Society for Metabolic and Bariatric Surgery recommends LMWH rather than unfractionated heparin (UFH) and refers to the Bariatric Outcomes Longitudinal Database (BOLD), which shows that 73% of venous thromboembolism (VTE) events occur after discharge. It therefore recommends extended VTE prophylaxis be considered for high-risk patients, but does not offer dosage or duration recommendations.[66] The AACE/TOS/ASMBS Clinical Practice Guidelines recommend either UFH or LMWH to be started within 24 hours postoperatively and consideration of extended chemoprophylaxis in high-risk patients, but also does not give dosage or duration recommendations.[31]

Literature exists to support that BMI or weight-based dosing, monitored by factor Xa levels, is superior to standard dosage, and that 0.5 mg/kg actual body weight subcutaneously daily is an appropriate dosage for morbidly obese patients.[68–70] The target factor Xa level used was 0.2 to 0.4 IU/mL.[68] Singh and colleagues[71] found in their small retrospective study that preoperative and postoperative LMWH is well tolerated. However, randomized controlled trials are lacking. Also in the literature, an extended prophylaxis duration of 28 to 35 days is recommended in high-risk patients.[68]

The use of prophylactic inferior vena cava (IVC) filter placement routinely in obese patients before surgery is controversial. Although no consensus definition of high risk exists, recommendations exist for IVC filters for obese patients with prior venous stasis disease, previous PE/DVT, patients who are superobese or have BMI greater than 55 kg/m^2, or patients with known hypercoagulable conditions.[3,15,18,72,73] The ASMBS does not support the use of IVC filters as the sole method of prophylaxis but as an adjunct to pharmacologic and mechanical prophylaxis in high-risk obese patients.[66] The AACE/TOS/ASMBS mention the Michigan Bariatric Collaborative study, which found that prophylactic IVC filter placement did not decrease VTE-related events or death, as well as the BOLD database, which reported that the risk of VTE was greater with IVC filters and therefore do not recommend it in the guidelines.[31] If a filter is placed, timing of removal is preferably within 3 months to have the best chance for successful removal.[72,73]

SUMMARY

It is hoped that this article explains the complex issues in the management of obese patients who require an integrative and multidisciplinary team for a successful hospital stay and offers a good reference for practicing surgeons in the perioperative management of this challenging, but increasingly common, patient population.

REFERENCES

1. Flegal KM, Carroll MD, Kit BK, et al. Prevalence of obesity and trends in the distribution of body mass index among US adults, 1999-2010. JAMA 2012;307:491–7.
2. Ogden CL, Lamb MM, Carroll MD, et al. Obesity and socioeconomic status in adults: United States, 2005-2008. NCHS Data Brief 2010;1–8.
3. Kuruba R, Koche LS, Murr MM. Preoperative assessment and perioperative care of patients undergoing bariatric surgery. Med Clin North Am 2007;91:339–51, ix.
4. Livingston EH. The incidence of bariatric surgery has plateaued in the US. Am J Surg 2010;200:378–85.
5. Buchwald H, Oien DM. Metabolic/bariatric surgery worldwide 2008. Obes Surg 2009;19:1605–11.
6. Obesity: preventing and managing the global epidemic. Report of a WHO consultation. World Health Organ Tech Rep Ser 2000;894:i–xii, 1–253.
7. Cullen A, Ferguson A. Perioperative management of the severely obese patient: a selective pathophysiological review. Can J Anaesth 2012;59:974–96.
8. Levin PD, Weissman C. Obesity, metabolic syndrome, and the surgical patient. Med Clin North Am 2009;93:1049–63.
9. Abir F, Bell R. Assessment and management of the obese patient. Crit Care Med 2004;32:S87–91.
10. DeMaria EJ, Carmody BJ. Perioperative management of special populations: obesity. Surg Clin North Am 2005;85:1283–9, xii.
11. Glance LG, Wissler R, Mukamel DB, et al. Perioperative outcomes among patients with the modified metabolic syndrome who are undergoing noncardiac surgery. Anesthesiology 2010;113:859–72.
12. Ramchandani L, Belani K. Anesthesia considerations in the obese. In: Buchwald H, Cowan G, Pories WJ, editors. Surgical management of obesity. 1st edition. Philadelphia: Saunders Elsevier; 2007. p. 108–18.
13. Adesanya AO, Lee W, Greilich NB, et al. Perioperative management of obstructive sleep apnea. Chest 2010;138:1489–98.
14. Al-Benna S. Perioperative management of morbid obesity. J Perioper Pract 2011;21:225–33.
15. Kaw R, Aboussouan L, Auckley D, et al. Challenges in pulmonary risk assessment and perioperative management in bariatric surgery patients. Obes Surg 2008;18:134–8.
16. Mickelson SA. Preoperative and postoperative management of obstructive sleep apnea patients. Otolaryngol Clin North Am 2007;40:877–89.
17. Huschak G, Busch T, Kaisers UX. Obesity in anesthesia and intensive care. Best Pract Res Clin Endocrinol Metab 2013;27:247–60.
18. McGlinch BP, Que FG, Nelson JL, et al. Perioperative care of patients undergoing bariatric surgery. Mayo Clin Proc 2006;81:S25–33.
19. O'Leary J, Paige J, Martin L. Perioperative management of the bariatric surgery patient. In: Buchwald H, Cowan G, Pories WJ, editors. Surgical management of obesity. 1st edition. Philadelphia: Saunders Elsevier; 2007. p. 119–30.
20. Poirier P, Alpert MA, Fleisher LA, et al. Cardiovascular evaluation and management of severely obese patients undergoing surgery: a science advisory from the American Heart Association. Circulation 2009;120:86–95.
21. Servin F. Ambulatory anesthesia for the obese patient. Curr Opin Anaesthesiol 2006;19:597–9.
22. Porhomayon J, Leissner KB, El-Solh AA, et al. Strategies in postoperative analgesia in the obese obstructive sleep apnea patient. Clin J Pain 2013;29:998–1005.

23. Chand B, Gugliotti D, Schauer P, et al. Perioperative management of the bariatric surgery patient: focus on cardiac and anesthesia considerations. Cleve Clin J Med 2006;73(Suppl 1):S51–6.
24. Chakravartty S, Sarma DR, Patel AG. Rhabdomyolysis in bariatric surgery: a systematic review. Obes Surg 2013;23:1333–40.
25. Schumann R, Jones SB, Ortiz VE, et al. Best practice recommendations for anesthetic perioperative care and pain management in weight loss surgery. Obes Res 2005;13:254–66.
26. Leykin Y, Pellis T, Del Mestro E, et al. Anesthetic management of morbidly obese and super-morbidly obese patients undergoing bariatric operations: hospital course and outcomes. Obes Surg 2006;16:1563–9.
27. Pelosi P, Gregoretti C. Perioperative management of obese patients. Best Pract Res Clin Anaesthesiol 2010;24:211–25.
28. Benotti P, Rodriguez H. Preoperative preparation of the bariatric surgery patient. In: Buchwald H, Cowan G, Pories WJ, editors. Surgical management of obesity. 1st edition. Philadelphia: Saunders Elsevier; 2007. p. 102–7.
29. Murphy C, Wong DT. Airway management and oxygenation in obese patients. Can J Anaesth 2013;60:929–45.
30. Schachter L. Respiratory assessment and management in bariatric surgery. Respirology 2012;17:1039–47.
31. Mechanick JI, Youdim A, Jones DB, et al. Clinical practice guidelines for the perioperative nutritional, metabolic, and nonsurgical support of the bariatric surgery patient–2013 update: cosponsored by American Association of Clinical Endocrinologists, the Obesity Society, and American Society for Metabolic & Bariatric Surgery. Surg Obes Relat Dis 2013;9:159–91.
32. Tung A. Anaesthetic considerations with the metabolic syndrome. Br J Anaesth 2010;105(Suppl 1):i24–33.
33. Katkhouda N, Mason RJ, Wu B, et al. Evaluation and treatment of patients with cardiac disease undergoing bariatric surgery. Surg Obes Relat Dis 2012;8:634–40.
34. Guss D, Bhattacharyya T. Perioperative management of the obese orthopaedic patient. J Am Acad Orthop Surg 2006;14:425–32.
35. Apovian CM, Cummings S, Anderson W, et al. Best practice updates for multidisciplinary care in weight loss surgery. Obesity (Silver Spring) 2009;17:871–9.
36. Fleisher LA, Beckman JA, Brown KA, et al. ACC/AHA 2007 guidelines on perioperative cardiovascular evaluation and care for noncardiac surgery: a report of the American College of Cardiology/American Heart Association Task Force on Practice Guidelines (Writing Committee to Revise the 2002 Guidelines on Perioperative Cardiovascular Evaluation for Noncardiac Surgery): developed in collaboration with the American Society of Echocardiography, American Society of Nuclear Cardiology, Heart Rhythm Society, Society of Cardiovascular Anesthesiologists, Society for Cardiovascular Angiography and Interventions, Society for Vascular Medicine and Biology, and Society for Vascular Surgery. Circulation 2007;116:e418–99.
37. Watson K. Surgical risk in patients with metabolic syndrome: focus on lipids and hypertension. Curr Cardiol Rep 2006;8:433–8.
38. Lugli AK, Wykes L, Carli F. Strategies for perioperative nutrition support in obese, diabetic and geriatric patients. Clin Nutr 2008;27:16–24.
39. Choban P, Dickerson R, Malone A, et al. A.S.P.E.N. clinical guidelines: nutrition support of hospitalized adult patients with obesity. JPEN J Parenter Enteral Nutr 2013;37:714–44.

40. Jensen MD, Ryan DH, Apovian CM, et al. 2013 AHA/ACC/TOS guideline for the management of overweight and obesity in adults: a report of the American College of Cardiology/American Heart Association Task Force on Practice Guidelines and The Obesity Society. Circulation 2014;129:S102–38.
41. Currie A, Chetwood A, Ahmed AR. Bariatric surgery and renal function. Obes Surg 2011;21:528–39.
42. Kelz RR, Reinke CE, Zubizarreta JR, et al. Acute kidney injury, renal function, and the elderly obese surgical patient: a matched case-control study. Ann Surg 2013; 258:359–63.
43. Suneja M, Kumar AB. Obesity and perioperative acute kidney injury: a focused review. J Crit Care 2014;29:694.e1–6.
44. Thethi T, Kamiyama M, Kobori H. The link between the renin-angiotensin-aldosterone system and renal injury in obesity and the metabolic syndrome. Curr Hypertens Rep 2012;14:160–9.
45. Thakar CV, Kharat V, Blanck S, et al. Acute kidney injury after gastric bypass surgery. Clin J Am Soc Nephrol 2007;2:426–30.
46. Weingarten TN, Gurrieri C, McCaffrey JM, et al. Acute kidney injury following bariatric surgery. Obes Surg 2013;23:64–70.
47. Billings FT, Pretorius M, Schildcrout JS, et al. Obesity and oxidative stress predict AKI after cardiac surgery. J Am Soc Nephrol 2012;23:1221–8.
48. Bucaloiu ID, Perkins RM, DiFilippo W, et al. Acute kidney injury in the critically ill, morbidly obese patient: diagnostic and therapeutic challenges in a unique patient population. Crit Care Clin 2010;26:607–24.
49. McCullough PA, Gallagher MJ, Dejong AT, et al. Cardiorespiratory fitness and short-term complications after bariatric surgery. Chest 2006;130:517–25.
50. Ettinger JE, Marcilio de Souza CA, Azaro E, et al. Clinical features of rhabdomyolysis after open and laparoscopic Roux-en-Y gastric bypass. Obes Surg 2008;18: 635–43.
51. Ingrande J, Brodsky JB. Intraoperative fluid management and bariatric surgery. Int Anesthesiol Clin 2013;51:80–9.
52. Matot I, Paskaleva R, Eid L, et al. Effect of the volume of fluids administered on intraoperative oliguria in laparoscopic bariatric surgery: a randomized controlled trial. Arch Surg 2012;147:228–34.
53. Bratzler DW, Dellinger EP, Olsen KM, et al. Clinical practice guidelines for antimicrobial prophylaxis in surgery. Surg Infect (Larchmt) 2013;14:73–156.
54. Cardosi RJ, Drake J, Holmes S, et al. Subcutaneous management of vertical incisions with 3 or more centimeters of subcutaneous fat. Am J Obstet Gynecol 2006;195:607–14 [discussion: 614–6].
55. Kabon B, Nagele A, Reddy D, et al. Obesity decreases perioperative tissue oxygenation. Anesthesiology 2004;100:274–80.
56. Mullen JT, Davenport DL, Hutter MM, et al. Impact of body mass index on perioperative outcomes in patients undergoing major intra-abdominal cancer surgery. Ann Surg Oncol 2008;15:2164–72.
57. Wiedemann D, Schachner T, Bonaros N, et al. Does obesity affect operative times and perioperative outcome of patients undergoing totally endoscopic coronary artery bypass surgery? Interact Cardiovasc Thorac Surg 2009;9:214–7.
58. Fischer MI, Dias C, Stein A, et al. Antibiotic prophylaxis in obese patients submitted to bariatric surgery. A systematic review. Acta Cir Bras 2014;29:209–17.
59. Sturm AW, Allen N, Rafferty KD, et al. Pharmacokinetic analysis of piperacillin administered with tazobactam in critically ill, morbidly obese surgical patients. Pharmacotherapy 2014;34:28–35.

60. Li Z, Bowerman S, Heber D. Health ramifications of the obesity epidemic. Surg Clin North Am 2005;85:681–701, v.
61. Resources for optimal care of the metabolic and bariatric surgery patient 2014. Metabolic and Bariatric Surgery Accreditation and Quality Improvement Program standards and pathway manual. 2014. Available at: http://www.mbsaqip.org/docs/Resources%20for%20Optimal%20Care%20of%20the%20MBS%20Patient.pdf. Accessed June 1, 2014.
62. Davidson JE, Callery C. Care of the obesity surgery patient requiring immediate-level care or intensive care. Obes Surg 2001;11:93–7.
63. Hospital-acquired conditions. 2012. Available at: http://www.cms.gov/Medicare/Medicare-Fee-for-Service-Payment/HospitalAcqCond/Hospital-Acquired_Conditions.html. Accessed June 1, 2014.
64. Desciak MC, Martin DE. Perioperative pulmonary embolism: diagnosis and anesthetic management. J Clin Anesth 2011;23:153–65.
65. Kehl-Pruett W. Deep vein thrombosis in hospitalized patients: a review of evidence-based guidelines for prevention. Dimens Crit Care Nurs 2006;25:53–9 [quiz: 60–1].
66. American Society for Metabolic and Bariatric Surgery Clinical Issues Committee. ASMBS updated position statement on prophylactic measures to reduce the risk of venous thromboembolism in bariatric surgery patients. Surg Obes Relat Dis 2013;9:493–7.
67. Huo MH, Spyropoulos AC. The eighth American College of Chest Physicians guidelines on venous thromboembolism prevention: implications for hospital prophylaxis strategies. J Thromb Thrombolysis 2011;31:196–208.
68. Borkgren-Okonek MJ, Hart RW, Pantano JE, et al. Enoxaparin thromboprophylaxis in gastric bypass patients: extended duration, dose stratification, and antifactor Xa activity. Surg Obes Relat Dis 2008;4:625–31.
69. Ludwig KP, Simons HJ, Mone M, et al. Implementation of an enoxaparin protocol for venous thromboembolism prophylaxis in obese surgical intensive care unit patients. Ann Pharmacother 2011;45:1356–62.
70. Rondina MT, Wheeler M, Rodgers GM, et al. Weight-based dosing of enoxaparin for VTE prophylaxis in morbidly obese, medically-Ill patients. Thromb Res 2010;125:220–3.
71. Singh K, Podolsky ER, Um S, et al. Evaluating the safety and efficacy of BMI-based preoperative administration of low-molecular-weight heparin in morbidly obese patients undergoing Roux-en-Y gastric bypass surgery. Obes Surg 2012;22:47–51.
72. Shamian B, Chamberlain RS. The role for prophylaxis inferior vena cava filters in patients undergoing bariatric surgery: replacing anecdote with evidence. Am Surg 2012;78:1349–61.
73. Vaziri K, Devin Watson J, Harper AP, et al. Prophylactic inferior vena cava filters in high-risk bariatric surgery. Obes Surg 2011;21:1580–4.

Perioperative Management of Elderly Patients

Lisa L. Schlitzkus, MD, Alyson A. Melin, DO, Jason M. Johanning, MD, Paul J. Schenarts, MD*

KEYWORDS

- Elderly • Geriatric • Perioperative management • Surgery • Frailty
- Preoperative care • Postoperative care

KEY POINTS

- The older population is rapidly growing and living longer, and this growth is expected to drastically increase surgical demand for both elective and emergent cases.
- The elderly population undergoes significant changes of numerous organ systems as a result of the aging process; their tenuous homeostasis can be drastically unraveled by minor changes in the perioperative period.
- The perioperative management of the elderly population is complex and requires a multidisciplinary team focusing on education, frequent assessment, functional status, and quality-of-life outcomes as well as traditional outcome measures.
- There remains a paucity of best-practice guidelines and randomized control trials focusing on the elderly; there are growing data investigating frailty indices as predictors of outcomes in perioperative elderly patients.

INTRODUCTION

Because of longer life expectancies and the aging baby boomer generation, the growth of the aging American population at this time is unprecedented.[1–3] One out of every 7 Americans is older than 65 years, and there has been a 21% increase in this age group over the past 10 years.[1] With a life expectancy of about 20 years, the older population (65+ years) is becoming older. Since 1900, the 65- to 74-year age group is 10 times larger; the 75- to 84-year group is 17 times larger; and the group aged 85 years and older is 48 times larger.[1] The centenarian population has had a 93% increase since 1980, a larger percentage increase than the total population.[1]

None of the undersigned authors have any conflict of interests to report.

Department of Surgery, University of Nebraska Medical Center, 983280 Nebraska Medical Center, Omaha, NE 68198-3280, USA
* Corresponding author.
E-mail address: Paul.Schenarts@unmc.edu

Surg Clin N Am 95 (2015) 391–415
http://dx.doi.org/10.1016/j.suc.2014.12.001 surgical.theclinics.com
0039-6109/15/$ – see front matter

Moreover, the older population has the highest incidence rate for 60% of operations compared with other age groups.[4] It is predicted that the amount of procedure-based work in general surgery will grow by 31% by 2020 because of the growing older patient population.[4] These patients often are not the healthiest, with multiple comorbidities, malnutrition, frailty, and little reserve. As the elderly become our primary surgical population, we will need to understand the differences in their physiology as we are challenged with their perioperative care.

ASSESSMENT OF OPERATIVE RISK

Geriatric patients now compose a significant number of patients undergoing surgical intervention in the United States,[5] and many of these patients undergo operative procedures in the last year of their life.[6] The geriatric surgical population with its unique physiology and response to surgical insult poses challenges in perioperative assessment. It is now well established that frailty is a strong predictor of perioperative complication and mortality in surgical patients. Frailty is a recognized geriatric syndrome with no agreed on or recognized definition unfortunately.[7–9] For the sake of surgical understanding, the most important definition would be an inability to tolerate physiologic insult. What is better known, however, is that frailty can be defined by specific indicators, including cognitive, functional, social, and nutritional function. Varying measures of these functional areas are now recognized as strong predictors of perioperative outcomes.[10,11]

As frailty is now recognized as a strong predictor of postoperative outcomes in multiple specialties, it is imperative to recognize frailty in geriatric surgical patients. Therefore, one must be able to assess frailty before operations and be familiar with the tools to assess frailty. A stepwise approach to assessing frailty will be the accepted approach in the future. This approach will consist of a screening tool to identify those patients who are potentially frail based on a bedside screen of frailty characteristics. If patients have findings consistent with frailty, a more formal assessment in the form of the comprehensive geriatric assessment would be in order to provide for a more detailed workup and provide for shared decision making, surgical buy-in, discussion about increased morbidity and mortality compared with younger patients, and ultimately bring the surgical team together to increase communication in high-risk patients. The comprehensive geriatric assessment is a multidisciplinary process that serves to identify limitations in frail patients in an effort to develop a coordinated treatment plan to optimize their management.[10,12] The assessment accounts for functional independence—caring for themselves in their environment, which is usually the most important factor to geriatric patients—maintaining quality of life. This multidisciplinary assessment results in patients less likely to require nursing home admission as demonstrated in a randomized controlled trial.[13] Fried and colleagues[9] describe a phenotype (Fried-Hopkins frailty index):

- Shrinking
- Weakness
- Poor endurance and energy
- Slowness
- Low physical activity level

When combined with other standard prediction models (American Society of Anesthesiologists, Lee, and Eagle scores), the Fried phenotype improved the predictive power of the usual models[11]; when used alone for elective operations, it showed an increased risk of complications, length of stay, and discharge to facility.[11] Other assessment tools to date include the Rockwood-Robinson frailty index[7,14] and assessments of gait speed,[15] grip strength,[16] and initiation of movement.[17] These specific tools help clinicians to recognize additional risk factors compared with younger, nonfrail surgical patients. It is imperative that risk factors be defined preoperatively using an appropriate geriatric risk assessment to allow for a candid and a more accurate discussion with elderly patients regarding their risk of surgical intervention and outcomes.

Another related but distinct concept to be aware of in geriatric patients is that of sarcopenia. Sarcopenia is distinctly different from frailty with areas of overlap in the relationship primarily with regard to nutrition with markedly decreased muscle mass compared with age-matched controls. This decreased muscle mass similar to frailty is correlated with markedly increased risks of mortality and complications.[18,19] Sarcopenia, in contrast to frailty, has more defined measurement tools consisting of hand grip strength and psoas or total abdominal muscle area as measured by computed tomography scan. Similar to frailty, sarcopenia seems reasonable to assess, specifically in specialties whereby frail patients are not routinely considered for major surgical intervention (transplant, cardiac surgery). Cachexia is a metabolic syndrome associated with underlying illness leading to muscle loss. An upregulation of interleukin 1 (IL-1), IL-6, and tumor necrosis factor–alpha is observed leading to lipolysis, muscle breakdown, and anorexia.[20,21] Sarcopenia, present in half of patients older than 80 years,[22] not only involves the loss of muscle mass but also the loss of strength and functionality.[23,24]

PHARMACOKINETICS

The normal aging process results in changes in body composition and essentially all tissues. These changes significantly influence the pharmacologic effects and dosing of analgesic and anesthetic medications.

As the body ages, there is a shift in body mass from muscle to adipose tissue. This progressive adiposity is also associated with a loss of lean body mass and a decrease in total body water, making appropriate dosing of medications challenging. The expansion of adipose tissue increases the reservoir of lipid-soluble agents, contributing to the protracted clearance and increased duration of action for benzodiazepines, volatile agents, narcotics, and sedative-hyponotics.[25] In addition, the decrease in total body water decreases the volume of distribution for water-soluble medications, resulting in higher average and peak plasma concentrations.[26] This condition ultimately results in an exaggerated drug effect. For example, the initial volume of distribution for thiopental in patients aged 20 to 40 years is 15 to 30 L; however, this decreases to 3 to 7 L in patients aged 60 to 90 years.[27] The end result is that the dosing of many anesthetic drugs needs to be reduced. Complicating matters further, geriatric patients frequently suffer from malnutrition. Medications such as propofol and diazepam are highly bound to albumin. Low albumin levels can result in increased levels of free drug and subsequent increased sensitivity to these drugs.[28]

In addition to changes in body composition, age-related changes to the anatomy and physiology of various organs also influence the use of various medications. The kidneys lose approximately 10% of parenchymal thickness per decade of life.[29] Between 20 and 90 years of age, a 50% decrease in renal blood flow contributes to a 30% to 50% decrease in glomerular filtration rate.[26,29] Simultaneously, there is a decrease in hepatic mass by 20% to 40% and a decline in hepatic blood flow with advancing age.[30] This age-related impairment in renal and hepatic function affects the metabolism and excretion of multiple analgesic, sedative, and anesthetic agents.

The loss of neurons and decline in cognitive function in the elderly may increase the sensitivity to certain medications. These neuronal changes result in increased sedation and cardiorespiratory depression at lower blood concentration levels.[31] In contradistinction, the elderly may also have a higher threshold for pain perception.[32] Another consideration in the elderly is delayed drug absorption from the gastrointestinal tract, which leads to an inconsistent dose response relationship.[28]

It has been estimated that 40% of elderly patients take 5 or more different medications per week, and up to 19% use 10 or more medications per week.[33] This polypharmacy and drug-drug interactions are additive to the age-related changes in body composition and organ function rendering pharmacologic management in the elderly very challenging.

ANALGESIA IN THE ELDERLY

Narcotics are the mainstay of pain control. As a result of age-related increases in adipose tissue, narcotics and other lipophilic medications have a relatively larger reservoir and should be anticipated to have a prolonged or inconsistent effect. Elderly patients have been shown to have a 2-fold higher sensitivity to ventilatory depressive effects of opiates compared with younger patients.[34] Therefore, in the elderly, it is recommended to use a balanced (or multimodal) analgesic approach, which can minimize the adverse effects of opioids. Using a combination of local anesthetics, acetaminophen, nonsteroidal antiinflammatory drugs (NSAIDs), steroids, and nontraditional analgesic agents is safe and efficacious in this age group. White and colleagues[28] have compressively reviewed the use of this strategy in the elderly.

Local Anesthetics

The preemptive, adjunctive use of a subcutaneous or intra-articular local anesthetic has been demonstrated to reduce narcotic use.[35,36] The utility of adding epinephrine to prolong the duration is well known. However, the addition of clonidine, ketorolac, methylprednisolone, or dexamethasone also prolongs the duration of the local analgesic effect.[28,37–39]

Acetaminophen

Despite reduced hepatic function, acetaminophen has been shown to be safe in the elderly and does not require dosage adjustment compared with younger patients.[40,41]

Nonsteroidal Antiinflammatory Drugs

The effectiveness of NSAIDs for prevention of postoperative pain and reducing narcotic requirement is well known. However, the complications of these agents, such as platelet dysfunction, gastrointestinal bleeding, and kidney injury deserve special attention in the elderly.

Steroids

In addition to combining steroids with local anesthetics, steroids alone or as part of a multimodal regimen also have a beneficial effect on pain control.[42–44] Although there were no increased bleeding complications with this strategy, there may be an additional benefit of decreasing postoperative nausea and vomiting.[44–46]

Nontraditional Analgesic Drugs

Several nontraditional agents have been shown to improve pain management in the postoperative period. Ketamine (in a single dose, as an infusion during surgery, or as part of a multimodal approach) has been demonstrated to reduce postoperative pain and narcotic consumption and decrease the development of chronic pain.[47,48] The efficacy of adding gabapentin to a multimodal strategy for pain control may be useful, but the associated sedation and dizziness may limit its use in the elderly.[49,50] Alpha-2-agonists (ie, dexmedetomidine) have long been known to have an anesthetic-sparing effect but are now being used in the perioperative period where they have decreased fentanyl use, improved postanesthesia care unit length of stay, and decreased postoperative emesis.[51,52] Although not frequently considered to augment pain control, esmolol infusions have also been demonstrated to decrease opioid usage in the postoperative period.[53,54]

ANESTHESIA CONSIDERATIONS IN THE ELDERLY

Peripheral Nerve Blocks

Properly done, this approach is an excellent anesthetic in the elderly because it is site specific with few side effects. The use of peripheral nerve block offers better post-operative pain control, decreased opioid requirement, and increased patient satisfaction.[28] One potential downside of this approach is a documented higher risk of permanent nerve damage in elderly patients.[55]

General Anesthesia

Although fragile patients with multiple comorbidities may be best served by local or regional anesthesia, this is not true for most elderly patients. In a study of 800,000 patients, Arbous and colleagues[56] found that advanced age was not an independent risk factor for serious morbidity or mortality in patients undergoing general anesthesia. However, anesthetic management needs to be individualized for elderly patients. For example, when using propofol in the elderly, a lower induction dose is needed[57]; the slower blood-brain circulation results in a slower onset and delayed maximal cardiopulmonary depressive effect.[58] As a result of less compliant vasculature, the elderly are also more prone to develop hypotension with this agent.[28] The use of inhalational anesthetics also needs to be adjusted in the elderly. For every decade after 30 years of age, there is a 7% increase in the potency of inhalational agents.[59] In particular, desflurane offers more rapid recovery than other agents in this age group.[28,60]

Spinal and Epidural Anesthesia

The use of spinal or epidural techniques may be appropriate in the elderly; but the side effects of hypotension, dizziness, and delayed ambulation may especially have negative impacts in the elderly.[55] Additionally, given that prostatic hypertrophy is nearly universal in elderly men, this approach may be problematic.

POSTOPERATIVE COGNITIVE IMPAIRMENT IN THE ELDERLY

The importance of postoperative central nervous system dysfunction after surgery in the elderly is coming into greater focus. The basic science mechanisms underlying this are complex and beyond the scope of this publication. However, the work by Hussain and colleagues[61] provides an excellent overview of the topic. Two cognitive syndromes have been described in elderly postoperative patients: postoperative delirium (POD) and postoperative cognitive dysfunction, which differ with respect to onset, manifestations, and permanency.

Postoperative Delirium

POD occurs shortly after surgery and is an acute change in cognitive status characterized by fluctuating attention and consciousness as well as abnormalities in memory and perception.[62,63] It is estimated that the incidence of POD in older adults occurs between 36.8% and 73.5%.[62,64] Although common, this well-recognized clinical entity is associated with a prolonged hospital stay, delayed functional recovery, and increased morbidity and mortality.[65]

Pathophysiology

In general the pathophysiology of delirium is caused by an absolute or relative lack of the neurotransmitter acetylcholine or an excess of dopamine.[66,67] There are, however, multiple other contributing factors in play, including hypoglycemia; hypoxia; cytokines associated with the stress response; medications, such as penicillin, vasoactive agents, and tranquilizers; as well as histamine (type 2) blockers.[68] Dehydration and hypoperfusion are frequent causes of delirium in the elderly.[69] Delirium may also be the only finding in the elderly suffering from a postoperative infection.

The relative contributions of the surgical procedure and the type of anesthetic used yield interesting results. The inflammatory response and the resultant cognitive deficits are caused more by the operation than the use of a general anesthetic.[61] Likewise, the use of a general anesthetic did not confer a higher risk of POD compared with regional anesthesia in a meta-analysis.[70]

Risk Factors

Although preexisting psychiatric diseases, withdrawal from alcohol, nutritional deficiencies, and anticholinergic medications predispose the elderly to delirium, many of these are interrelated; it is difficult to identify the specific culprit.[65] Inouye and colleagues[71] have identified 5 independent risk factors in the elderly: baseline dementia, vision impairment, physical restraints, functional impairment, and several comorbidities.

Diagnosis

Delirium is chiefly characterized by acute onset, disorientation, disorganized thought and speech, disrupted sleep-wake cycle, memory disturbance, clouded consciousness, and hallucinations and elusions that last for days to weeks.[72] Several bedside cognitive function tests, such as the Mini-Mental Status Examination, the Abbreviated Mental Test, and the Confusion Assessment Method are easy to perform and are useful in confirming the diagnosis and following the level of improvement or decline.[65]

Prevention and Treatment

To reduce dopamine levels in order to prevent delirium, it would be reasonable to give haloperidol preoperatively. The prophylactic use of haloperidol demonstrated a reduction in the duration and severity of delirium but unfortunately not the incidence.[73] Rapid correction of dehydration and infectious cause will be beneficial in preventing delirium from developing. Continuation of eyeglasses and hearing aids should also be of utmost importance.

Once delirium has developed, the best acute treatment is haloperidol. This drug can be dosed starting at 0.5 mg and repeated every 15 to 30 minutes to a maximum dosage of 20 mg every 24 hours. If this is not effective, the addition of low-dose lorazepam, 0.5 mg up to 6 mg per 24 hours, can be used.[68] In addition to medication, frequent reorientation, normalization of the sleep-wake cycle, and increased daytime activities may also be beneficial.

Postoperative Cognitive Dysfunction

Unlike POD, postoperative cognitive dysfunction (POCD) occurs days to weeks after surgery and is characterized by impairment of memory, concentration, and social integration. Also unlike POD, POCD is milder but may remain a permanent disorder.[65] As a result, the implications of POCD have significant socioeconomic implications because of the increased need for long-term care.[65] Following noncardiac surgery, 25% of patients were demonstrated to have POCD. Although this improved to 10% at 3 months postoperatively, this is still a significant percentage far out from an operation.[74] Like POD, POCD is also associated with an increased mortality.[75]

Pathophysiology

Little is understood about the pathophysiologic mechanisms that cause POCD.

Risk Factors

The specific risk factors for the development of POCD are still under investigation. It is likely that there are multiple contributing factors. Unlike POD, there is an increased risk associated with general anesthesia[70] and inhalational anesthetics but no difference between desflurane versus servoflurane.[76] Similar to POD, patients with multiple medical problems and poor functional status are at an increased risk.[65]

Diagnosis

Diagnosis of POCD remains difficult because of the lack of uniform criteria and unreliable neuropsychological tests capable of detecting mild functional impairment.[65] POCD also shares several features of Alzheimer disease that further confounds the diagnosis.[61] Of note, POCD is not recognized in the *Diagnostic and Statistical Manual of Mental Disorders* (Fourth Edition).

Treatment

Unfortunately, there is no evidence that once POCD is diagnosed it can be successfully treated.[65]

PULMONARY

Pulmonary function is most notably affected by anatomic changes in the elderly. Kyphosis, vertebral compression, calcification of the costal cartilage, and contracture of the intercostal muscles lead to decreased chest wall compliance.[77] Loss of intercostal muscle strength alone can decrease maximum inspiratory and expiratory force by as much as 50%.[77,78] The loss of the elasticity of the lung parenchyma collapses small airways, leading to increased alveolar compliance with uneven ventilation and air trapping.[77,78] This perfusion mismatch results in a 0.3- to 0.4-mm Hg decrease per year in arterial oxygen tension.[78] Although total lung capacity remains unchanged, there is a mild increase in functional residual capacity (FRC; 1%–3% per decade) and an increase in residual volume (5%–10% per decade).[77,78] Thus, vital capacity decreases 20 to 30 mL per year.[77] Mucociliary clearance decreases, whereas swallowing dysfunction, loss of cough reflex, and oropharyngeal colonization contribute to aspiration.[79] Additionally, the neurologic autonomic response to hypoxia and hypercapnia is decreased by 40% and 50%, respectively.[79]

Just before extubation and in the immediate postoperative period, respiratory drive may be decreased because of the incomplete elimination of inhalational anesthetics, opioids, and benzodiazepines.[80] These medication side effects may be more prominent in the elderly because of altered pharmacokinetics and pharmacodynamics.[77]

Aggressive pulmonary toilet using incentive spirometry, early mobilization, and upright positioning, which increases FRC, are absolutes for elderly patients to prevent atelectasis.[77,80] Voluntary movement of the chest wall muscles may be limited by pain or physically disrupted with an incision.[77] Thoracic and abdominal operations are associated with higher rates of pulmonary complications,[79] and it is postulated that manipulation in these cavities results in afferent nerve inhibition of respiratory muscle function.[77]

Noninvasive ventilation has not been studied in elderly surgical patients; but in other patient populations, it has reduced intubation rates. Although noninvasive ventilation may initially be attempted in the elderly struggling after extubation, the failure rate is still about 30%.[79] A study of 330,000 patients demonstrates an exponential increase in the incident of acute respiratory failure each decade until 85 years of age.[81] Unfortunately, we as providers are inaccurate in identifying respiratory failure, attributing confusion, agitation, delirium, and altered level of consciousness to dementia and previous stroke rather than hypoxia and hypercarbia.[82] Our patients' self-perception of dyspnea and bronchoconstriction also decreases with age.[83]

Mechanical ventilation should not be withheld because of age alone.[84,85] After adjusting for severity of illness, Ely and colleagues[84] demonstrated that the 75-years-of-age-and-older cohort had an equivalent number of ventilator days, intensive care unit and hospital length of stay, and mortality rate compared with their younger counterparts. Theoretically we would expect the aforementioned physiologic changes with age to affect ventilator weaning.[86] Readiness to extubate may be as difficult to assess as need for intubation. Usual tools such as frequency-tidal volume ratio, negative inspiratory force, and minute ventilation are not predictive of extubation failure in the elderly.[84,87] For those intubated greater than 7 days, one prospective study of critically ill medical patients found that a rapid shallow breathing index less than 130 may improve the accuracy in predicting successful extubation.[88] Once an elderly patient has been on the ventilator for greater than 6 hours per day for more than 21 days, long-term ventilator dependence increases proportionately in those aged 70 years and older.[89]

Age is not an independent risk factor for perioperative pulmonary complications; comorbidities, especially chronic obstructive pulmonary disease (COPD), have a greater risk association with perioperative pulmonary complications.[90] COPD is the single most important predictor of perioperative pulmonary complications in the elderly with a 3- to 4-fold increased risk.[90]

CARDIOVASCULAR

The most common cause of death in perioperative elderly patients is cardiac.[91] In the elderly, it is difficult to decipher if complications arise because of cardiac disease versus the physiologic changes that accompany the normal aging process.

Specific anatomic changes are noted in the heart as aging occurs. The overall weight of the heart increases in women, the ventricular septum thickens proportionally more than the left ventricle wall, and the left atria dilates.[91–95] The diameter of the aortic root increases[94]; although the valves may become sclerosed and calcified, this has a minor impact on their function.[96] In fact, all 4 valves may become dilated,[97] explaining the multi-valvular regurgitation in healthy older adults. The actual shape changes from elliptical to spheroid.[95] The epicardium's fat content, especially overlying the right ventricle, increases.[91] On a cellular level, the actual number of myocytes decreases, whereas the size of those remaining increases.[98] There is an increase in intracellular lipofuscin, the degenerative pigment, amyloid, collagen, and elastin.[91,99,100] Within the conduction system, 90% of the sinus node cells are replaced by fat and connective tissue, and the tracts become fibrosed.[101] These changes also affect the cardiac vasculature, resulting in dilation, intimal thickening, and calcification independent of atherosclerosis.[91,93,100] The vessels become less compliant and reactive to nitric oxide and the renin-angiotensin system, resulting in increased systolic blood pressure and pulse pressure, turbulent flow, and elevated pulse wave velocities.[91,93,100] In fact, Roman and colleagues[102] demonstrated that the pulse pressure is a better predictor of cardiovascular events than systolic or diastolic blood pressure. Overall, these structural changes result in a stiff heart with decrease contractility and compliance and at risk for sick sinus syndrome, arrhythmias, and bundle branch blocks.

The impact of these structural changes on the function of the heart is difficult to assess with age, frailty, metabolic changes, overall cardiac health, and atherosclerotic disease complicating the picture. Generally, function is divided into systolic and diastolic function. Systolic function is usually preserved as the heart ages.[91,93,100] In diastole, the heart is slower to relax, so it fills slower and later in the phase.[93] However, as flow demand is increased, the aged heart is less responsive to catecholamines. Maximum heart rate is decreased. End diastolic volume and stroke volume increase. There is no change in end systolic volume. Peak ejection fraction and cardiac output decrease; overall, the size of the left ventricle increases, leading to decreased or nil reserve with greater risk for cardiac failure.[91,93,100]

Fifty percent of the elderly have abnormal resting electrocardiograms frequently caused by the aforementioned anatomic changes.[103] Echocardiograms are excellent in assessing chamber size and function, but can be difficult in the elderly because of chest wall deformities.[103] Likewise, exercise stress tests are limited by the physical ability of older patients. The sensitivity and specificity of dobutamine stress echocardiography to detect myocardia ischemia have not been studied in the elderly,[103] but myocardial perfusion scintigraphy using dipyridamole (Persantine) is well tolerated, with sensitivity, specificity, and safety equivalent to those less than 65 years old.[104]

Myocardial infarction mortality is increased in the elderly: 17.8% in those 75 years and older versus 2.0% in those less than 55 years.[105] In the perioperative period, it is important to remember that only one-third of those older than 85 years will present with classic chest pain.[103] Older patients may present with vague, nonspecific, nonclassic signs and symptoms caused by comorbidities and altered pain sensitivity,[103] such as

- Shortness of breath
- Heart failure
- Pulmonary edema
- Nausea
- Emesis
- Syncope
- Confusion
- Delirium
- Agitation
- Stroke

When assessing perioperative elderly surgical patients in failure, precipitants include anemia, infection, thyroid dysfunction, atrial fibrillation, dietary, and medications. A quick review of the overall picture can be insightful. First, determine if the failure is systolic or diastolic. Systolic failure presents with an insidious onset in patients with hypertension, history of myocardial infarction, diabetes, and chronic valvular insufficiency. They present with progressive shortness of breath, displaced point of maximal impulse (PMI), cardiomegaly, q waves on electrocardiogram, and decreased left ventricular ejection fraction on echocardiogram.[106] Although diastolic failure occurs in patients with similar histories, they have acute pulmonary edema and congestion, an S4 gallop with PMI unchanged, a normal-sized heart with left ventricular hypertrophy on electrocardiogram, and a normal or even increased left ventricular ejection fraction on echocardiogram.[106] Treatment varies depending on the cause. Although venodilators like digitalis and diuretics are mainstays in systolic heart failure, they may exacerbate diastolic dysfunction that responds to medications that improve preload and ventricular relaxation like calcium channel blockers, angiotensin-converting enzyme inhibitors, and beta-adrenergic antagonists.[106] Unfortunately, the elderly are highly susceptible to the side effects of these medications, which include dehydration, electrolytes disturbances, and further conduction slowing resulting in bradyarrhythmias to name a few.[103] As a result, the elderly frequently need lower doses because of impaired excretion.

Arrhythmias are also frequently encountered in perioperative elderly surgical patients. They may present as syncope or as mental status changes, but significant arrhythmias may present without symptoms or with palpitations.[103] A syncopal episode with a cardiovascular cause carries a 24% 1-year mortality rate.[107] Single supraventricular premature beats are present in almost all individuals older than 80 years, are usually asymptomatic, and do not require treatment.[103] Atrial fibrillation is present in 10% of patients older than 80 years.[108] Unfortunately in the elderly, antiarrhythmic adverse drug reactions caused by altered metabolic function, drug elimination, and polypharmacy can potentiate conduction abnormalities and ventricular dysfunction.[103]

Given the elderly's tenuous nature and sometimes unpredictable response to cardiac medications, more frequent monitoring, follow-up, and closer surveillance to ensure compliance and recognize early signs and symptoms of toxicity and progressing disease are imperative. Truly a multidisciplinary approach is needed involving education, frequent assessment, and careful management. A team approach has proven to reduce readmissions, improve medication compliance, be more cost-effective, and ultimately improve the functional status of patients.[109,110] In fact, lack of emotional support is a strong independent predictor of fatal and nonfatal cardiovascular events following a hospitalization in elderly women.[111]

GASTROINTESTINAL AND NUTRITION

The gastrointestinal tract is one of the systems relatively unchanged functionally by aging.[112–115] Dysphagia is a common elderly problem leading to aspiration in the perioperative period. This problem may be caused by decreased senses (olfactory, taste), decreased tongue muscle mass and strength, medications and as a result of neurologic disorders and neurovascular disease.[116] Treatment is multidisciplinary involving nursing care, speech therapists, and medical and surgical specialists. There is an increased incidence of certain gastrointestinal disorders in the elderly. Gastroesophageal reflux disease (GERD) is present in about 30% of the elderly.[117,118] There are conflicting data about whether gastric acid secretion and gastric emptying decrease or remain normal in the elderly.[116] What is proven extensively through epidemiologic studies is that *Helicobacter pylori* and subsequently gastric ulcer incidence increases with age,[119] such that half of all adults are seropositive by 50 years of age. Gastritis and gastric atrophy are 2 of the most common gastrointestinal disorders in the elderly, placing them at risk for gastrointestinal bleeding. The stress in the perioperative period, along with the use of NSAIDs that deplete mucosal prostaglandins may incite bleeding and ulceration.[116] Particularly at risk are women,[120–122] those patients with a prior history of peptic ulcer disease, and patients with increased age.[123,124] The treatment of GERD and peptic ulcer disease is the same in the elderly: antacids, H_2 receptor antagonists, proton pump inhibitors, sucralfate, misoprostol, and antibiotics for *H pylori* eradiation. Care must be taken as elderly are prone to side effects and medication interactions, altering absorption. Antacids may increase sodium and magnesium, affecting the kidneys and causing diarrhea, and alter absorption (antibiotics, quinidine)[125,126] as can proton pump inhibitors. Cimetidine may cause confusion with high doses or parenteral administration.[125,126] Sucralfate can cause constipation.[127,128] Misoprostol may cause diarrhea.[128]

If an elderly patient develops a gastrointestinal bleed, upper or lower, independent of cause, then mortality can range from 10% to 25%.[129,130] Bleeds are approached in the same manner in the elderly: assessment, resuscitation, identification of source, and treatment. Vascular ectasias of the colon are primarily a recurrent and subacute elderly disease (two-thirds of patients older than 70 years), but 15% present with severe hemorrhage.[116] Additionally, vascular disease in the elderly often involves the mesenteric vasculature. Despite significant collaterals, embolic disease, ischemic colitis, or severe disease (involving 2 main mesenteric trunks) complicating the perioperative period may be encountered because of arrhythmias or hypotension. Presentation may be subtle, such as a postoperative ileus, or as severe as shock caused by acute intestinal infarction or gastrointestinal bleed in ischemic colitis.[116]

The liver decreases in weight and number of hepatocytes with age,[116] impacting pharmacokinetics. Alcoholic cirrhosis may be encountered in elderly surgical patients without previous knowledge of its existence, impacting surgical and perioperative management.[116] More importantly, providers must be cognizant of acetaminophen toxicity, with multiple medications containing acetaminophen and attempts to avoid opioids. As a result of cardiovascular failure in the perioperative period, patients may develop hepatic ischemia or congestion. Although pancreatic function is not altered by age, the main duct increases in size 8% per decade.[131]

One of the most commonly encountered perioperative issues arising in the elderly is constipation. Although 60% to 70% of the functional elderly have a daily bowel movement, 15% to 30% take laxatives on a regular basis.[132,133] It is important to identify those at risk and ask daily about bowel function. Opioid use, immobility, decreased oral water intake, and dietary changes while hospitalized contribute to perioperative constipation. In patients naïve to over-the-counter constipation regimens, treatment involves laxatives (milk of magnesia, lactulose, sorbitol, anthraquinones, saline laxatives, combination preparations of polyethylene glycol 3350 and electrolytes [GoLYTELY]) and mild stimulants (senna and bisacodyl).[116] Mineral oil is discouraged in those with dysphagia because of the aspiration pneumonitis risk. The elderly should be assessed for impaction if there is no output or diarrhea and manually disimpacted on identification. Enemas may soften the stool in the rectal vault and reach fecal material above manual manipulation.

Finally, chronic vascular occlusion may contribute to abdominal angina, leading to weight loss and malnourishment. Additionally with age, the villi of the small intestine shorten and become clubbed, decreasing the surface area, which is also thought to contribute to malnutrition.[113,134,135] More than 70% of hospitalized elderly patients are malnourished or at an increased nutritional risk, which is associated with increased mortality.[136,137] The Academy of Nutrition and Dietetics and the American Society for Parenteral and Enteral Nutrition has provided a consensus for the diagnosis of malnutrition including insufficient nutritional intake, weight, muscle mass and subcutaneous fat loss, fluid overload, and decreased handgrip strength.[138] They recommend regular and consistent weight measurements for hospitalized and high-risk patients.[138]

Unintentional weight loss and decreased appetite in older community-dwelling patients is associated with increased mortality.[139] Similar results are also observed in obese patients older than 70 years.[140] Although a variety of definitions of weight loss exist, it is considered clinically significant if there is a 5% decrease in weight over 1 month's time period (>5% considered severe), 7.5% decrease in weight over 3 months' time period (>7.5% considered severe), or 10% decrease in weight over 6 months' time period (>10% severe).[141] There are several nutrition screening tools available for malnutrition and nutritional risk in older patients. The Mini Nutritional Assessment and the Malnutrition Screening Tool have the highest sensitivity and specificity.[142] Although these are formal tools, data suggest even a simple question such as presence of a good appetite can be predictive of outcomes.

Involuntary weight loss is multifactorial but ultimately is attributed to inadequate intake. Inadequate oral intake is similarly multifactorial because of social, psychiatric, and medical factors.[143,144] Malignancy and depression are identified as the most frequent causes of malnutrition in elderly patients.[145,146] Dysphagia, reportedly present in up to 10% of older patients, is also a contributing factor.[147] Nutritional supplementation is often used in elderly patients; however, data suggest morbidity and mortality was noted to improve only in malnourished hospitalized patients older than 75 years.[148] Results of appetite stimulants, such as megestrol, dronabinol, and mirtazapine, are mixed and not definitive for clinically significant and sustained weight gain. This subject is an obvious area ripe for research in the future to determine the impact of intensive preoperative or targeted nutritional supplementation.

RENAL

Total body water is reduced by 10% to 15% in older patients.[149] In contrast, they have a reduced glomerular filtration rate and reduced ability to concentrate urine, which predisposes them to fluid retention and volume overload.[150] Elderly patients are susceptible to acute kidney injury or acute on chronic kidney injury and electrolyte abnormalities. However, the older patient population is unique in that they are at an increased risk of electrolyte disturbances without underlying renal dysfunction, dehydration, and polypharmacy simply as a result of physiologic aging.[151,152] These disturbances result in increased morbidity and mortality and readmission rates in surgical patients particularly.[149,153–155] This condition is further exacerbated by age-related physiologic changes, including renal senescence defined as irreversible functional and structural changes associated with the kidneys of aging patients.[152]

Dehydration with a loss as little as 2% of total body water can result in a significant impairment of physical and cognitive performance.[156] Elderly patients are also more susceptible to water retention and associated electrolyte abnormalities that are exacerbated in the perioperative period, a time of increased physiologic stress.[157] Positive fluid balance is an independent risk factor for mortality in critically ill patients with acute kidney injury.[158,159]

Glomerular sclerosis leads to a decrease in glomerular mass in the elderly.[160,161] Creatinine clearance is also reduced.[150] Tubular dysfunction impairs the ability to concentrate urine, leading to electrolyte disturbances.[150] Furthermore, ischemia has also been noted to contribute to nephron loss.[162–164] Hormonal alterations have been noted to similarly affect fluid and electrolyte balance, particularly reduced levels of renin and aldosterone caused by increased atrial natriuretic peptide secondary to hypertension and increased right atrial filling at baseline.[165] There is also a decreased tubular response to hormones predisposing patients again to fluid and electrolyte abnormalities.[164]

Thirst response is blunted in older patients, resulting in a persistent hyperosmolar state that is further heightened by a reduction in the ability of the kidney to concentrate urine. Dysnatremia in older patients is of particular concern, and age is noted to be an independent risk factor.[166] It has been shown reproducibly that particularly hypernatremia is a risk factor for increased mortality.[167–169] Hyponatremia, which is more common, is noted to be a risk factor for bone fracture.[170–172] Hyperkalemia is a concern as tubular dysfunction impairs the secretion of potassium.[173–175] Hyperkalemia is further exacerbated by a decreased response to aldosterone and renin.[176] Furthermore, polypharmacy and physiologic stress increase the risk of abrupt alterations in potassium balance. Patients on angiotensin-converting enzyme inhibitors, diuretics, and NSAIDs are particularly susceptible.[177,178]

Physiologic changes in the perioperative period include systemic neurologic, hormonal, immune, and hematologic responses. Cognitive decline is a risk factor for dehydration.[179] Increased secretion of antidiuretic hormone, renin, and aldosterone during stress results in fluid retention. Older patients are increasingly susceptible given their underlying age-related physiologic changes at baseline.[157] Salt and water retention has been associated with increased risk of infection, cardiopulmonary complications, and impaired gastrointestinal function as well as a prolonged hospital stay.[180–185] Other studies report improved perioperative outcomes with zero fluid balance in the perioperative period.[186–189] Positive fluid balance was noted to be an independent factor for immediate perioperative mortality.[159] More recent data suggest that surgical patients are often noted to have a hyperchloremic acidosis secondary to the use of normal saline.[190,191] Data suggest that chloride-restricted intravenous fluid resuscitation in the perioperative period reduces the incidence of acute kidney injury, improves gastrointestinal blood flow, decreases salt and water retention, and overall decreases the risk of morbidity and mortality, particularly important as this age group is increasingly susceptible to these physiologic changes.[192–194] Additionally, studies report in older adults and high-risk patients small boluses of colloid to optimize stroke volume result in improved outcomes and decreased morbidity and mortality.[195–200]

Knowledge of age-related physiologic changes, particularly renal senescence and hormonal alterations that directly affect the fluid and electrolyte balance in older patients, is key in the perioperative period as even the slightest change in this delicate balance in this patient population can have significant effects on morbidity and mortality. Age-related changes in fluid and electrolyte homeostasis greatly affects the ability of these patients to adapt to situations that exacerbate this homeostasis, like surgical intervention and hospitalization.

OUTCOMES

When reviewing guidelines pertaining to the elderly in perioperative period, there is a paucity. Many guidelines are based on multiple randomized controlled trials that generally exclude the elderly. Furthermore, they are unable to account for the multiple comorbidities the elderly have and the statistical impact the morbidities have on outcomes.[201]

Selective use of routine studies guided by the patients' history (complete blood count, basic blood chemistries, chest radiograph, and electrocardiogram) is supported by the American Society of Anesthesiologists and Cochrane review.[202–204] Several cardiovascular risk indices, the American Heart Association, The New England Vascular Surgery Group, and others, attempt to risk stratify the elderly's cardiovascular risk. While looking at quantitative traditional outcomes, they fail to account for things the elderly cherish the most: independence, functional capacity, and quality of life. The American Diabetes Association leads the way in recognizing the limitations of its guidelines with respect to the elderly, strongly recommending individualized treatment.[205] The American College of Surgeons in collaboration with the American Geriatrics Society has created best-practice guidelines to help surgeons identify high-risk patients, prevent complications, and achieve best outcomes in elderly surgical patients[17]; unfortunately, these are labor intensive, require extensive financial resources, and are not usually feasible in the emergent setting.

Overall surgical mortality in the elderly has been on the decline even in the most complex, risky operations.[206] Furthermore, even in those patients older than 90 years, long-term survival does not seem to be affected by surgical intervention.[207] The death rate for elective operations ranges from 0% to 5.4%, with 7.0% to 20.0% suffering a nonfatal complication[208–210]; these statistics hold true with age-matched cohorts.[211,212] Unfortunately, many operations are of the emergent nature in the elderly when they do not fair as well. The percentage of emergent operations increases with age: 14.5% aged 65 to 74 years, 27.9% aged 75 years and older,[209] 69.0% aged 90 years and older.[210] Usually the emergent cases are related to infection, intestinal obstruction, incarcerated hernias, and hemorrhage.[210,213] Because of the emergent nature, morbidity rates range from 30% to 68% and mortality 13.6% to 31.0%.[209,210,213] In fact, Rigberg and colleagues[210] found that all postoperative deaths in patients older than 90 years were emergent operations. With regard to oncologic operations, Dekker and colleagues[214] demonstrated that elderly patients who survive the first year following resection of their colorectal cancer have the same cancer survival rate as younger patients. Long-term survival is related to early morbidity and mortality.

As previously mentioned outcomes in elderly patients are not just about morbidity and mortality; independence, functional capacity, and quality of life play a major role. Postoperative cognitive dysfunction impairs nearly 13% of the elderly 3 months after an operation, double the rate of other age groups.[215] In a cohort of elderly patients aged 75 years and older independent at admission, 75% were not independent at discharge, 15% of whom were discharged to a nursing home[216]; they do not leave the nursing homes, 33% of those sent to a nursing home after a hip fracture remain there a year later.[217] Kemper found that of those who enter nursing homes, 55% will spend at least 1 year of total lifetime and 21% will spend 5 years or more.[218] Many die, are sent to other hospitals, rehabilitation facilities, and other long-term care facilities. In fact, only 12% ever return home.[219]

SUMMARY

The older population continues to grow at an unprecedented rate and is living longer. Thus, surgeons are encountering older patients more frequently and can expect an increase in surgical demand because of this rapidly growing population. This article highlights some of the anatomic and physiologic changes that are a result of aging. These changes can sometimes drastically alter the perioperative care of the elderly, leaving the surgeon to face challenging, complex treatment decisions and ethical questions. Clearly, the management of the older patient population requires meticulous management with a multidisciplinary approach.

REFERENCES

1. U.S. Department of Health and Human Services Administration on Aging. Available at: http://www.aoa.gov/Aging_Statistics/Profile/2013/2.aspx. Accessed November 17, 2014.

2. Centers for Disease Control and Prevention. The state of aging and health in America 2013. Atlanta (GA): Centers for Disease Control and Prevention, US Dept of Health and Human Services; 2013. Available at: http://www.cdc.gov/features/agingandhealth/state_of_aging_and_health_in_america_2013.pdf.
3. U.S. Department of Health and Human Services Administration on Aging. Available at: http://www.aoa.acl.gov/Aging_Statistics/Profile/2013/3.aspx. Accessed November 17, 2014.
4. Etzioni DA, Liu JH, Maggard MA, et al. The aging population and its impact on the surgery workforce. Ann Surg 2003;238:170–7.
5. Neuman MD, Bosk CL. The redefinition of aging in American surgery. Milbank Q 2013;91:288–315.
6. Kwok AC, Semel ME, Lipsitz SR, et al. The intensity and variation of surgical care at the end of life: a retrospective cohort study. Lancet 2011;378:1408–13.
7. Rockwood K, Mitnitski A. Frailty defined by deficit accumulation and geriatric medicine defined by frailty. Clin Geriatr Med 2011;27:17–26.
8. Fried LP, Ferrucci L, Darer J, et al. Untangling the concepts of disability, frailty, and comorbidity: implications for improved targeting and care. J Gerontol A Biol Sci Med Sci 2004;59:255–63.
9. Fried LP, Tangen CM, Walston J, et al. Frailty in older adults: evidence for a phenotype. J Gerontol A Biol Sci Med Sci 2001;56(3):M146–56.
10. Stuck AE, Siu AL, Wieland GD, et al. Comprehensive geriatric assessment: a meta-analysis of controlled trials. Lancet 1993;342(8878):1032–6.
11. Makary MA, Segev DL, Pronovost PJ, et al. Frailty as a predictor of surgical outcomes in older patients. J Am Coll Surg 2010;210:901–8.
12. Devons CA. Comprehensive geriatric assessment: making the most of the aging years. Curr Opin Clin Nutr Metab Care 2002;5:19–24.
13. Rubenstein LZ, Josephson KR, Wieland GD, et al. Effectiveness of a geriatric evaluation unit: a randomized trial. N Engl J Med 1984;311:1664–70.
14. Robinson TN, Wu DS, Pointer L, et al. Simple frailty score predicts postoperative complications across surgical specialties. Am J Surg 2013;206:544–50.
15. Afilalo J, Eisenberg MJ, Morin JF, et al. Gait speed as an incremental predictor of mortality and major morbidity in elderly patients undergoing cardiac surgery. J Am Coll Cardiol 2010;56:1668–76.
16. Chung CJ, Wu C, Jones M, et al. Reduced handgrip strength as a marker of frailty predicts clinical outcomes in patients with heart failure undergoing ventricular assist device placement. J Card Fail 2014;20:310–5.
17. Chow WB, Rosenthal RA, Merkow RP, et al. Optimal preoperative assessment of the geriatric surgical patient: a best practices guideline from the American College of Surgeons National Surgical Quality Improvement Program and the American Geriatrics Society. J Am Coll Surg 2012;215:453–66.
18. Malafarina V, Uriz-Otano F, Iniesta R, et al. Sarcopenia in the elderly: diagnosis, physiopathology and treatment. Maturitas 2012;71:109–14.
19. Pahor M, Kritchevsky S. Research hypotheses on muscle wasting, aging, loss of function and disability. J Nutr Health Aging 1998;2:97–100.
20. Evans WJ, Morley JE, Argiles J, et al. Cachexia: a new definition. Clin Nutr 2008;27:793–9.
21. Martinez M, Arnalich F, Hernanz A. Alterations of anorectic cytokine levels from plasma and cerebrospinal fluid in idiopathic senile anorexia. Mech Ageing Dev 1993;72:145–53.

22. Lindle RS, Metter EJ, Lynch NA, et al. Age and gender comparisons of muscle strength in 654 women and men aged 20–93 yr. J Appl Physiol (1985) 1997;83: 1581–7.
23. Roubenoff R. Origins and clinical relevance of sarcopenia. Can J Appl Physiol 2001;26:78–89.
24. Janssen I. The epidemiology of sarcopenia. Clin Geriatr Med 2011;27:355–63.
25. Vuky J. Pharmacodynamics in the elderly. Best Pract Res Clin Anaesthesiol 2003;17:207–18.
26. Aymanns C, Keller F, Maus S, et al. Review on pharmacokinetics and pharmacodynamics and the aging kidney. Clin J Am Soc Nephrol 2010;5:314–27.
27. Homer TD, Stanski DR. The effect of increasing age on thiopental disposition and anesthetic requirement. Anesthesiology 1985;62:714–24.
28. White PF, White LM, Monk T, et al. Perioperative care for older outpatient undergoing ambulatory surgery. Anesth Analg 2012;114:1190–215.
29. Gourtsoyiannis N, Prassopoulos P, Cavouras D, et al. The thickness of renal parenchyma decreases with age: a CT study of 360 patients. Am J Roentgenol 1990;155:541–4.
30. Schmucker DL. Age-related changes in liver structure and function: implications for disease? Exp Gerontol 2005;40:650–9.
31. Tang J, Eckenhoff MF, Eckenhoff RG. Anesthesia and the old brain. Anesth Analg 2010;110:421–6.
32. Gibson SJ, Helme RD. Age-related differences in pain perception and report. Clin Geriatr Med 2001;17:433–56.
33. Barnett SR. Polypharmacy and perioperative medications in the elderly. Anesthesiol Clin 2009;27:377–89.
34. Minto CF, Schider TW, Egan TD, et al. Influence of age and gender on the pharmacokinetics and pharmacodynamics of remifentanil: I model development. Anesthesiology 1997;80:143–8.
35. Ong CK, Lirk P, Seymour RA, et al. The efficacy of preemptive analgesia for acute post-operative pain management: a meta-analysis. Anesth Analg 2005; 100:757–73.
36. Moinche S, Mikkelsen S, Wetterslev J, et al. A systematic review of intra-articular local anesthesia for post-operative pain relief after arthroscopic knee surgery. Reg Anesth Pain Med 1999;24:430–7.
37. Popping DM, Elia N, Marret E, et al. Clonidine as an adjuvant to local anesthetics, for peripheral nerve and plexus blocks: a meta-analysis of randomized trials. Anesthesiology 2009;111:406–15.
38. Essving P, Axelsson K, Kjellberg J, et al. Reduced hospital stay, morphine consumption and pain intensity with local infiltration analgesia (LIA) following total knee arthroplasty. Acta Orthop 2010;81:354–60.
39. Vieira P, Pulai I, Tsao GC, et al. Dexamethasone with bupivacaine increases duration of analgesia with ultrasound guided brachial plexus blockade. Eur J Anaesthesiol 2010;27:285–8.
40. Toms L, McQuay HJ, Derry S, et al. Single dose oral paracetamol (acetaminophen) for postoperative pain in adults. Cochrane Database Syst Rev 2008;(4): CD004602.
41. Miners JO, Penhall R, Robson RA, et al. Comparison of paracetamol metabolism in young adult and elderly males. Eur J Clin Pharmacol 1988;35:157–60.
42. Bisgaard T, Klarskov B, Kehlet H, et al. Preoperative dexamethasone improves surgical outcomes after laparoscopic cholecystectomy: a randomized double-blind placebo-controlled trial. Ann Surg 2003;238:651–60.

43. Hval K, Thagaard K, Schlichting E, et al. The prolonged postoperative analgesic effect when dexamethasone is added to a nonsteroidal anti-inflammatory drug (rofecoxib) before breast surgery. Anesth Analg 2007;105:481–6.
44. Rommundstad L, Brevik H, Roald H, et al. Methylprednisolone reduces pain, emesis, and fatigue after breast augmentation surgery: a single dose, randomized, parallel-group study with methylprednisolone 125 mg, parecoxib 40 mg, and placebo. Anesth Analg 2006;102:419–25.
45. Whitlock RP, Chan S, Devereaux PJ, et al. Clinical benefit of steroid use in patients undergoing cardiopulmonary bypass: a meta-analysis of randomized trials. Eur Heart J 2008;29:2592–600.
46. Henzi I, Walder B, Tramer MR. Dexamethasone for the prevention of postoperative nausea and vomiting: a quantitative systematic review. Anesth Analg 2000;90:186–94.
47. Loftus RW, Yeager MP, Clark JA, et al. Intraoperative ketamine reduces perioperative opiate consumption in opiate-dependent patients with chronic back pain undergoing back surgery. Anesthesiology 2010;113:639–46.
48. Remerand F, Le Tendre C, Baud A, et al. The early and delayed analgesic effects of ketamine after total hip arthroplasty: a prospective, randomized, controlled, double-blind study. Anesth Analg 2009;109:1963–71.
49. Gilron I, Orr E, Tu D, et al. A randomized double-blind, controlled trial of perioperative administration of gabapentin, meloxicam and their combination for spontaneous and movement-evoked pain after ambulatory laparoscopic cholecystectomy. Anesth Analg 2009;108:623–30.
50. Turan A, White PF, Karamanlioglu D, et al. Gabapentin-an alternative to COX-2 inhibitors for perioperative pain management. Anesth Analg 2006; 102:175–81.
51. Erola O, Kortila K, Aho M, et al. Comparison of intramuscular dexmedetomidine and midazolam premedication for elective abdominal hysterectomy. Anesth Analg 1994;79:646–53.
52. Tufanogullari B, White PF, Peixoto MP, et al. Dexmedetomidine infusion during laparoscopic bariatric surgery: the effect on recovery room outcome variables. Anesth Analg 2008;106:1741–8.
53. Coloma M, Chiu JW, White PF, et al. The use of esmolol as an alternative to remifentanil during desflurane anesthesia for fast-track outpatient gynecologic laparoscopic surgery. Anesth Analg 2001;92:352–7.
54. Lee SJ, Lee JN. The effect of perioperative esmolol infusion on postoperative nausea, vomiting and pain after laparoscopic appendectomy. Korean J Anesthesiol 2010;59:179–84.
55. Auroy Y, Benhamou D, Bargues L, et al. Major complications of regional anesthesia in France: the SOS regional anesthesia hotline service. Anesthesiology 2002;97:1274–80.
56. Arbous MS, Meursing AE, van Kleef JW, et al. Impact of anesthesia management characteristics on severe morbidity and mortality. Anesthesiology 2005; 102:257–68.
57. Schnider TW, Minto CF, Shafer SL, et al. The influence of age on propofol pharmacodynamics. Anesthesiology 1999;90:1502–16.
58. Kazama T, Ikeda K, Morita K, et al. Comparison of the effect-site k(eO)s of propofol for blood pressure and EEG bispectral index in elderly and younger patients. Anesthesiology 1999;90:1517–27.
59. Eger EL. Age, minimal alveolar anesthetic concentration and minimum alveolar anesthetic concentration-awake. Anesth Analg 2001;93:947–53.

60. Chen X, Zhao M, White PF, et al. The recovery of cognitive function after general anesthesia in elderly patients: a comparison of desflurane and sevoflurane. Anesth Analg 2001;93:1489–95.
61. Hussain M, Berger M, Eckenhoff RG, et al. General anesthetic and the risk of dementia in the elderly: current insight. Clin Interv Aging 2014;4:1619–28.
62. Dyer CB, Aston CM, Teasdale TA. Postoperative delirium: a review of 80 primary data-collection studies. Arch Intern Med 1995;155:461–5.
63. Practice guidelines for the treatment of patients with delirium. American Psychiatric Association. Am J Psychiatry 1999;156:1–20.
64. Kimball CP. The experience of open heart surgery. 3. Toward a definition and understanding of postcardiotomy delirium. Arch Gen Psychiatry 1972;27:57–63.
65. Bekker AY, Weeks EJ. Cognitive function after anaesthesia in the elderly. Best Pract Res Clin Anaesthesiol 2003;17:259–72.
66. Flacker JM, Cummings V, Mach JR Jr, et al. The association of serum anticholinergic activity with delirium in elderly medical patients. Am J Geriatr Psychiatry 1998;6:31–41.
67. Trzepacz PT. Is there a final common pathway in delirium? Focus on acetylcholine and dopamine. Semin Clin Neuropsychiatry 2000;5:132–48.
68. Hamrick I, Meyer F. Perioperative management of delirium and dementia in the geriatric surgical patient. Langenbecks Arch Surg 2013;298:947–55.
69. Inouye SK, Bogardus ST Jr, Charpentier PA, et al. A multicomponent intervention to prevent delirium in hospitalized older patients. N Engl J Med 1999;340:669–76.
70. Mason SE, Noel-Storr A, Ritchie CW. The impact of general and regional anesthesia on the incidence of post-operative cognitive dysfunction and post-operative delirium: a systematic review with meta-analysis. J Alzheimers Dis 2010;22:67–79.
71. Inouye SK, Zhang Y, Jones RN, et al. Risk factors for delirium at discharge: development and validation of a predictive model. Arch Intern Med 2007;167: 1406–13.
72. American Psychiatric Association. Diagnostic and statistical manual of mental disorders. IV-TR ed. Washington, DC: American Psychiatric Association; 2000.
73. Kalsvaart KJ, de Jonghe JF, Bogaards MJ, et al. Haloperidol prophylaxis for elderly hip fracture patients at risk for delirium: a randomized placebo-controlled study. J Am Geriatr Soc 2005;53:1658–66.
74. Moller JT, Cluitmans P, Raqssmussen LS, et al. Long-term postoperative cognitive dysfunction in the elderly ISPOCD1 study. ISPOCD investigators. International Study of Post-Operative Cognitive Dysfunction. Lancet 1998;351:857–61.
75. Steinmetz J, Christensen KB, Lund T, et al. Long-term consequences of post-operative cognitive dysfunction. Anesthesiology 2009;110:548–55.
76. Rortgen D, Kloos J, Fries M, et al. Comparison of early cognitive function and recovery after desflurane or sevoflurane anaesthesia in the elderly: a double-blinded randomized controlled trial. Br J Anaesth 2010;104:167–74.
77. Rosenthal RA, Kavic SM. Assessment and management of the geriatric patient. Crit Care Med 2004;32:S92–105.
78. Sprung J, Gajic O, Warner DO. Review article: age related alteration in respiratory function – anesthestic considerations. Can J Anaesth 2006;53:1244–57.
79. Antonelli M, Conti G, Moro ML, et al. Predictors of failure of noninvasive positive pressure ventilation in patients with acute hypoxemic respiratory failure: a multi-center study. Intensive Care Med 2001;27:1718–28.
80. Warner DO. Preventing postoperative pulmonary complications. Anesthesiology 2000;92:1467–72.

81. Behrendt CE. Acute respiratory failure in the United States. Chest 2000;118:1100–5.
82. Solh AA, Ramadan FH. Overview of respiratory failure in older adults. J Intensive Care Med 2006;21:345–51.
83. Connolly MJ, Crowley JJ, Charan NB, et al. Reduced subjective awareness of bronchoconstriction provoked by methacholine in elderly asthmatic and normal subjects as measured on a simple awareness scale. Thorax 1992;47:410–3.
84. Ely EW, Evans GW, Haponik EF. Mechanical ventilation in a cohort of elderly patients admitted to an intensive care unit. Ann Intern Med 1999;131:96–104.
85. Pesau B, Falger S, Berger E, et al. Influence of age on outcome of mechanically ventilated patients in an intensive care unit. Crit Care Med 1992;20:489–92.
86. Thompson LF. Failure to wean: exploring the influence of age-related pulmonary changes. Crit Care Nurs Clin North Am 1996;8:7–16.
87. Krieger BP, Ershowsky PF, Becker DA, et al. Evaluation of conventional criteria for predicting successful weaning from mechanical ventilator support in elderly patients. Crit Care Med 1989;17:858–61.
88. Krieger BP, Isber J, Breitenbucher A, et al. Serial measurements of the rapid-shallow-breathing index as a predictor of weaning outcome in elderly medical patients. Chest 1997;112:1029–34.
89. Kleinhenz ME, Lewis CY. Chronic ventilator dependence in elderly patients. Clin Geriatr Med 2000;16:735–56.
90. Smetana G. Preoperative pulmonary evaluation. N Engl J Med 1999;340:937–44.
91. Rosenthal RA, Perkal MF. Physiologic considerations in the elderly surgical patient. In: Miller TA, editor. Modern surgical care: physiologic foundations and clinical applications. 2nd edition. New York: Informa; 2006. p. 1129–48.
92. Kitzman DW, Edwards WD. Age-related changes in the anatomy of the normal human heart. J Gerontol 1990;45:M33–9.
93. Strait JB, Lakatta EG. Aging-associated cardiovascular changes and their relationship to heart failure. Heart Fail Clin 2012;8:143–64.
94. Gerstenblith G, Frederiksen J, Yin FC, et al. Echocardiographic assessment of a normal adult aging population. Circulation 1977;56:273–8.
95. Hees PS, Fleg JL, Lakatta EG, et al. Left ventricular remodeling with age in normal men versus women: novel insights using three-dimensional magnetic resonance imaging. Am J Cardiol 2002;90:1231–6.
96. Sahasakul Y, Edwards WD, Naessens JM, et al. Age-related changes in aortic and mitral valve thickness: implications for two-dimensional echocardiography based on an autopsy study of 200 normal human hearts. Am J Cardiol 1988;62:424–30.
97. Kitzman DW, Scholz DG, Hagen PT, et al. Age-related changes in normal human hearts during the first 10 decades of life. Part II (maturity): a quantitative anatomic study of 765 specimens from subjects 20 to 99 years old. Mayo Clin Proc 1988;63:137–46.
98. Olivetti G, Melissari M, Capasso JM, et al. Cardiomyopathy of the aging human heart. Myocyte loss and reactive cellular hypertrophy. Circ Res 1991;68:1560–8.
99. Lakatta EG, Mitchell JH, Pomerance A, et al. Human aging: changes in structure and function. J Am Coll Cardiol 1987;10:42A–7A.
100. Priebe HJ. The aged cardiovascular risk patient. Br J Anaesth 2000;85:763–78.
101. Davies MJ. Pathology of the conduction system. In: Caird FL, Dalle JL, Kennedy RD, editors. Cardiology in old age. New York: Plenum Press; 1976. p. 57–9.

102. Roman MJ, Devereux RB, Kizer JR, et al. High central pulse pressure is independently associated with adverse cardiovascular outcome the strong heart study. J Am Coll Cardiol 2009;54:1730–4.
103. Wenger NK. Cardiovascular disease. In: Cassell CK, Leipzig RM, Cohen HJ, et al, editors. Geriatric medicine. 4th edition. New York: Springer; 2003. p. 509–43.
104. Lam JY, Chaitman BR, Glaenzer M. Safety and diagnostic accuracy in dipyridamole-thallium imaging in the elderly. J Am Coll Cardiol 1988;11:585–9.
105. Weaver WD, Litwin PE, Marte JS, et al. Effect of age on use of thrombolytic therapy and mortality in acute myocardial infarction. J Am Coll Cardiol 1991;18: 657–62.
106. Tresch DD, McGough MF. Heart failure with normal systolic function: a common disorder in older people. J Am Geriatr Soc 1995;43:1035–42.
107. Lipsitz LA, Wei JY, Rowe JQ. Syncope in an elderly, institutionalized population: prevalence, incidence, and associated risk. Q J Med 1985;55:45–54.
108. Ryder KM, Benjamin EJ. Epidemiology and significance of atrial fibrillation. Am J Cardiol 1999;84:131R–8R.
109. Rich MW, Beckham V, Wittenberg C, et al. A multidisciplinary intervention to prevent the readmission of elderly patients with congestive heart failure. N Engl J Med 1995;333:1190–5.
110. Rich MW, Gray DB, Beckham V, et al. Effect of a multidisciplinary intervention on medication compliance in elderly patients with congestive heart failure. Am J Med 1996;101:270–6.
111. Krumholz HM, Butler J, Miller J, et al. Prognostic importance of emotional support for elderly patients hospitalized with heart failure. Circulation 1998;97:958–64.
112. Shamburek RD, Farrar J. Disorders of the digestive system in the elderly. N Engl J Med 1990;322:438–43.
113. Holt PR. Gastrointestinal system: changes in morphology and cell proliferation. Aging 1991;3:392–4.
114. Russell RM. Change in gastrointestinal function attributed to aging. Am J Clin Nutr 1992;55:1203S–7S.
115. Blechman MB, Gelb AM. Aging and gastrointestinal physiology. Clin Geriatr Med 1999;15:429–38.
116. Wilson JAP. Gastroenterologic disorders. In: Cassell CK, Leipzig RM, Cohen HJ, et al, editors. Geriatric medicine. 4th edition. New York: Springer; 2003. p. 835–51.
117. Ellis FH. Current concepts. Esophageal hiatal hernia. N Engl J Med 1972;287: 646–69.
118. Spechler SJ. Epidemiology and natural history of gastro-oesophageal reflux disease. Digestion 1992;51:24–9.
119. Perez-Perez GI, Dworkin BM, Chodos JE, et al. *Campylobacter pylori* antibodies in humans. Ann Intern Med 1988;109:11–7.
120. Allison MC, Torrance CJ, Russell RI. Non-steroidal anti-inflammatory drugs, gastroduodenal ulcers and their complications: prospective controlled autopsy study. N Engl J Med 1992;327:749–54.
121. Skander MP, Ryan FP. Non-steroidal anti-inflammatory drugs and pain-free peptic ulceration in the elderly. BMJ 1988;297:833–4.
122. Gabriel SE, Jaakkimainen L, Bombardier C. Risk for serious gastrointestinal complications related to use of NSAIDs: a meta-analysis. Ann Intern Med 1991;115:787–96.
123. Griffin MR, Piper JM, Daughtery MS, et al. Nonsteroidal anti-inflammatory drug use and increased risk for peptic ulcer disease in elderly persons. Ann Intern Med 1991;114:257–63.

124. Borum MA. Peptic-ulcer disease in the elderly. Clin Geriatr Med 1999;15: 457–71.
125. Walt RP, Langman MJ. Antacids and ulcer healing. A review of the evidence. Drugs 1991;42:205–12.
126. Freston JW. Overview of medical therapy of peptic ulcer disease. Gastroenterol Clin North Am 1990;19:121–40.
127. Rees WD. Mechanisms of gastroduodenal protection by sucralfate. Am J Med 1991;91:58S–63S.
128. Scheiman JM. Pathogeneses of gastroduodenal injury due to nonsteroidal anti-inflammatory drugs: implications for prevention and therapy. Semin Arthritis Rheum 1992;21:201–10.
129. Reinus JF, Brandt LJ. Lower intestinal bleeding in the elderly. Clin Geriatr Med 1991;7:301–19.
130. Rosen AM. Gastrointestinal bleeding in the elderly. Clin Geriatr Med 1999;15: 511–25.
131. Gullo L, Ventrucci M, Naldoni P, et al. Aging and exocrine pancreatic function. J Am Geriatr Soc 1986;34:790–2.
132. Wilson JA. Constipation in the elderly. Clin Geriatr Med 1999;15:499–510.
133. Whitehead WE, Drinkwater D, Cheskin LJ, et al. Constipation in the elderly living at home—definition, prevalence, and relationship to lifestyle and health status. J Am Geriatr Soc 1989;37:423–9.
134. Holt PR, Tierney AR, Kotler DP. Delayed enzyme expression: a defect of aging rat gut. Gastroenterology 1985;89:1026–34.
135. Holt PR. Gastrointestinal disorders in the elderly: the small intestine. Clin Gastroenterol 1985;14:689–723.
136. de Luis D, Lopez GA. Nutritional status of adult patients admitted to internal medicine departments in public hospitals in Castilla y Leon, Spain: a multi-center study. Eur J Intern Med 2006;17:556–60.
137. Wallace JI, Schwartz RS, LaCroix AZ, et al. Involuntary weight loss in older outpatients: incidence and clinical significance. J Am Geriatr Soc 1995;43:329–37.
138. White JV, Guenter P, Jensen G, et al. Consensus statement of the Academy of Nutrition and Dietetics/American Society for Parenteral and Enteral Nutrition: characteristics recommended for the identification and documentation of adult malnutrition (undernutrition). J Acad Nutr Diet 2012;112:730–8.
139. Wannamethee SG, Shaper AG, Lennon L. Reasons for intentional weight loss, unintentional weight loss, and mortality in older men. Arch Intern Med 2005; 165:1035–40.
140. Allison DB, Gallagher D, Heo M, et al. Body mass index and all-cause mortality among people age 70 and over: the longitudinal study of aging. Int J Obes Relat Metab Disord 1997;21:424–31.
141. Health Care Financing Administration. Long term care facility resident assessment user's manual, minimum data set, version 2. Natick (MA): Elior Press; 1999.
142. Skipper A, Ferguson M, Thompson K, et al. Nutrition screening tools: an analysis of the evidence. JPEN J Parenter Enteral Nutr 2012;36:292–8.
143. de Castro JM, Brewer EM. The amount eaten in meals by humans is a power function of the number of people present. Physiol Behav 1992;51:121–5.
144. Locher JL, Robinson CO, Roth DL, et al. The effect of the presence of others on caloric intake in homebound older adults. J Gerontol A Biol Sci Med Sci 2005; 60:1475–8.
145. Wilson MM, Vaswani S, Liu D, et al. Prevalence and causes of undernutrition in medical outpatients. Am J Med 1998;104:56–63.

146. Thompson MP, Morris LK. Unexplained weight loss in the ambulatory elderly. J Am Geriatr Soc 1991;39:497–500.
147. Achem SR, Devault KR. Dysphagia in aging. J Clin Gastroenterol 2005;39: 357–71.
148. Milne AC, Avenell A, Potter J. Meta-analysis: protein and energy supplementation in older people. Ann Intern Med 2006;144:37–48.
149. Allison SP, Lobo DN. Fluid and electrolytes in the elderly. Curr Opin Clin Nutr Metab Care 2004;7:27–33.
150. Lindeman RD, Tobin J, Shock NW. Longitudinal studies on the rate of decline in renal function with age. J Am Geriatr Soc 1985;33:278–85.
151. Schlanger LE, Bailey JL, Sands JM. Electrolytes in the aging. Adv Chronic Kidney Dis 2010;17:308–19.
152. Melk A. Senescence of renal cells: molecular basis and clinical implications. Nephrol Dial Transplant 2003;18:2474–8.
153. Hari M, Rosenzweig M. Incidence of preventable postoperative readmissions following pancreaticoduodenectomy: implications for patient education. Oncol Nurs Forum 2012;39:408–12.
154. Khan MA, Hossain FS, Dashti Z, et al. Causes and predictors of early readmission after surgery for a fracture of the hip. J Bone Joint Surg Br 2012; 94:690–7.
155. Messaris E, Sehgal R, Deiling S, et al. Dehydration is the most common indication for readmission after diverting ileostomy creation. Dis Colon Rectum 2012; 55:175–80.
156. Grandjean AC, Grandjean NR. Dehydration and cognitive performance. J Am Coll Nutr 2007;26:S549–54.
157. Desborough J. The stress response to trauma and surgery. Br J Anaesth 2000; 85:109–17.
158. Bagshaw SM, Brophy PD, Cruz D, et al. Fluid balance as a biomarker: impact of fluid overload on outcome in critically ill patients with acute kidney injury. Crit Care 2008;12:169.
159. Payen D, de Pont AC, Sakr Y, et al. A positive fluid balance is associated with a worse outcome in patients with acute renal failure. Crit Care 2008;12:R74.
160. Nyengaard JR, Bendtsen TF. Glomerular number and size in relation to age, kidney weight, and body surface in normal man. Anat Rec 1992;232:194–201.
161. Epstein M. Aging and the kidney. J Am Soc Nephrol 1996;7:1106–22.
162. Messerli FH, Sundgaard-Riise K, Ventura HO, et al. Essential hypertension in the elderly: haemodynamics, intravascular volume, plasma renin activity, and circulating catecholamine levels. Lancet 1983;2:983–6.
163. Hollenberg NK, Adams DF, Solomon HS, et al. Senescence and the renal vasculature in normal man. Circ Res 1974;34:309–16.
164. Beck LH. The aging kidney. Defending a delicate balance of fluid and electrolytes. Geriatrics 2000;55:26–8, 31–2.
165. Lobo DN, Stanga Z, Aloysius MM, et al. Effect of volume loading with 1 liter intravenous infusions of 0.9% saline, 4% succinylated gelatine (Gelofusine) and 6% hydroxyethyl starch (Voluven) on blood volume and endocrine responses: a randomized, three-way crossover study in healthy volunteers. Crit Care Med 2010; 38:464–70.
166. Hawkins RC. Age and gender as risk factors for hyponatremia and hypernatremia. Clin Chim Acta 2003;337:169–72.
167. Alshayeb HM, Showkat A, Babar F, et al. Severe hypernatremia correction rate and mortality in hospitalized patients. Am J Med Sci 2011;341:356–60.

168. Snyder NA, Feigal DW, Arieff AI. Hypernatremia in elderly patients. A heterogeneous, morbid, and iatrogenic entity. Ann Intern Med 1987;107:309–19.
169. Herrod PJ, Awad S, Redfern A, et al. Hypo- and hypernatraemia in surgical patients: is there room for improvement? World J Surg 2010;34:495–9.
170. Gankam Kengne F, Andres C, Sattar L, et al. Mild hyponatremia and risk of fracture in the ambulatory elderly. QJM 2008;101:583–8.
171. Zilberberg MD, Exuzides A, Spalding J, et al. Epidemiology, clinical and economic outcomes of admission hyponatremia among hospitalized patients. Curr Med Res Opin 2008;24:1601–8.
172. Kinsella S, Moran S, Sullivan MO, et al. Hyponatremia independent of osteoporosis is associated with fracture occurrence. Clin J Am Soc Nephrol 2010;5:275–80.
173. Musso C, Liakopoulos V, De Miguel R, et al. Transtubular potassium concentration gradient: comparison between healthy old people and chronic renal failure patients. Int Urol Nephrol 2006;38:387–90.
174. Frassetto L, Sebastian A. Age and systemic acid-base equilibrium: analysis of published data. J Gerontol A Biol Sci Med Sci 1996;51:B91–9.
175. Berkemeyer S, Vormann J, Gunther AL, et al. Renal net acid excretion capacity is comparable in prepubescence, adolescence, and young adulthood but falls with aging. J Am Geriatr Soc 2008;56:1442–8.
176. Mulkerrin E, Epstein FH, Clark BA. Aldosterone responses to hyperkalemia in healthy elderly humans. J Am Soc Nephrol 1995;6:1459–62.
177. Gurwitz JH, Field TS, Harrold LR, et al. Incidence and preventability of adverse drug events among older persons in the ambulatory setting. JAMA 2003;289:1107–16.
178. Chapman MD, Hanrahan R, McEwen J, et al. Hyponatraemia and hypokalaemia due to indapamide. Med J Aust 2002;176:219–21.
179. Adan A. Cognitive performance and dehydration. J Am Coll Nutr 2012;31:71–8.
180. Arieff AI. Fatal postoperative pulmonary edema: pathogenesis and literature review. Chest 1999;115:1371–7.
181. Lobo DN, Macafee DA, Allison SP. How perioperative fluid balance influences postoperative outcomes. Best Pract Res Clin Anaesthesiol 2006;20:439–55.
182. Holte K, Sharrock NE, Kehlet H. Pathophysiology and clinical implications of perioperative fluid excess. Br J Anaesth 2002;89:622–32.
183. Michell AR. Diuresis and diarrhea: is the gut a misunderstood nephron? Perspect Biol Med 2000;43:399–405.
184. Lobo DN, Bostock KA, Neal KR, et al. Effect of salt and water balance on recovery of gastrointestinal function after elective colonic resection: a randomised controlled trial. Lancet 2002;359:1812–8.
185. Chowdhury AH, Lobo DN. Fluids and gastrointestinal function. Curr Opin Clin Nutr Metab Care 2011;14:469–76.
186. Brandstrup B, Tonnesen H, Beier-Holgersen R, et al. Effects of intravenous fluid restriction on postoperative complications: comparison of two perioperative fluid regimens: a randomized assessor-blinded multicenter trial. Ann Surg 2003;238:641–8.
187. McArdle GT, McAuley DF, McKinley A, et al. Preliminary results of a prospective randomized trial of restrictive versus standard fluid regime in elective open abdominal aortic aneurysm repair. Ann Surg 2009;250:28–34.
188. Neal JM, Wilcox RR, Allen HW, et al. Near-total esophagectomy: the influence of standardized multimodal management and intraoperative fluid restriction. Reg Anesth Pain Med 2003;28:328–34.
189. Varadhan KK, Lobo DN. A meta-analysis of randomized controlled trials of intravenous fluid therapy in major elective open abdominal surgery: getting the balance right. Proc Nutr Soc 2010;69:488–98.

190. Reid F, Lobo DN, Williams RN, et al. (Ab)normal saline and physiological Hartmann's solution: a randomized double-blind crossover study. Clin Sci (Lond) 2003;104:17–24.
191. Williams EL, Hildebrand KL, McCormick SA, et al. The effect of intravenous lactated Ringer's solution versus 0.9% sodium chloride solution on serum osmolality in human volunteers. Anesth Analg 1999;88:999–1003.
192. Yunos NN, Bellomo R, Hegarty C, et al. Association between a chloride-liberal vs chloride-restrictive intravenous fluid administration strategy and kidney injury in critically ill adults. JAMA 2012;308:1566–72.
193. McCluskey SA, Karkouti K, Wijeysundera D, et al. Hyperchloremia after noncardiac surgery is independently associated with increased morbidity and mortality: a propensity-matched cohort study. Anesth Analg 2013;117:412–21.
194. Shaw AD, Bagshaw SM, Goldstein SL, et al. Major complications, mortality, and resource utilization after open abdominal surgery: 0.9% saline compared to plasma-lyte. Ann Surg 2012;255:821–9.
195. Sinclair S, James S, Singer M. Intraoperative intravascular volume optimization and length of hospital stay after repair of proximal femoral fracture: randomized controlled trial. BMJ 1997;315:909–12.
196. Venn R, Steele A, Richardson P, et al. Randomized controlled trial to investigate influence of the fluid challenge on duration of hospital stay and perioperative morbidity in patients with hip fractures. Br J Anaesth 2002;88:65–71.
197. Noblett SE, Snowden CP, Shenton BK, et al. Randomized clinical trial assessing the effect of Doppler-optimized fluid management on outcome after elective colorectal resection. Br J Surg 2006;93:1069–76.
198. Gan TJ, Soppitt A, Maroof M, et al. Goal-directed intraoperative fluid administration reduces length of hospital stay after major surgery. Anesthesiology 2002;97:820–6.
199. Mythen MG, Webb AR. Intraoperative gut mucosal hypoperfusion is associated with increased post-operative complications and cost. Intensive Care Med 1994;20:99–104.
200. Walsh SR, Tang T, Bass S, et al. Doppler-guided intra-operative fluid management during major abdominal surgery: systematic review and meta- analysis. Int J Clin Pract 2008;62:466–70.
201. Akhtar S. Guidelines and perioperative care of the elderly. Int Anesthesiol Clin 2014;52:64–76.
202. Committee on Standard and Practice Parameters, Apfelbaum JJ, Connis RT, et al. Practice advisory for preanesthesia evaluation: an updated report by the American Society of Anesthesiologists Task Force on Preanesthesia Evaluation. Anesthesiology 2012;116:522–38.
203. Benarrock-Gampel J, Sheffied KM, Duncan CB, et al. Preoperative laboratory testing in patients undergoing elective, low-risk ambulatory surgery. Ann Surg 2012;256:518–28.
204. Keay K, Lindsley K, Tielsch J, et al. Routine preoperative medical testing for cataract surgery. Cochrane Database Syst Rev 2012;(3):CD007293.
205. American Diabetes Association. Standards of medical care in diabetes – 2013. Diabetes Care 2013;36:S11–66.
206. Thomas DR, Ritchie DS. Preoperative assessment of older adults. J Am Geriatr Soc 1995;43:211–5.
207. Hosking MP, Warner MA, Lobdell CM, et al. Outcomes of surgery in patients 90 years of age and older. JAMA 1989;261:1909–15.

208. Keller SM, Markovitz LJ, Wilder JR, et al. Emergency and elective surgery in patients over age 70. Am Surg 1987;53:636–40.
209. Barlow AP, Zarifa Z, Shillito RG, et al. Surgery in a geriatric population. Ann R Coll Surg Engl 1989;71:110–4.
210. Rigberg D, Cole M, Hiyama D, et al. Surgery in the nineties. Am Surg 2000;66: 813–6.
211. Warner MA, Hosking MP, Lobdell CM, et al. Surgical procedures among those greater than or equal to 90 years of age. A population-based study in Olmsted County, Minnesota, 1975–85. Ann Surg 1988;207:380–6.
212. Edwards AE, Seymour DG, McCarthy JM, et al. A 5-year survival study of general surgical patients aged 65 years and over. Anaesthesia 1996;51:3–10.
213. Keller SM, Markovitz LJ, Wilder JR, et al. Emergency surgery in patients aged over 70 years. Mt Sinai J Med 1987;54:25–8.
214. Dekker JW, van den Broek CB, Bastiaannet E, et al. Importance of the first postoperative year in the prognosis of elderly colorectal cancer patients. Ann Surg Oncol 2011;18:1533–9.
215. Monk TG, Weldon BC, Garvan CW, et al. Predictors of cognitive dysfunction after major noncardiac surgery. Anesthesiology 2008;108:18–30.
216. Lamont CT, Sampson S, Matthias R, et al. The outcome of hospitalization for acute illness in the elderly. J Am Geriatr Soc 1983;31:282–8.
217. Fitzgerald JF, Moore PS, Dittus RS. The care of elderly patients with hip fracture. Changes since implementation of the prospective payment system. N Engl J Med 1988;319:1392–7.
218. Kemper P, Murtaugh CM. Lifetime use of nursing home care. N Engl J Med 1991;324:595–600.
219. Sloane PD, Pickasrd CG. Custodial nursing home care. Setting realistic goals. J Am Geriatr Soc 1985;33:864–8.

Perioperative Management in the Patient with Substance Abuse

Sharon Moran, MD*, Jason Isa, MD, Susan Steinemann, MD

KEYWORDS

• Drug screening • Substance abuse • Perioperative management

KEY POINTS

- Chronic substance use and acute intoxication may affect all aspects of perioperative care, including starting an intravenous line, securing an airway, intraoperative management, and postoperative pain control.
- The clinician should screen for alcohol and drug use in all patients and obtain serum or urine tests on those who are likely by history, physical examination, or circumstances to be intoxicated.
- Operations on acutely intoxicated patients should be delayed, if possible, because of the potential for hemodynamic instability.
- Those caring for a substance user postoperatively should be wary of the potential for hemodynamic compromise, poor wound healing, altered consciousness, and difficulty with pain management.

INTRODUCTION

Alcohol and drug use and abuse have been an increasing problem in the United States. The major categories of drugs of abuse include alcohol, stimulants, opiates, cannabinoids, and hallucinogens. Both acute intoxication and chronic abuse of these substances present challenges for anesthetic management during and after an operation. Whereas some procedures may be delayed while the issue is addressed, others are urgent or emergent and the surgeon and anesthesiologist must be able to deal with the physiologic changes that may occur in these patients.

According to the 2012 National Survey on Drug Use and Health,[1] which interviews persons aged 12 or older, 23.9 million Americans, or 9.2% of the population, were current users of illicit drugs (**Fig. 1**). This was an increase compared with 2008. Current

The authors have nothing to disclose.
Department of surgery, The Queen's Medical Center, University of Hawaii, 1356 Lusitana 6th floor, Honolulu, HI 96813, USA
* Corresponding author.
E-mail address: sharonemoran@gmail.com

Surg Clin N Am 95 (2015) 417–428
http://dx.doi.org/10.1016/j.suc.2014.11.001
surgical.theclinics.com

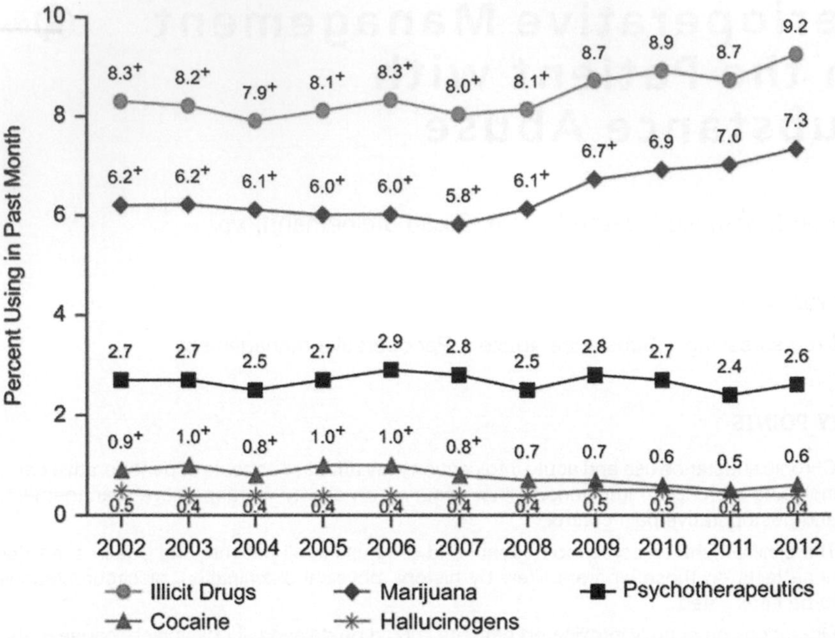

Fig. 1. Past month use of selected illicit drugs among persons aged 12 or older: 2002–2012. (*From* National Survey on Drug Use and Health (US), United States, Substance Abuse and Mental Health Services Administration, Office of Applied Studies, Center for Behavioral Health Statistics and Quality (US). Results from the 2012 National Survey on Drug Use and Health: summary of national findings, NSDUH Series H-46, HHS Publication No. (SMA) 13-4795. Rockville (MD): Substance Abuse and Mental Health Services Administration; 2013.)

drinkers of alcohol represent 52.1% of the population, with 6.5% reporting heavy use (**Fig. 2**). Those rates are similar to 2008. A total of 8.5% were considered to have a substance dependence or abuse disorder.

SCREENING FOR SUBSTANCE USE

Questions regarding alcohol and drug use should be part of any history and physical. The surgeon and anesthesiologist should emphasize that the question allows them to better take care of the patient and is not meant to be judgmental or to be used for criminal charges. Most patients are honest with the provider, but testing should be considered in the unconscious patient and in certain populations.[2,3] Substance abuse has been well studied in the trauma population because screening and intervention programs are required elements for a trauma center. Cost-benefit analysis supports testing those who arrive meeting trauma team activation criteria.[4] Patients seeking liver transplants are often enrolled in routine testing, but other organ transplant patients can be at risk for substance use disorders.[5] The bariatric surgery population has also been studied for increased substance use.[6] Features of the physical examination, such as tachycardia, tremors, a smell of alcohol, and poor dentition, may lead the physician to suspect substance use.

Results of urine testing are typically reported within a half hour of the sample being received. Serum alcohol results may take an hour to process. There are several different drug screen panels available, but most test for marijuana, amphetamines/methamphetamines, phencyclidine (PCP), cocaine, opioids, barbiturates, and benzodiazepines

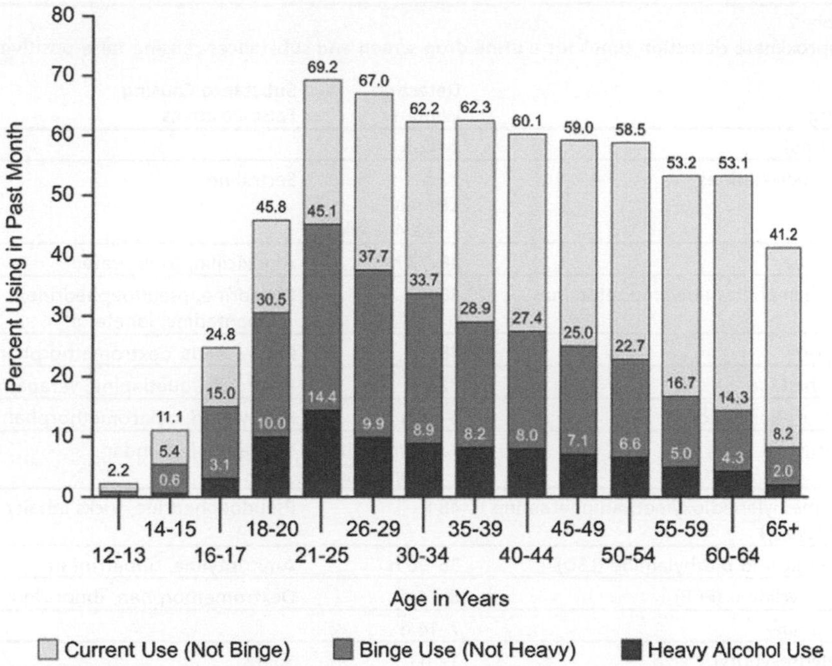

Fig. 2. Current, binge, and heavy alcohol use among persons aged 12 or older, by age: 2012. (*From* Substance Abuse and Mental Health Services Administration. Results from the 2012 National Survey on Drug Use and Health: summary of national findings, NSDUH Series H-46, HHS Publication No. (SMA) 13-4795. Rockville (MD): Substance Abuse and Mental Health Services Administration; 2013.)

(**Table 1**). If the patient screens positive for acute intoxication by history or laboratory testing and the operation is not urgent, the procedure should be delayed. The patient should be informed of the anesthetic risks particular to the substance used. If use is chronic, referral to treatment should be provided.

ALCOHOL

Depending on the screening tool used, up to 28.5% of patients presenting for an operation have an alcohol use disorder.[7] Blood levels decrease by approximately 0.015 g/dL per hour.

Airway: Aspiration Risk and Lung Injury

The intoxicated patient with a full stomach presents an aspiration risk. In addition, alcohol decreases lower esophageal sphincter pressure.[8] Chronic alcoholics have more airway colonization with pathologic bacteria, increasing the risk for pneumonia.[9] Even without aspirating, an injured patient with elevated blood alcohol content has been shown to be at increased risk for acute respiratory distress syndrome.[10] The chronic user is also at risk because of impaired cellular mechanisms and a decrease in antioxidants.[11,12]

Intraoperative Management

Anesthetic requirements vary widely, depending on degree of intoxication and degree of liver and other organ damage. Care should be taken when titrating oxygen because acutely intoxicated patients have less tolerance for hypoxia.[13] The patient with

Table 1
Approximate detection times for a urine drug screen and substances causing false-positives

Drug	Detection Window	Substance Causing False-Positives
Alcohol	2–12 h	
Benzodiazepines	72 h Chronic use 4–6 wk	Sertraline
Cocaine	48–72 h	Amoxicillin, tonic water
Methamphetamine/amphetamines	48 h	Ephedrine, pseudoephedrine, amantadine, labetalol
Heroin	48 h	Poppy seeds, dextromethorphan
Methadone	72 h	Ibuprofen, quetiapine, verapamil
Prescription opioids	6–96 h	Poppy seed, dextromethorphan
Marijuana	7 d–2 mo with chronic use	Dronabinol, sulindac
3,4-methylenedioxymethamphetamine (ecstasy)	48 h	Pseudoephedrine, Vicks inhaler
Lysergic acid diethylamide (LSD)	36–96 h	Amitriptyline, sumatriptan
Phencyclidine (PCP)	8–14 d	Dextromethorphan, ibuprofen
Ketamine	7–14 d	
γ-Hydroxybutyric acid	12 h	Soaps

cirrhosis has special fluid and electrolyte needs, and is at risk for bleeding; blood products should be made available. Hypotension may result from dehydration, cardiomyopathy,[14] or a diminished adrenocortical response to stress.[15]

Postoperative Management

Sensitivity to pain varies widely depending on degree of alcohol use and underdosing or overdosing of pain medicine is a possibility. In addition to pulmonary complications, alcoholics are at risk for wound infections caused by immunosuppression.[16]

The most serious postoperative complications are alcohol withdrawal and delirium tremens, because they are life-threatening conditions. Incidence varies depending on type of operation, age, and comorbidities. Symptoms of withdrawal can vary from mild tremors, confusion, and fever to severe electrolyte abnormalities (hyponatremia, hypokalemia, hypocalcemia, hypophosphatemia, and hypomagnesemia), hemodynamic instability, and seizures.

Implementation of a symptom-triggered withdrawal prophylaxis practice guideline using lorazepam, haloperidol, or clonidine can decrease the development of withdrawal syndromes.[17] Dexmedetomidine has been investigated as an adjunct to benzodiazepine in the prevention of withdrawal.[18]

BENZODIAZEPINES

Benzodiazepines are available by prescriptions for the treatment of anxiety, posttraumatic stress disorder, and other psychiatric illnesses.

Airway

Because benzodiazepines are most often ingested, there are not usually airway concerns outside of overdose. If there has been an overdose, flumazenil can be used as a reversal agent. Although there have been concerns for using flumazenil in patients with concomitant tricyclic overdose or chronic benzodiazepine users, experimental studies have shown that with proper precautions, it can be used safely.[19]

Intraoperative Management

Intraoperative complications in benzodiazepine using patients are not widely reported.

Postoperative Management

Benzodiazepine withdrawal is manifested by anxiety, poor sleep, tremors, and in its most serious form, seizures. Patients who are preoperatively on benzodiazepine treatment should have their medication continued. Those who were abusing benzodiazepines may be started on a symptom-triggered or tapered dose withdrawal regimen using a long-acting benzodiazepine[20] or be treated with low-dose flumazenil.[21]

STIMULANTS

Stimulants include cocaine and amphetamines. Route of administration varies and influences the length of intoxication and the manifestations of chronic use.

Cocaine

Cocaine is still used as a topical anesthetic, especially in ear, nose, and throat surgery. It may be smoked, taken intranasally ("snorted"), or injected. Its effects last from 30 to 60 minutes. Toxicity is manifested by psychosis, dysphoria, paranoia, anxiety, and cerebral hemorrhage. Coronary vasoconstriction may occur because of inhibition of catecholamine reuptake and inhibition of nitric oxide synthesis.[22]

Airway

Chronic nasal cocaine use can cause septal destruction and soft palate necrosis.[23] Caution should be taken while intubating or placing a nasogastric or orogastric tube. Smoked, or crack, cocaine can cause a wide variety of pulmonary complications including interstitial fibrosis, barotrauma, alveolar hemorrhage, and pulmonary hypertension that may make oxygenation or ventilation difficult.[24]

Intraoperative management

If the patient has normal vital signs and the electrocardiogram is normal, anesthesia has been shown in one study to be used safely in chronic users[25]; however, others argue for more caution. β-Blockers, such as propranolol, may result in unopposed α-adrenergic stimulation.[26] Nitroprusside, nitroglycerin, or demedetomidine may be used to control blood pressure. Hemodynamic instability may occur during acute intoxication when the patient can be hypertensive and hyperthermic, or hypotensive as a result of catecholamine depletion.[27] The hypotension may be ephedrine resistant, in which case phenylephrine may be effective.[27] Ketamine and halothane may potentiate negative cardiac effects and should be avoided.[27]

Postoperative management

Withdrawal symptoms include anxiety, restlessness, and tremors. Animal studies have explored treatment with buspirone, ondansetron, and propranolol.[28]

Methamphetamine and Amphetamines

Amphetamines may be used or abused during treatment for such conditions as narcolepsy and attention-deficit disorder. Methamphetamine can be ingested, snorted, smoked, or injected. Cardiac pathology includes arrhythmias, aortic dissection, acute coronary syndrome, and cardiomyopathy.[29] An electrocardiogram should be obtained and, if time warrants, an echocardiogram in long-time users.

Airway

"Meth mouth" is caused by poor oral hygiene, xerostomia, and poor diet[30] and may lead to damaged and loose teeth that can be dislodged during intubation. Inhaled methamphetamine may lead to pulmonary toxicity including reduced number of alveolar sacs and arteriole remodeling[31] and to pulmonary hypertension.[32] Like cocaine, intranasal use can lead to septal necrosis and care should be taken with nasogastric tubes.

Intraoperative management

Like cocaine, the patient may become hypertensive or hypotensive, depending on the circulating catecholamines. Evidence supports continuing prescription amphetamines during the perioperative period[33] to prevent further instability. In addition, methamphetamine has been associated with cardiomyopathy[34,35] and myocardial ischemia,[36] and the clinician should be aware of potential hemodynamic compromise in the patient who was unable to undergo preoperative work-up.

Postoperative management

Methamphetamine withdrawal peaks at 24 hours after last use and is characterized by increased sleeping, eating, and depression symptoms.[37] There is no consensus on the treatment of methamphetamine withdrawal, although psychosocial support and medical treatments have been investigated.[38]

OPIOIDS

Opioids have therapeutic and illicit uses. Prescription drug abuse has been increasing. As pharmaceutical companies produce drugs that are resistant to crushing, and therefore injecting, and as states are better at monitoring opiate prescribing, heroin use may increase. Local, regional, and epidural analgesia should be considered in the opioid-tolerant patient. Opioids may be injected, inhaled, ingested, or snorted.

Heroin

Heroin is commonly injected or administered by "skin popping," either of which may make intravenous access difficult. Caution should be taken because intravenous drug abusers may have communicable diseases, such as HIV or hepatitis.

Airway

Several factors may compromise airway and oxygenation/ventilation. Pulmonary edema may occur in patients who have overdosed.[39] Chronic use may lead to pulmonary hemorrhage caused by hypoxia and to granulomatous infiltration.[40] Aspiration may occur because of delayed gastric emptying.

Intraoperative management

Like all opioids, anesthesia and analgesia may be difficult, especially in long-term users, who can have increased sensitivity to pain caused by opioid-induced hyperalgesia. The variability in purity makes it difficult to calculate an equianalgesic dose of a therapeutic opioid. Opioids need to be continued to prevent withdrawal, but other medications, such as acetaminophen, nonsteroidal anti-inflammatory drugs, gabapentin, and pregabaline, may be included in a multimodal therapy regimen. Ketamine has been used in the perioperative period to reduce the amount of narcotics needed and decrease hyperalgesia.[41]

Postoperative management

Withdrawal can begin within 6 to 18 hours. High doses of narcotics may be needed to prevent or alleviate symptoms. Opioid agonists-antagonists, such as nalbuphine, should not be given to chronic opioid users because they may precipitate withdrawal.[42] Although a good adjunct for pain management, epidural anesthesia alone can lead to withdrawal if oral or intravenous opioids are not also given. Some centers are able to transition the patient to a methadone maintenance program.

Methadone

Methadone is prescribed by specialized physicians for opioid addiction or any physician for pain. It is a very effective analgesic because it has a fairly rapid onset, long half-life, and is a *N*-methyl-D-aspartate antagonist and a mu receptor agonist. It also has a potential for abuse.

Airway

Methadone is usually taken orally without physical effects on the airway. Naive users may exhibit impaired ventilator response to hypercapnea that resolves with chronic use.

Intraoperative management

The management is similar to that for heroin.

Postoperative management

Withdrawal can begin within 24 to 48 hours. Management of pain and withdrawal is similar to that for heroin. If methadone is used for pain control, caution should be taken because a small dose increase can result in a toxic level.

Prescription Opioids

Prescription opioid use and abuse has been an increasing problem. New formulations of pills have been designed to prevent the nonoral use of medications, such as grinding pills for inhalation or injection.

Airway

Inhalation of crushed pills can lead to septal and soft palate necrosis.[43] Pulmonary talcosis and resulting cor pulmonale may occur with injection of ground pills.[44]

Intraoperative management

The management is similar to that for heroin. If the patient has been using a fentanyl patch, it should be removed because the distribution is altered by fluid shifts and temperature during the operation.[41]

Postoperative management

Time to withdrawal depends on the formulation of the drug used. There may be cross-tolerance between systemic and epidural morphine. Epidural bupivacaine/sufentanyl has been shown to be effective in chronic morphine users.[45] Otherwise, management of pain and withdrawal is similar to that for heroin.

MARIJUANA

Marijuana is the most commonly abused illicit drug. Marijuana has been legalized for medical use in many states and a few states have allowed sales for recreational use. Although traditionally smoked, marijuana dispensaries also dispense edible products with high concentrations of tetrahydrocannabinol that have been associated in the popular press with adverse events including psychosis and violent behavior.[46]

Airway

Compared with nicotine cigarettes, the airway effects of smoking marijuana are mild. Bronchodilation can happen in the short term, but a chronic cough and mild airflow obstruction can develop over long-term use.[47] Upper airway edema has been described because of smoking.[48] Also, there are reports of pneumothorax from frequent Valsalva-like maneuvers.[49]

Intraoperative Management

Marijuana may increase the stimulatory effects of amphetamines and cocaine and the depressant effects of alcohol and benzodiazepines. The cardiovascular effects are biphasic. Low doses result in sympathetic stimulation with tachycardia and slight hypertension.[50] High doses can inhibit sympathetic activity with unopposed parasympathetic activity leading to bradycardia and hypotension.[50]

Postoperative Management

Withdrawal symptoms include anxiety, irritability, depressed mood, and lack of appetite.[51] Patients with chronic cough are at risk for wound dehiscence. The patient should be observed for signs of stridor caused by upper airway edema.

CLUB DRUGS AND DESIGNER DRUGS

This is class that includes drugs that originally were used therapeutically and newer drugs that may not have consistent purity. Coingestion of multiple substances and use with alcohol are common. Some of the most popular drugs are ecstasy (methylenedioxymethamphetamine), lysergic acid diethylamide (LSD), PCP, ketamine, flunitrazepam (Rohypnol, "roofies") γ-hydroxybutyric acid, "bath salts," and "spice." There are few data on the effects of anesthesia on patients intoxicated with these substances, but physiologic and neurologic effects are well described.

Ecstasy/Methylenedioxymethamphetamine

The ecstasy high lasts about 6 hours and includes euphoria and relaxation. Toxicity is manifested by fever, hyponatremia, rhabdomyolysis, renal and liver failure, and death.[52] Nondepolarizing muscle relaxers, benzodiazepines, propofol, nitroprusside, and nitroglycerin are safe.[22] Atypical antipsychotics may lower the seizure threshold. Temperature should be controlled with cold fluid or a cooling blanket. Treatment with dantrolene is controversial, but has been used safely and effectively.[53] Hyponatremia should be corrected slowly to prevent central pontine myelinolysis. Creatine kinase or myoglobin levels can be used for suspected rhabdomyolysis. Ecstasy has also been associated with spontaneous pneumothorax and pneumomediastinum and should be suspected with any unexplained oxygenation or ventilation difficulty.[54]

Lysergic Acid Diethylamide

LSD was legal until the 1960s and there is new interest in its use as an adjunct to psychotherapy. Toxic effects include hallucinations, dilated pupils, synesthesia, tachycardia, tachypnea, fever, hypertonia, and hyperglycemia. Effects last from 6 to 10 hours.[55]

Phencyclidine

PCP ("angel dust") is typically inhaled, with effects lasting 4 to 8 hours. Toxic effects include nystagmus, violent behavior, tachycardia, hypertension, psychosis, coma, and cerebral hemorrhage. Supportive treatment includes benzodiazepines and atypical antipsychotics.[56] Ketamine is a derivative of PCP and should not be used in these patients.[57]

Ketamine

Ketamine, in its nontherapeutic use, is often snorted or ingested and called "Special K." It has a rapid onset, short duration, and induces a dissociative state. Adverse effects include confusion, apnea, nystagmus, cardiovascular dysfunction, and severe bladder toxicity.[58] Treatment is supportive. Benzodiazepines and haloperidol can be used.[22] Contrary to classic teaching, ketamine does not increase intracranial pressure in either traumatic or nontraumatic brain injury.[59,60]

Flunitrazepam

Flunitrazepam is a benzodiazepine used therapeutically in many countries. It has been used as a "date rape" drug for its sedative-hypnotic properties. Effects include slurred speech, bradycardia, respiratory depression, and coma. As with other benzodiazepines, there may be a withdrawal syndrome. Treatment may be started with a long-acting benzodiazepine, such as clonazepam. Flumazenil is used for overdoses.

γ-Hydroxybutyric Acid

γ-Hydroxybutyric acid is an analogue of γ-aminobutyric acid and has a history of use as an anesthetic and body building supplement. More recently it has also become known as a "date rape" drug. Euphoria lasts around 4 hours, but the undesired effects of respiratory and central nervous system depression may linger and require intubation or cause death.[61] A withdrawal syndrome is similar to that for alcohol, and should be treated accordingly.

Bath Salts

Bath salts cause tachycardia, hypertension, delusions, dilated pupils, and can be fatal in severe cases. Treatment with benzodiazepines and antipsychotics has been explored.[62]

Spice

Spice was originally marketed as legal marijuana and is a synthetic cannabinoid. Effects last 2 to 4 hours and can include hallucinations, tachycardia, and seizures.[63]

SUMMARY

Drug and alcohol use is a pervasive problem in the general population and in those requiring anesthesia for an operation. History and screening can help delineate those who may be acutely intoxicated or chronic users. The clinician should be aware of problems that may be encountered during any part of anesthesia or postoperative care.

REFERENCES

1. National Survey on Drug Use and Health (U.S.), United States, Substance Abuse and Mental Health Services Administration, Office of Applied Studies, Center for Behavioral Health Statistics and Quality (U.S.). Results from the 2012 National Survey on Drug Use and Health: summary of national findings. Rockville (MD): Substance Abuse and Mental Health Services Administration; 2013. p. 1 HHS publication no (SMA) 13-4795. Online resource.

2. Brown J, Kranzler HR, Del Boca FK. Self-reports by alcohol and drug abuse inpatients: factors affecting reliability and validity. Br J Addict 1992;87(7):1013–24.
3. Rockett IR, Putnam SL, Jia H, et al. Declared and undeclared substance use among emergency department patients: a population-based study. Addiction 2006;101(5):706–12.
4. Dunham CM, Chirichella TJ. Trauma activation patients: evidence for routine alcohol and illicit drug screening. PLoS One 2012;7(10):e47999.
5. Sirri L, Potena L, Masetti M, et al. Prevalence of substance-related disorders in heart transplantation candidates. Transplant Proc 2007;39(6):1970–2.
6. Kudsi OY, Huskey K, Grove S, et al. Prevalence of preoperative alcohol abuse among patients seeking weight-loss surgery. Surg Endosc 2013;27(4):1093–7.
7. Agabio R, Gessa GL, Montisci A, et al. Use of the screening suggested by the National Institute on Alcohol Abuse and Alcoholism and of a newly derived tool for the detection of unhealthy alcohol drinkers among surgical patients. J Stud Alcohol Drugs 2012;73(1):126–33.
8. Castell DO. The lower esophageal sphincter. Physiologic and clinical aspects. Ann Intern Med 1975;83(3):390–401.
9. Fernandez-Sola J, Junque A, Estruch R, et al. High alcohol intake as a risk and prognostic factor for community-acquired pneumonia. Arch Intern Med 1995; 155(15):1649–54.
10. Afshar M, Smith GS, Terrin ML, et al. Blood alcohol content, injury severity, and adult respiratory distress syndrome. J Trauma Acute Care Surg 2014;76(6):1447–55.
11. Guidot DM, Roman J. Chronic ethanol ingestion increases susceptibility to acute lung injury: role of oxidative stress and tissue remodeling. Chest 2002;122(Suppl 6):309S–14S.
12. Kaphalia L, Calhoun WJ. Alcoholic lung injury: metabolic, biochemical and immunological aspects. Toxicol Lett 2013;222(2):171–9.
13. Nettles JL, Olson RN. Effects of alcohol on hypoxia. JAMA 1965;194(11):1193–4.
14. Biancofiore G, Mandell MS, Rocca GD. Perioperative considerations in patients with cirrhotic cardiomyopathy. Curr Opin Anaesthesiol 2010;23(2):128–32.
15. Haxholdt OS, Johansson G. The alcoholic patient and surgical stress. Anaesthesia 1982;37(8):797–801.
16. Sander M, Irwin M, Sinha P, et al. Suppression of interleukin-6 to interleukin-10 ratio in chronic alcoholics: association with postoperative infections. Intensive Care Med 2002;28(3):285–92.
17. Stanley KM, Amabile CM, Simpson KN, et al. Impact of an alcohol withdrawal syndrome practice guideline on surgical patient outcomes. Pharmacotherapy 2003;23(7):843–54.
18. DeMuro JP, Botros DG, Wirkowski E, et al. Use of dexmedetomidine for the treatment of alcohol withdrawal syndrome in critically ill patients: a retrospective case series. J Anesth 2012;26(4):601–5.
19. Weinbroum A, Rudick V, Sorkine P, et al. Use of flumazenil in the treatment of drug overdose: a double-blind and open clinical study in 110 patients. Crit Care Med 1996;24(2):199–206.
20. McGregor C, Machin A, White JM. In-patient benzodiazepine withdrawal: comparison of fixed and symptom-triggered taper methods. Drug Alcohol Rev 2003;22(2):175–80.
21. Hood SD, Norman A, Hince DA, et al. Benzodiazepine dependence and its treatment with low dose flumazenil. Br J Clin Pharmacol 2014;77(2):285–94.
22. Demaria S Jr, Weinkauf JL. Cocaine and the club drugs. Int Anesthesiol Clin 2011;49(1):79–101.

23. Birchenough SA, Borowitz K, Lin KY. Complete soft palate necrosis and velopharyngeal insufficiency resulting from intranasal inhalation of prescription narcotics and cocaine. J Craniofac Surg 2007;18(6):1482–5.
24. Restrepo CS, Carrillo JA, Martinez S, et al. Pulmonary complications from cocaine and cocaine-based substances: imaging manifestations. Radiographics 2007; 27(4):941–56.
25. Hill GE, Ogunnaike BO, Johnson ER. General anaesthesia for the cocaine abusing patient. Is it safe? Br J Anaesth 2006;97(5):654–7.
26. Wong GT, Irwin MG. Poisoning with illicit substances: toxicology for the anaesthetist. Anaesthesia 2013;68(Suppl 1):117–24.
27. Hernandez M, Birnbach DJ, Van Zundert AA. Anesthetic management of the illicit-substance-using patient. Curr Opin Anaesthesiol 2005;18(3):315–24.
28. de Oliveira Cito Mdo C, da Silva FC, Silva MI, et al. Reversal of cocaine withdrawal-induced anxiety by ondansetron, buspirone and propranolol. Behav Brain Res 2012;231(1):116–23.
29. Kaye S, McKetin R, Duflou J, et al. Methamphetamine and cardiovascular pathology: a review of the evidence. Addiction 2007;102(8):1204–11.
30. Hamamoto DT, Rhodus NL. Methamphetamine abuse and dentistry. Oral Dis 2009;15(1):27–37.
31. Wang Y, Liu M, Wang HM, et al. Involvement of serotonin mechanism in methamphetamine-induced chronic pulmonary toxicity in rats. Hum Exp Toxicol 2013;32(7):736–46.
32. Chin KM, Channick RN, Rubin LJ. Is methamphetamine use associated with idiopathic pulmonary arterial hypertension? Chest 2006;130(6):1657–63.
33. Fischer SP, Schmiesing CA, Guta CG, et al. General anesthesia and chronic amphetamine use: should the drug be stopped preoperatively? Anesth Analg 2006;103(1):203–6. Table of contents.
34. Won S, Hong RA, Shohet RV, et al. Methamphetamine-associated cardiomyopathy. Clin Cardiol 2013;36(12):737–42.
35. Yeo KK, Wijetunga M, Ito H, et al. The association of methamphetamine use and cardiomyopathy in young patients. Am J Med 2007;120(2):165–71.
36. Hawley LA, Auten JD, Matteucci MJ, et al. Cardiac complications of adult methamphetamine exposures. J Emerg Med 2013;45(6):821–7.
37. McGregor C, Srisurapanont M, Jittiwutikarn J, et al. The nature, time course and severity of methamphetamine withdrawal. Addiction 2005;100(9):1320–9.
38. Pennay AE, Lee NK. Putting the call out for more research: the poor evidence base for treating methamphetamine withdrawal. Drug Alcohol Rev 2011;30(2):216–22.
39. Lynch K, Greenbaum E, O'Loughlin BJ. Pulmonary edema in heroin overdose. Radiology 1970;94(2):377–8.
40. Kringsholm B, Christoffersen P. Lung and heart pathology in fatal drug addiction. A consecutive autopsy study. Forensic Sci Int 1987;34(1–2):39–51.
41. Richebe P, Beaulieu P. Perioperative pain management in the patient treated with opioids: continuing professional development. Can J Anaesth 2009;56(12): 969–81.
42. Preston KL, Bigelow GE, Liebson IA. Antagonist effects of nalbuphine in opioid-dependent human volunteers. J Pharmacol Exp Ther 1989;248(3):929–37.
43. Greene D. Total necrosis of the intranasal structures and soft palate as a result of nasal inhalation of crushed OxyContin. Ear Nose Throat J 2005;84(8):512, 514, 516.
44. Griffith CC, Raval JS, Nichols L. Intravascular talcosis due to intravenous drug use is an underrecognized cause of pulmonary hypertension. Pulm Med 2012; 2012:617531.

45. de Leon-Casasola OA, Lema MJ. Epidural bupivacaine/sufentanil therapy for postoperative pain control in patients tolerant to opioid and unresponsive to epidural bupivacaine/morphine. Anesthesiology 1994;80(2):303–9.
46. Colorado to revisit edible marijuana rules after deaths. USA Today 2014.
47. Tashkin DP. Airway effects of marijuana, cocaine, and other inhaled illicit agents. Curr Opin Pulm Med 2001;7(2):43–61.
48. Mallat A, Roberson J, Brock-Utne JG. Preoperative marijuana inhalation–an airway concern. Can J Anaesth 1996;43(7):691–3.
49. Feldman AL, Sullivan JT, Passero MA, et al. Pneumothorax in polysubstance-abusing marijuana and tobacco smokers: three cases. J Subst Abuse 1993; 5(2):183–6.
50. Ghuran A, Nolan J. Recreational drug misuse: issues for the cardiologist. Heart 2000;83(6):627–33.
51. Kouri EM, Pope HG Jr. Abstinence symptoms during withdrawal from chronic marijuana use. Exp Clin Psychopharmacol 2000;8(4):483–92.
52. Ben-Abraham R, Szold O, Rudick V, et al. "Ecstasy" intoxication: life-threatening manifestations and resuscitative measures in the intensive care setting. Eur J Emerg Med 2003;10(4):309–13.
53. Grunau BE, Wiens MO, Brubacher JR. Dantrolene in the treatment of MDMA-related hyperpyrexia: a systematic review. CJEM 2010;12(5):435–42.
54. Mazur S, Hitchcock T. Spontaneous pneumomediastinum, pneumothorax and ecstasy abuse. Emerg Med 2001;13(1):121–3.
55. Passie T, Halpern JH, Stichtenoth DO, et al. The pharmacology of lysergic acid diethylamide: a review. CNS Neurosci Ther 2008;14(4):295–314.
56. Bey T, Patel A. Phencyclidine intoxication and adverse effects: a clinical and pharmacological review of an illicit drug. Cal J Emerg Med 2007;8(1):9–14.
57. Vadivelu N, Mitra S, Kaye AD, et al. Perioperative analgesia and challenges in the drug-addicted and drug-dependent patient. Best practice research. Best Pract Res Clin Anaesthesiol 2014;28(1):91–101.
58. Corazza O, Assi S, Schifano F. From "Special K" to "Special M": the evolution of the recreational use of ketamine and methoxetamine. CNS Neurosci Ther 2013; 19(6):454–60.
59. Zeiler FA, Teitelbaum J, West M, et al. The ketamine effect on intracranial pressure in nontraumatic neurological illness. J Crit Care 2014;29(6):1096–106.
60. Zeiler FA, Teitelbaum J, West M, et al. The ketamine effect on ICP in traumatic brain injury. Neurocrit Care 2014;21(1):163–73.
61. Mason PE, Kerns WP 2nd. Gamma hydroxybutyric acid (GHB) intoxication. Acad Emerg Med 2002;9(7):730–9.
62. Centers for Disease Control and Prevention (CDC). Emergency department visits after use of a drug sold as "bath salts"—Michigan, November 13, 2010-March 31, 2011. MMWR Morb Mortal Wkly Rep 2011;60(19):624–7.
63. Harris CR, Brown A. Synthetic cannabinoid intoxication: a case series and review. J Emerg Med 2013;44(2):360–6.

Management of Pregnant Patients Undergoing General Surgical Procedures

Melissa K. Stewart, MD, Kyla P. Terhune, MD*

KEYWORDS

• Pregnancy • Nonobstetric surgery • Perioperative care

KEY POINTS

- Physiologic changes during pregnancy span almost every organ system, influencing even laboratory values of pregnant patients, and must be understood in order to optimize perioperative and operative care.
- Diagnostic modalities are necessary but can have effects on fetuses and should be understood in order to minimize radiation exposure during pregnancy.
- Most preoperative considerations for pregnant patients are similar to those for nonpregnant patients; however, a basic knowledge of medications and anesthetic considerations is important in order to provide safe care.
- Surgical patients are surgical patients, whether pregnant or not. Surgical issues must be addressed, and delay of operative care can lead to worsened outcomes, despite gestational status and stage.

INTRODUCTION

Of women of reproductive age, 102.1 per 1000 women are pregnant in the United States at any given time.[1] Of those who are pregnant, approximately 0.2% to 0.75% require nonobstetric surgical intervention during pregnancy.[2,3] As in the general surgery population, the most common presenting conditions requiring nonobstetric operations during pregnancy are appendicitis and cholecystitis.[4] In general, the approach is the same: to address the surgical issue. However, there are a multitude of additional considerations for pregnant patients, one of which is recognizing the importance of multidisciplinary care. As stated in an American Congress of Obstetrics and Gynecology opinion in 2011, the management of a pregnant patient should be multifaceted, involving the coordination of the obstetrician, surgeon, anesthesiologist, and neonatologist, because concerns regarding both the fetus and the mother may require management modification.[5]

Disclosures: The authors have no financial disclosures.
Department of Surgery, Vanderbilt University Medical Center, 1161 21st Avenue South, Nashville, TN 37232, USA
* Corresponding author. D-4309 MCN, 1161 21st Avenue South, Nashville, TN 37232.
E-mail address: kyla.terhune@vanderbilt.edu

Surg Clin N Am 95 (2015) 429–442
http://dx.doi.org/10.1016/j.suc.2014.10.007
0039-6109/15/$ – see front matter Published by Elsevier Inc.

PHYSIOLOGIC CHANGES IN PREGNANCY

Physiologic changes during pregnancy are numerous and span most organ systems (**Fig. 1**). By recognizing and understanding these changes, surgeons may optimize

System:

Cardiovascular:

- Lateral displacement of heart apex
- Eccentric Hypertrophy (increased blood volume)
- Increased Stroke Volume
- Increased Heart Rate

→ Increased Cardiac Output

- Compression of IVC by gravid uterus → Positional Preload

Respiratory:

- Edematous and hyperemic nasopharynx
- Decreased TLC, FRC, and RV
- Increased respiratory rate

→ Chronic Respiratory Alkalosis

Hematologic:

- 40-50% increased blood volume
- 30% increased erythrocyte mass

→ Anemia

- Leukocytosis
- Venous Stasis
- Increased procoagulants

→ Increased risk of Thromboembolic events

Gastrointestinal:

- Relaxation of smooth muscle tone
  - -esophagus, stomach, bowel, gallbladder
- Mechanical gastric compression
- Increased intra-abdominal pressure

→ Reflux, Biliary stasis, Cholecystitis

Urological:

- Increased size of organs
- Dilation of pelvis, calyces and ureters
- Increased GFR

→ Decreased creatinine, BUN, and uric acid

- Structural changes of position and capacitance of bladder

Fig. 1. Physiologic changes during pregnancy by system. BUN, blood urea nitrogen; FRC, functional residual capacity; GFR, glomerular filtration rate; IVC, inferior vena cava; RV, residual volume; TLC, total lung capacity.

perioperative and intraoperative management. Each affected organ system is discussed separately later.

Cardiovascular System

With expansion of the gravid uterus and subsequent increased intra-abdominal pressure, the diaphragm is upwardly displaced and rib shape is changed. This change leads to longitudinal rotation and lateral displacement of the heart, which can result in false radiographic findings that suggest cardiomegaly.

The heart develops eccentric hypertrophy secondary to increased blood volume. This increased blood volume increases the cardiac output by increasing stroke volume. When combined with concomitant increased heart rate, cardiac output can increase by 30% to 50% in pregnant patients, peaking at 25 to 30 weeks' gestation. Despite this increase in cardiac output, maternal blood pressure is decreased secondary to decreased systemic vascular resistance. In addition, all of these balanced dynamics can be markedly affected by positional changes, most of which can be accounted for by inferior vena cava compression by the gravid uterus.[6,7]

Respiratory Changes

As in most systems, the respiratory effects are a combination of hormonal and mechanical changes. Increased estrogen causes the mucosa of the nasopharynx to become edematous and hyperemic, leading to both hypersecretion and an increased likelihood of spontaneous or induced epistaxis. Relaxation of the cartilaginous attachments between the ribs and sternum, as well as mechanical pressure from the gravid uterus, leads to structural changes of the thoracic cavity, including an increase in subcostal angle, increased chest diameter, and rise in the diaphragm. These changes result in decreased total lung capacity, decreased functional residual capacity, and decreased residual volume. In addition, secondary to progesterone, an increased respiratory rate occurs. Combined with decreased capacities and volumes, this results in increased alveolar ventilation and a chronic respiratory alkalosis.[6,7]

Hematologic Changes

Changes in maternal blood volume begin to occur as early as the first month of pregnancy. Throughout the pregnancy, blood volume increases progressively, expanding by 40% to 50%, until about 30 to 34 weeks' gestation. Erythrocyte mass also increases by approximately 30%. The differential increase in blood volume versus erythrocyte mass leads to an overall net decrease in hematocrit; a condition that is called physiologic anemia of pregnancy.

The white blood cell count also progressively increases. The cause of this leukocytosis is unclear but may be related to increased cortisol and estrogen levels. Moreover, because of relative venous stasis secondary to compression of the inferior vena cava and concomitant hypercoagulability secondary to an increase in procoagulants, a state thought to be protective against peripartum hemorrhage, pregnancy results in a 5-fold to 6-fold increased risk of thromboembolic events.[6,7]

Gastrointestinal Changes

Secondary to relaxant effects of estrogen and progesterone on smooth muscle, the tone and the motility of the esophagus and stomach are decreased. This change, in conjunction with mechanical gastric compression from an enlarged uterus, leads to a marked increase in gastroesophageal reflux during pregnancy. Approximately 30% to 50% of pregnant women report having dyspepsia and reflux. In addition, 30% to 40% complain of changes in bowel habits, ranging from constipation to diarrhea. Similar to the alimentary tract, the gallbladder is affected by hormone-induced changes. Such changes lead to decreased ejection fraction and increased biliary cholesterol saturation, making biliary sludge and stones more likely.[6,7]

Renal/Urinary Changes

The kidney and renal collection system increase in size during pregnancy with dilatation of the renal pelvis, calyces, and ureters. Renal plasma flow and, subsequently, glomerular filtration rate are markedly increased during pregnancy; nearly 50% within the first trimester alone. This hyperfiltration leads to a physiologic decrease in serum creatinine level, blood urea nitrogen level, and uric acid concentration. Other anatomic changes include increase in the bladder trigone and potentially increased vascular tortuosity resulting in increased microhematuria. Also of note, secondary to outward pressure by the expanding uterus, bladder capacitance decreases over time, resulting in urinary frequency, urgency, and incontinence.[6,7]

PREOPERATIVE EVALUATION

A principle that underpins the work-up of a patient was aptly stated by Sir Zachary Cope: "Earlier diagnosis means better prognosis."[8] This mantra holds true especially in pregnancy, in relation to both the prognosis of the mother and fetus. For example, 36% of women with perforated appendicitis, which can often be attributed to delayed diagnosis, experience fetal loss, compared with 1.5% to 9% in those with nonperforated appendicitis.[9]

Although the evaluation of pregnant patients carries a unique set of dilemmas, the work-up should be initiated in the same manner as that of nonpregnant patients, beginning with a detailed history and physical examination. In the physical examination, the clinician must consider that the organ in question, such as the appendix, may be significantly displaced secondary to the gravid uterus. Subsequently, the clinician must carefully consider the use of adjunctive diagnostic modalities, because effects on both the patient and fetus must be considered. Evaluation by both laboratory and radiographic techniques, with accompanying description of the modality and specific risks/benefits, are described later.

Biochemical Evaluation

Based on the anatomic and physiologic changes described earlier, altered laboratory values may be seen in pregnant patients compared with normal values.[10] A summarization of these changes is shown in **Table 1**.[11]

Imaging Techniques

Computed tomography

Computed tomography (CT) uses ionizing radiation: high-energy photons capable of damaging DNA and generating caustic free radicals (summarized in **Table 2**).[12] Given this, fetal exposure carries potential risks of gene mutations, which could lead to teratogenesis or malignancy. Although causality has been established in the literature, the risk remains small. Most usual diagnostic examinations used in the work-up of general surgical patients (ie, CT abdomen, CT pelvis, and CT pyelogram) are all below the proposed maximum radiation level.[13] As stated by the American College of Radiology, "No single diagnostic procedure results in a radiation dose that threatens the well-being of the developing embryo and fetus."[12] Note that the effect is cumulative, and the recommended level of exposure to the fetus should not exceed 5 rad.[14]

Table 1
Summary of expected laboratory values during pregnancy across trimesters

	Nonpregnant	First Trimester	Second Trimester	Third Trimester
Complete Blood Count				
Hemoglobin (g/dL)	12.0–15.8	11.6–13.9	9.7–14.8	9.5–15.0
Hematocrit (%)	35.4–44.4	31.0–41.0	30.0–39.0	28.0–40.0
Platelet ($\times 10^9$/L)	165–415	174–391	155–409	146–429
White blood cell count ($\times 10^3$/mm^3)	3.5–9.1	5.7–13.6	5.6–14.8	5.9–16.9
Coagulation Profile				
Prothrombin time (s)	12.7–15.4	9.7–13.5	9.5–13.4	9.6–12.9
International Normalized Ratio	0.9–1.04	0.85–1.08	0.83–1.02	0,80–1.09
Partial thromboplastin time (s)	26.3–39.4	23–38.9	22.9–38.1	22.6–35.0
Complete Metabolic Panel				
Sodium (mEq/L)	136–146	133–148	129–148	130–148
Potassium (mEq/L)	3.5–5.0	3.6–5.0	3.3–5.0	3.3–5.1
Chloride (mEq/L)	102–109	101–105	97–109	97–109
Bicarbonate (mmol/L)	22–30	20–24	20–24	20–24
Urea nitrogen (mg/dL)	7–20	7–12	3–13	3–11
Creatinine (mg/dL)	0.5–0.9	0.4–0.7	0.4–0.8	0.4–0.9
Alanine transaminase (U/L)	7–41	3–30	2–33	2–25
Aspartate transaminase (U/L)	12–38	2023	3–33	4–32
Bilirubin, total (mg/dL)	0.3–4.8	0–4.9	0–9.1	0–11.3
Bilirubin, unconjugated (mg/dL)	0.2–0.9	0.1–0.5	0.1–0.4	0.1–0.5
Bilirubin, conjugated (mg/dL)	0.1–0.4	0–0.1	0–9.1	0–0.1
Alkaline phosphatase (U/L)	33–96	17–88	25–126	38–229
Amylase (U/L)	20–96	24–83	16–73	15–81
Lipase (U/L)	3–43	21–76	26–100	41–112
Magnesium (mg/dL)	1.5–2.3	1.6–2.2	1.5–2.2	1.1–2.2
Phosphate (mg/dL)	2.4–4.3	3.1–4.6	2.5–4.6	2.8–4.6

Data from Cunningham F. Normal reference ranges for laboratory values in pregnancy. In: Post TW, editor. UpToDate; 2014. [cited August 1, 2014].

Ultrasonography

Sound waves, not ionizing radiation, are used in ultrasonography. These waves are generally thought to be safe to the fetus. Although no documentation of adverse fetal effects from diagnostic ultrasonography procedures exists, the US Food and Drug Administration recommends limiting ultrasonography energy exposure to

Table 2
Summary of imaging modalities

Modality		Risk	Potential Effects	Limit
Radiograph, fluoroscopy, CT	Ionizing radiation	Gene mutation	Teratogenesis, malignancy	5 rad
Ultrasonography	Sound waves	—	—	94 mW/cm^2
MRI	Magnetic energy	Acoustic noise, heat	—	—

94 mW/cm^2.[15] Because of the improved safety profile of ultrasonography, it has gained popularity and largely replaced radiographic diagnostic modalities using ionizing radiation.[16] However, it is limited by body habitus and can be highly operator dependent. Hence, reliability and precision may be decreased. For example, in multiple studies analyzing identification of acute appendicitis during pregnancy with the use of ultrasonography, sensitivities ranged from 50% to 100% and specificity from 96% to 100%.[17–19] These values are markedly less than the nearly 98% sensitivity, specificity, and diagnostic accuracy of CT and MRI.[20,21]

MRI

Like ultrasonography, MRI provides a nonionizing radiation imaging alternative. MRI uses magnetic energy to alter the state of hydrogen protons.[16] Although it is postulated that the acoustic noise and heat produced may be detrimental to a developing fetus, no specific adverse fetal effects of MRI have been reported.[22,23] Although fetal effects have yet to be elucidated, intravenous gadolinium agents, which are used to increase definition in certain MRI studies, can cross the placenta.[24] Because of this and the potential risk of nephrogenic systemic fibrosis, its use is not recommended in pregnant patients.[25]

Cholangiography: intraoperative and endoscopic retrograde cholangiopancreatography

The potential ill effects of cholangiography are secondary to radiation exposure. Typical intraoperative cholangiography exposure is estimated to be between 0.2 and 0.5 rad/s.[26] It is recommended that the fetus be shielded by placing a protective barrier between the patient and the radiation source. In fluoroscopy, this radiation source is generally beneath the operating table, necessitating the placement of lead directly on the table and the patient on the lead. This placement is not instinctive because the tendency is to cover the patient with lead, which would provide no protection. Other methods of protection should also be used. Rather than using so-called live fluoroscopy, clinicians could inject the contrast agent and obtain a single completion cholangiogram, thus minimizing radiation exposure. Endoscopic retrograde cholangiopancreatography (ERCP) radiation exposure can be significantly higher than that of intraoperative cholangiography, averaging between 2 and 12 rad/s.[27] Moreover, ERCP carries the additional risks of bleeding and pancreatitis.

In summary, the same potential diagnostic studies are available to pregnant patients and should be used when necessary. When deciding on a modality, clinicians must consider the risks and benefits. The risk of a missed or incorrect diagnosis almost always outweighs the risk of any of the aforementioned studies. It is of utmost importance that physicians communicate said risks to their patients, allowing an active, informed conversation and joint decision making.

PATIENT SELECTION/PREOPERATIVE PREPARATION

If a condition requiring surgical intervention is diagnosed, such as appendicitis or cholecystitis, an urgent operation should be performed regardless of the trimester. In contrast, if a condition is deemed elective, it should be scheduled for after delivery, when the impact to the fetus is no longer a concern. This timing confers the added advantage of maternal physiology returning to normalcy. If a condition is deemed necessary but semielective, the second trimester is considered the safest time.[5] This recommendation stems from a multitude of available data. During the second trimester, after organ system differentiation has occurred, the risk for anesthetic-induced malformation or spontaneous abortion declines significantly.[28] Although the differential between first and second trimesters is genetically based, the preference for second versus third trimester is mechanically based. In the second trimester, the uterus size does not greatly crowd the abdominal operative domain. Moreover, the risk of preterm labor is lower during the second trimester.[4] Specific preoperative considerations include the following.

Fasting Guidelines/Aspiration Precautions

Based on guidelines presented by the American Society of Anesthesiologist Task Force on Obstetric Anesthesia in 2007, the fasting guidelines for pregnant patients mimic the guidelines set forth for standard adults. Recommendations suggest abstaining from solids for at least 6 hours before surgery and from clear liquids for at least 2 hours before surgery.[29] Although it is known that the incidence of gastroesophageal reflux is increased in pregnancy, no specific intervention has been shown to improve clinical outcomes with regard to aspiration prevention. However, most providers practice rapid sequence intubation to minimize the risk of aspiration.[30]

Thromboprophylaxis

As described earlier, the risk of thromboembolic events is markedly increased during pregnancy. The American College of Chest Physicians recommends mechanical and/or pharmacologic thromboprophylaxis for all pregnant patients undergoing an operation. Low-molecular-weight heparin is the recommended modality and is a safe drug choice during pregnancy. Early mobilization should be encouraged, and prophylaxis should be continued until the patient is mobilized postoperatively.[31]

Antibiotic Prophylaxis

The need for antibiotic prophylaxis during pregnancy depends on the specific operative procedure and is similar to the guidelines set forth for standard surgical patients. In generic terms, penicillins, cephalosporins, azithromycin, clindamycin, and erythromycin have good safety profiles. However, there are some classes of antibiotics to avoid. Aminoglycosides carry a risk of fetal and maternal ototoxicity and nephrotoxicity. Tetracyclines have been associated with suppression of bone growth and staining of developing teeth in fetuses. Fluoroquinolones are known to have toxic effects on developing cartilage. Given the possible toxicities described earlier, before antibiotic prescription, the specific safety profile must be explored and understood, and pharmacologic consultation obtained if needed.[28]

Preterm Labor Prophylaxis: Glucocorticoids and Tocolytics

Preterm labor risk in the perioperative period is notably increased. If preterm birth is anticipated or deemed a high risk, and the fetus is deemed potentially viable, prophylaxis with glucocorticoids should be considered. If preterm labor occurs, administration of glucocorticoids 24 to 48 hours before surgery markedly reduces perinatal morbidity and mortality. However, antenatal glucocorticoids may impair the maternal immune response to the underlying disorder. Consultation should be obtained from an obstetrics service to help project the risk of preterm birth. Prophylactic use of tocolytic agents has not proved to be beneficial.[32–36] From a physical standpoint, minimizing uterine manipulation may reduce the risk of uterine contraction and subsequent preterm labor.[37,38]

ANESTHESIA

Plausible risks of anesthesia to fetuses include direct teratogenic effects of medications and anesthetic agents, decreased uteroplacental blood flow secondary to changing maternal physiology, and preterm labor. Although this list is not complete, basic anesthetic considerations are discussed later.

Positioning

Secondary to possible hemodynamic consequences of vena cava compression from an enlarged uterus, it is recommended that pregnant patients be positioned with a 15% left lateral tilt when possible.[28,39,40]

Fetal Heart Rate Monitoring

Coordinating obstetricians and neonatologists can be helpful in determining the need and technique for fetal monitoring. The American College of Obstetricians and Gynecologists has stated that the decision to use intermittent or continuous intraoperative fetal monitoring should be based on the type of surgery, available resources, and gestational age. During the first and early second trimester, fetal heart tones are typically monitored before and after anesthesia exposure and operative intervention, but not during the case. During the late second and third trimester, secondary to the viability of the fetus, continuous intraoperative fetal monitoring via transabdominal ultrasonography is generally used. If the surgical field involves the abdomen, transvaginal ultrasonography can be used.[16] Despite this recommendation, multiple studies have shown that it is likely unnecessary to use continuous monitoring, because the risk of ill effect and/or the need for intervention is minimal.[28,41]

Type of Anesthetic

Decisions regarding the type of anesthetic to be used should involve consideration of the planned intervention, the projected risk of maternal physiologic changes, and the predicted teratogenesis. Despite this recommendation, no studies exist that show a significant difference in outcomes. Choices and considerations based on our physiologic understanding of the effects are listed here:

Monitored anesthesia care

Monitored anesthesia care (MAC) involves intermittent administration of analgesics and anxiolytics, combined with continuous monitoring of the patient. Much of the concern surrounding the use of MAC during pregnancy is derived from the possibility of induced hypoventilation with subsequent acidosis and decreased placental circulation. The risk of aspiration secondary to positioning and induced smooth muscle relaxation may also be increased.[42] However, because most operations completed during pregnancy are intra-abdominal, the use of MAC is generally not an option.

Regional anesthesia

Regional anesthesia via peripheral nerve and neuroaxial blocks is considered safe during pregnancy. Such blocks are particularly useful and encouraged during extremity operations. Moreover, neuroaxial blocks may be used for surgery of the lower abdomen, pelvis, and lower extremities. If neuroaxial blocks are used, the provider must be cautious of the potential for induced maternal hypotension from a sympathetic block. Systemic hypotension can lead to reduction in placental perfusion and subsequent fetal compromise.[42]

General anesthesia

As noted earlier, most operations performed during pregnancy involve laparoscopy or laparotomy, thus requiring general anesthesia. Anesthesia induction involves preoxygenation, medication administration (anesthesia/analgesia/paralytic), and intubation. Preoxygenation is vital in pregnant patients, because hypoxia can lead to compromised placental blood flow. Per the physiologic discussion earlier, pregnant patients have less reserve and can desaturate in less time than nonpregnant women.[43]

Once preoxygenation is complete, propofol is generally used as the induction agent of choice, although no induction agent has been shown to be teratogenic. Hemodynamic effects of induction must be anticipated and mitigated in order to maintain placental blood flow.[28]

For muscle relaxation, nondepolarizing neuromuscular blocking agents are thought to be safe, because they do not cross the placenta. Succinylcholine is the medication most often used, because it facilitates rapid sequence intubation (RSI).[28] Despite these general practices, no data have shown differences in outcomes secondary to RSI.[44]

Hemodynamic and Fluid Management

In pregnant and nonpregnant patients alike, the goal is to maintain perfusion and oxygenation of vital organs. During pregnancy, vital organs also include the uterus and placenta. Much of the effect of medications on the fetus is not a direct effect but is secondary to an effect on maternal physiology and subsequent uterine perfusion.[45,46] The effect is further compounded because uterine circulation is not autoregulated in the same manner as circulation to other vital organs. Thus, vasopressors may have little or no direct effect on uterine circulation. Physical maneuvers, such as fluid bolus, Trendelenburg position, compression stockings, and leg elevation, may have larger impacts on increasing uterine blood flow.[28]

Mechanical Ventilation

Both hyperventilation and hypoventilation can have detrimental effects, so clinicians must be vigilant with pregnant women under general anesthesia. As discussed earlier, pregnancy is associated with a chronic respiratory alkalosis secondary to increased alveolar ventilation. Higher levels of carbon dioxide in hypoventilation may lead to an increased gradient across the placenta and cause acidosis and myocardial depression of the fetus. In contrast, hyperventilation may lead to severe alkalosis and compromise of fetal blood flow and oxygenation.[47–50] Thus, mechanical ventilation during anesthesia should maintain the normal physiologic respiratory alkalosis when breathing spontaneously rather than attempt to correct it to usual normal parameters.

SURGICAL APPROACH

Once a diagnosis is confirmed and the decision to operate is made, the surgical approach is based on the disorder, surgical skill, and the availability of equipment and staff. When plausible, the benefits of laparoscopy in pregnancy seem to mimic the benefits seen in nonpregnant patients, including decreased postoperative pain and narcotic use, decreased rate of postoperative ileus, decreased length of hospital stay, and quicker return to work.[51–55]

Laparoscopy

Initial port placement

Given the concern for possible uterine or fetal injury, laparoscopic abdominal access in pregnant patients has been debated in the literature. Because the intra-abdominal domain is significantly altered during the second and third trimesters, access via a subcostal approach has been advocated. If the site of initial access is adjusted based on consideration of fundal height, the Hasson technique, Veress needle, and optical trocar all seem to provide safe entry options.[37,41,56–58] Surgeons should assess their own comfort levels with these approaches and proceed with the safest means possible.

Carbon dioxide insufflation

The concern regarding carbon dioxide insufflation in pregnant patients stems from the potential for respiratory compromise secondary to diaphragm displacement and the possibility of peritoneal absorption of carbon dioxide. A pressure of 15 mm Hg is typically used in nonpregnant patients and has been routinely used without increasing adverse maternal/fetal outcomes.[3,41,56] With regard to carbon dioxide exchange and possible fetal acidosis, no data exist showing detrimental effects to the fetus.[4] As noted earlier, clinicians should consider monitoring in the situation of a viable fetus, and this may provide some guidance with regard to intraoperative effects.

Open Approach

If an open approach is chosen, the type of incision depends on the surgical procedure and gestational age. A vertical incision is used for ease of incisional extension if needed to facilitate exposure.

POSTOPERATIVE PAIN MANAGEMENT

Pain control in the postoperative period is also important. Nonsteroidal antiinflammatory drugs should not be used in pregnancy because of the risk for premature closure of the ductus arteriosis.[28,59] Therefore, opioids, intravenous and oral, are the pain medications of choice. If intravenous opioids must be used, a patient-controlled analgesia pump may be the best initial option, given its low associated risk of maternal respiratory depression. As in all patients, intravenous pain medications should be converted to oral forms as soon as possible. It is recommended that patients be weaned off all narcotics as soon as possible to avoid fetal dependence. Babies born with opioid dependency can manifest decreased birth weight, respiratory depression, and extreme drowsiness, which can lead to feeding problems.[28] However, this consideration should not deter the surgeon from providing adequate perioperative pain control for pregnant women.

OUTCOMES/SUMMARY

The goals of treating pregnant patients in the perioperative setting are the same as with any patient: to provide safe preoperative, operative, and postoperative care. This task is complicated by the need to consider the well-being of both of the mother and the fetus. Moreover, the primary patient, the mother, has altered physiology. Surgeons must be aware of the physiologic and anatomic changes of pregnancy and recognize the surgical and anesthetic modifications necessary for safe care. Providers can be encouraged that surgical outcomes in pregnant patients have been shown to be similar to those of nonpregnant patients. A review article published in 2005 based on studies from 1966 to 2001 (the largest available) reveals that the overall rate of miscarriage in pregnant women exposed to surgical intervention in the first trimester is 10.5%, which is similar to the rate of miscarriage in the general obstetric population. Moreover, the overall rate of birth defects (approximately 2%) was not significantly increased compared with the general obstetric population. The aforementioned study also quantified the risk of delivery related to surgery (3.5%) and the risk of fetal loss (0.8%–2.5%).[60] It is also important to note, as validated in a study of 720,000 patients, that specific types of anesthesia or surgical procedures were not associated with different outcomes. The rates of stillbirths and congenital malformations were similar in pregnant women who underwent operations during pregnancy compared with pregnant women who did not. The only significant differences were increased rates of low birth weight infants and early neonatal death, with relative risks of 2.0 and 2.1 respectively. Even in these situations, it is difficult to determine whether these findings were secondary to the procedures or to the disorders.[2] In conclusion, surgical diseases arise in pregnant and nonpregnant patients alike. Delayed diagnosis and management, secondary to avoidance of fetal risk of diagnostic or therapeutic interventions, pose a greater risk to the mother and fetus than radiation, anesthesia, or operative intervention.

REFERENCES

1. Curtin SC, Abma JC, Ventura SJ, et al. Pregnancy rates for U.S. women continue to drop. NCHS Data Brief 2013;(136):1–8.
2. Mazze RI, Kallen B. Reproductive outcome after anesthesia and operation during pregnancy: a registry study of 5405 cases. Am J Obstet Gynecol 1989;161(5): 1178–85.
3. Soper NJ. SAGES' guidelines for diagnosis, treatment, and use of laparoscopy for surgical problems during pregnancy. Surg Endosc 2011;25(11):3477–8.
4. Fatum M, Rojansky N. Laparoscopic surgery during pregnancy. Obstet Gynecol Surv 2001;56(1):50–9.
5. ACOG Committee on Obstetric Practice. ACOG committee opinion no. 474: Non-obstetric surgery during pregnancy. Obstet Gynecol 2011;117(2 Pt 1):420–1.
6. Chesnutt AN. Physiology of normal pregnancy. Crit Care Clin 2004;20(4):609–15.
7. Gabbe SG, Niebyl JR, Galan HL, et al. Obstetrics: normal and problem pregnancies. Elsevier Health Sciences; 2012.
8. Cope Z, Silen W. Cope's early diagnosis of the acute abdomen. Oxford University Press; 1983.
9. Hee P, Viktrup L. The diagnosis of appendicitis during pregnancy and maternal and fetal outcome after appendectomy. Int J Gynaecol Obstet 1999;65(2):129–35.
10. Larsson A, Palm M, Hansson LO, et al. Reference values for clinical chemistry tests during normal pregnancy. BJOG 2008;115(7):874–81.
11. Cunningham F. Normal reference ranges for laboratory values in pregnancy. In: Post TW, editor. UpToDate; 2014 [cited August 1, 2014].
12. Hall EJ. Scientific view of low-level radiation risks. Radiographics 1991;11(3): 509–18.
13. Toppenberg KS, Hill DA, Miller DP. Safety of radiographic imaging during pregnancy. Am Fam Physician 1999;59(7):1813–8, 1820.
14. Karam PA. Determining and reporting fetal radiation exposure from diagnostic radiation. Health Phys 2000;79(5 Suppl):S85–90.
15. Barnett SB. Routine ultrasound scanning in first trimester: what are the risks? Semin Ultrasound CT MR 2002;23(5):387–91.
16. ACOG Committee on Obstetric Practice. ACOG committee opinion. Number 299, September 2004 (replaces no. 158, September 1995). Guidelines for diagnostic imaging during pregnancy. Obstet Gynecol 2004;104(3):647–51.
17. Lim HK, Bae SH, Seo GS. Diagnosis of acute appendicitis in pregnant women: value of sonography. AJR Am J Roentgenol 1992;159(3):539–42.
18. Israel GM, Malguria N, McCarthy S, et al. MRI vs. ultrasound for suspected appendicitis during pregnancy. J Magn Reson Imaging 2008;28(2):428–33.
19. Khandelwal A, Fasih N, Kielar A. Imaging of acute abdomen in pregnancy. Radiol Clin North Am 2013;51(6):1005–22.

20. Ames Castro M, Shipp TD, Castro EE, et al. The use of helical computed tomography in pregnancy for the diagnosis of acute appendicitis. Am J Obstet Gynecol 2001;184(5):954–7.
21. Rao PM, Rhea JT, Novelline RA, et al. Effect of computed tomography of the appendix on treatment of patients and use of hospital resources. N Engl J Med 1998;338(3):141–6.
22. Patel SJ, Reede DL, Katz DS, et al. Imaging the pregnant patient for nonobstetric conditions: algorithms and radiation dose considerations. Radiographics 2007; 27(6):1705–22.
23. De Wilde JP, Rivers AW, Price DL. A review of the current use of magnetic resonance imaging in pregnancy and safety implications for the fetus. Prog Biophys Mol Biol 2005;87(2–3):335–53.
24. Birchard KR, Brown MA, Hyslop WB, et al. MRI of acute abdominal and pelvic pain in pregnant patients. AJR Am J Roentgenol 2005;184(2):452–8.
25. Media, ACoRCoDaC. ACR manual on contrast media. Reston (VA): American College of Radiology; 2013.
26. Karthikesalingam A, Markar SR, Weerakkody R, et al. Radiation exposure during laparoscopic cholecystectomy with routine intraoperative cholangiography. Surg Endosc 2009;23(8):1845–8.
27. Jorgensen JE, Rubenstein JH, Goodsitt MM, et al. Radiation doses to ERCP patients are significantly lower with experienced endoscopists. Gastrointest Endosc 2010;72(1):58–65.
28. Sabiston DC, Townsend CM, Beauchamp RD, et al. Sabiston textbook of surgery: the biological basis of modern surgical practice. Elsevier Saunders; 2012.
29. American Society of Anesthesiologists Task Force on Obstetric Anesthesia. Practice guidelines for obstetric anesthesia: an updated report by the American Society of Anesthesiologists Task Force on Obstetric Anesthesia. Anesthesiology 2007;106(4):843–63.
30. Paranjothy S, Griffiths JD, Broughton HK, et al. Interventions at caesarean section for reducing the risk of aspiration pneumonitis. Cochrane Database Syst Rev 2010;(1):CD004943.
31. Guyatt GH, Akl EA, Crowther M, et al. Executive summary: Antithrombotic Therapy and Prevention of Thrombosis, 9th ed: American College of Chest Physicians Evidence-Based Clinical Practice Guidelines. Chest 2012;141(2 Suppl):7s–47s.
32. Roberts D, Dalziel S. Antenatal corticosteroids for accelerating fetal lung maturation for women at risk of preterm birth. Cochrane Database Syst Rev 2006;(3):CD004454.
33. Katz VL, Farmer RM. Controversies in tocolytic therapy. Clin Obstet Gynecol 1999;42(4):802–19.
34. Berkman ND, Thorp JM Jr, Lohr KN, et al. Tocolytic treatment for the management of preterm labor: a review of the evidence. Am J Obstet Gynecol 2003;188(6): 1648–59.
35. Tan TC, Devendra K, Tan LK, et al. Tocolytic treatment for the management of preterm labour: a systematic review. Singapore Med J 2006;47(5):361–6.
36. Romero R, Sibai BM, Sanchez-Ramos L, et al. An oxytocin receptor antagonist (atosiban) in the treatment of preterm labor: a randomized, double-blind, placebo-controlled trial with tocolytic rescue. Am J Obstet Gynecol 2000;182(5): 1173–83.
37. Soriano D, Yefet Y, Seidman DS, et al. Laparoscopy versus laparotomy in the management of adnexal masses during pregnancy. Fertil Steril 1999;71(5): 955–60.

38. Curet MJ. Special problems in laparoscopic surgery. Previous abdominal surgery, obesity, and pregnancy. Surg Clin North Am 2000;80(4):1093–110.
39. Clark SL, Cotton DB, Pivarnik JM, et al. Position change and central hemodynamic profile during normal third-trimester pregnancy and post partum. Am J Obstet Gynecol 1991;164(3):883–7.
40. Elkayam U, Gleicher N. Cardiac problems in pregnancy: diagnosis and management of maternal and fetal heart disease. Wiley; 1998.
41. Rollins MD, Chan KJ, Price RR. Laparoscopy for appendicitis and cholelithiasis during pregnancy: a new standard of care. Surg Endosc 2004;18(2):237–41.
42. Reitman E, Flood P. Anaesthetic considerations for non-obstetric surgery during pregnancy. Br J Anaesth 2011;107(Suppl 1):i72–8.
43. Baraka AS, Hanna MT, Jabbour SI, et al. Preoxygenation of pregnant and nonpregnant women in the head-up versus supine position. Anesth Analg 1992;75(5):757–9.
44. Neilipovitz DT, Crosby ET. No evidence for decreased incidence of aspiration after rapid sequence induction. Can J Anaesth 2007;54(9):748–64.
45. Alon E, Ball RH, Gillie MH, et al. Effects of propofol and thiopental on maternal and fetal cardiovascular and acid-base variables in the pregnant ewe. Anesthesiology 1993;78(3):562–76.
46. Okutomi T, Whittington RA, Stein DJ, et al. Comparison of the effects of sevoflurane and isoflurane anesthesia on the maternal-fetal unit in sheep. J Anesth 2009;23(3):392–8.
47. Haruta M, Funato T, Naka Y, et al. Effects of maternal hyperventilation and oxygen inhalation during labor on fetal blood-gas status. Nihon Sanka Fujinka Gakkai Zasshi 1988;40(9):1377–84 [in Japanese].
48. Muller G, Huber JC, Salzer H, et al. Maternal hyperventilation as a possible cause of fetal tachycardia sub partu. A clinical and experimental study. Gynecol Obstet Invest 1984;17(5):270–5.
49. Hohimer AR, Bissonnette JM, Metcalfe J, et al. Effect of exercise on uterine blood flow in the pregnant Pygmy goat. Am J Physiol 1984;246(2 Pt 2):H207–12.
50. Levinson G, Shnider SM, DeLorimier AA, et al. Effects of maternal hyperventilation on uterine blood flow and fetal oxygenation and acid-base status. Anesthesiology 1974;40(4):340–7.
51. Reedy MB, Galan HL, Richards WE, et al. Laparoscopy during pregnancy. A survey of laparoendoscopic surgeons. J Reprod Med 1997;42(1):33–8.
52. Al-Fozan H, Tulandi T. Safety and risks of laparoscopy in pregnancy. Curr Opin Obstet Gynecol 2002;14(4):375–9.
53. Shay DC, Bhavani-Shankar K, Datta S. Laparoscopic surgery during pregnancy. Anesthesiol Clin North America 2001;19(1):57–67.
54. Oelsner G, Stockheim D, Soriano D, et al. Pregnancy outcome after laparoscopy or laparotomy in pregnancy. J Am Assoc Gynecol Laparosc 2003;10(2):200–4.
55. Andreoli M, Servakov M, Meyers P, et al. Laparoscopic surgery during pregnancy. J Am Assoc Gynecol Laparosc 1999;6(2):229–33.
56. Affleck DG, Handrahan DL, Egger MJ, et al. The laparoscopic management of appendicitis and cholelithiasis during pregnancy. Am J Surg 1999;178(6):523–9.
57. Geisler JP, Rose SL, Mernitz CS, et al. Non-gynecologic laparoscopy in second and third trimester pregnancy: obstetric implications. JSLS 1998;2(3):235–8.
58. Lemaire BM, van Erp WF. Laparoscopic surgery during pregnancy. Surg Endosc 1997;11(1):15–8.

59. Schecter WP, Farmer D, Horn JK, et al. Special considerations in perioperative pain management: audiovisual distraction, geriatrics, pediatrics, and pregnancy. J Am Coll Surg 2005;201(4):612–8.
60. Cohen-Kerem R, Railton C, Oren D, et al. Pregnancy outcome following non-obstetric surgical intervention. Am J Surg 2005;190(3):467–73.

Advance Directives, Living Wills, and Futility in Perioperative Care

Matthew Goede, MD*, Matthew Wheeler, MD

KEYWORDS

- Advance directives • Living will • Durable power of attorney for health care • Futility
- Do not resuscitate • Perioperative

KEY POINTS

- Living wills and durable power of attorney for health care (DPOA-HC) have different implications for perioperative care.
- Patients can maintain do-not-resuscitate (DNR) orders while in an operating room (OR); however, these orders are fundamentally different from the standard DNR orders and require significant preoperative clarification.
- Futility has many different definitions, mostly because it is difficult to clearly define.
- There are several common cases where futility directly affects surgical care.

Advance directives have been considered essential to any hospital admission for more than 20 years. In the United States, the Patient Self-Determination Act of 1990 made it a requirement that all patients entering a health care institution have an inquiry into patients' advance directives and that information be provided about advance directives if patients have none. The major impetus behind this movement was the increased priority of patient autonomy in medical decision making and decrease in physician paternalism. It was realized that many medical decisions were being made when patients had been incapacitated by illness, and some means of honoring patients' wishes in those situations was required. Incapacitated patients have been subjected to interventions that they did not desire according to previously expressed wishes simply because they did not have written advance directives. In some US states, however, advance directives still only apply if patients are terminally ill; and terminally ill is narrowly defined as a person dying in a relatively short period of time regardless of life-supporting therapy. This strict legal definition can add confusion and complexity

Department of Surgery, College of Medicine, University of Nebraska, 983280 Nebraska Medical Center, Omaha, NE 68198-3280, USA
* Corresponding author.
E-mail address: mgoede@unmc.edu

Surg Clin N Am 95 (2015) 443–451
http://dx.doi.org/10.1016/j.suc.2014.10.005
0039-6109/15/$ – see front matter Published by Elsevier Inc.

and eliminates the application of advance directives from other situations in which an advance directive would be beneficial.

Initially, few patients had advance directives on admission and then, over the years, as awareness was increased about the necessity of such directives, patients made their advance directives known to their treatment team. Today, however, few patients have printed advance directives placed in the medical record, and discussions regarding a patient's advance directives take place with fewer than 25% of patients.[1,2] Frequently, in surgery, advance directives are implied. In the surgical literature, the concept of "patient buy-in" has been used to describe the implied advance directives that accompany informed consent.[3] After recording more than 50 informed consent discussions, Pencanac and colleagues[4] identified that although surgical risk and the possibility of a difficult recovery requiring invasive postoperative care are discussed, explicit discussion of advance directives is seldom performed. Instead, surgeons seem to rely on assuming that patients understand surgery is high risk and assent that they require difficult postoperative care after a major procedure. This may account for the perception that surgeons are overly aggressive in prolonging life in postoperative care, because a surgeon has had a discussion with a patient and told the patient what to expect intraoperatively and postoperatively, and the patient agreed to pursue the intervention. Some investigators who perform high-risk procedures have identified a greater need for written advance directives in these cases and emphasize the importance of these discussions taking place preoperatively.[2] Barnet and colleagues[5] looked at a series of patients who died within 1 year of their surgery. Only half had an advance directive at the time of their operation.

Studies have looked at surgeons' perspectives on advance directives' impact on end-of-life care. Schwarze and colleagues[6] found that 60% of surgeons who replied to a survey endorse sometimes or always refusing to operate on patients with preferences to limit life support. Interviews with surgeons and nonsurgical intensivists have revealed that advance directive discussions are the framework by which they make end-of-life decisions with patients and families. Written advance directives do not necessarily reflect the reality of what patients want in their end-of-life care.[7]

Even in circumstances in which it seems obvious that advance directives should be used, frequently they are not. Swetz and colleagues[8] looked at the use of advance directives in patients receiving left ventricular assist devices (LVADs). Only approximately 35% of LVAD patients had an advance directive prior to insertion of the LVAD, and only approximately 45% of LVAD patients ever created an advance directive. The advance directives that were present on the patients' charts addressed issues, such as tube feeding, cardiopulmonary resuscitation (CPR), mechanical ventilation, and hemodialysis. Most surprising, however, was that none of the advance directives in the study addressed the LVAD or conditions in which the LVAD should be withdrawn.

ADVANCE DIRECTIVES: LIVING WILLS AND DURABLE POWER OF ATTORNEY

Living wills are legal documents with the purpose of outlining a patient's goals of care and what type and to what extent the patient desires intervention. These documents are created when patients are in a state in which they can make decisions for the future if they would become incapacitated. These documents vary a great deal in content and range from a simple checkbox form that indicates which treatments are permissible to discussing decision making in elaborate hypothetical situations. Initially, living wills were a simple statement along the lines of, "if there is no possibility for recovery from physical or mental disability, I request no extraordinary or heroic means to prolong my life."[9] It was quickly realized that single statements like these are unmanageably vague, did not help define a patient's wishes, and were open to broad interpretations. The importance of living wills is in making a patient's wishes known, and, therefore, more thorough documents have been developed. Despite this, the major problem with living wills is that they are difficult to apply because a patient's generalized wishes have to be applied to specific circumstances by interpretation. A study by Mirarchi and colleagues[10] showed that trainees make significant errors in applying living wills.

DPOA-HC appoints a decision maker to act on behalf of a patient once the patient becomes unable to make decisions. DPOA-HC documents do not have to contain parameters or guidance to the appointed decision maker on what are acceptable treatment options. Frequently this is left to informal discussions that the DPOA-HC and the patient have had over time. Surrogate should act in the way they think patients would have proceeded, even if the DPOA-HC themselves disagree with that decision. It is infrequent, however, to find a surrogate who has that level of sophisticated thought process or even the formal explanation of the legal role of a DPOA-HC. A DPOA-HC supersedes other surrogate decision makers (eg, next of kin) and makes the named person the sole decision maker for the patient. Therefore, although it is always best to obtain broad consensus, in the end, the decision is left to the appointed DPOA-HC alone. It is possible to remove a surrogate if the physician believes that the DPOA-HC is not acting in the patient's interest; however, the legal bar for doing so is exceptionally high and it is usually more advantageous to try to resolve the conflict of opinion with the surrogate.

It is usually most helpful when living wills and DPOA-HC are both present so that a treatment paradigm and surrogate are both defined. Living wills are not binding documents, however, and, therefore, a DPOA-HC may choose not to honor the parameters laid out in a living will or cannot, due to the uniqueness of the situation that does not allow itself to a yes-or-no answer that can be predefined in a living will. In survey of the members of the Eastern Association for the Surgery of Trauma, only 55% of the health care providers thought that families follow patients' advance directives most or all of the time and 80% that family members are rarely or only sometimes in appropriate emotional states to make such choices.[11]

DO NOT RESUSCITATE

Discussion of a patient's wish to be resuscitated with advance cardiovascular life support (ACLS) in the event of cardiac arrest has become an essential part of any hospital admission and many advance directives. Research has long been present demonstrating dismal outcomes from CPR in patients in hospitals and skilled care facilities.[12] In the media, however, successful resuscitation from cardiac arrest is presented in an unrealistic way. Diem and colleagues[13] showed that the portrayed success rate after CPR was approximately 75% in popular television shows. This discrepancy between perception and reality has made the need to discuss DNR orders even more paramount.

DNR orders can be complex because the term, *do not resuscitate*, means different things to different patients and physicians. Frequently, DNR orders are broken down into subsequent components: do not intubate, no CPR, no cardioversion, and no antiarrhythmic medications. The fragmentation of DNR orders, however, is of no benefit because, even with the full ACLS complement, the outcomes are poor, and providing only a portion of ACLS likely provides for no physiologic benefit to patients and likely only supplies minimal psychological benefits for patients, families, and health care providers.

Another frequent issue is confusing DNR orders with comfort care orders or care limitation orders. DNR orders at most institutions apply to cardiopulmonary arrest. DNR orders do not limit the aggressiveness of the treatments prior to the point of cardiopulmonary arrest.[14] Care limitation orders are frequently formal extensions of a patient's living will. Care limitations are the orders that reflect the boundaries or exceptions that patients place on their care: for instance, a chronic obstructive pulmonary disease patient who does not want to be intubated or a patient who does not want dialysis or artificial nutrition. Comfort care orders specify a change in the course of treatment from a focus on cure to a focus on comfort, both physical and psychological.

These concepts are far more complicated in the circumstances of operative and perioperative care. The American College of Surgeons and American Society of Anesthesiologists have practice guidelines relating the suspension of DNR orders as a part of operative and anesthesia care.[1,15] Nurok and colleagues[16] found, however, that many anesthesiologists are unfamiliar with the content of these guidelines. To some, surgical procedures can reflect a suspension of DNR orders because patients have requested a significant intervention to reverse a condition and to prolong life. It should also be noted, however, that patient autonomy should not be limited solely because patients want to proceed with a surgical intervention. Cohen and Cohen[17] proposed the concept of "required reconsideration" when possible prior to surgery. This concept contains 5 tenets. First, does surgery achieve a beneficial objective? Is the surgery for palliation, or does it improve quality of life unrelated to patients' underlying condition for which they request a DNR status? Second, "resuscitation" needs to be clearly defined. Many things done by anesthesiologists occupy a gray zone that makes it essential to clarify with patients what resuscitation means in the OR. Intubation, mechanical ventilation, administering vasoactive and antiarrhythmic medications, and administering blood products are all necessary interventions to provide an adequate and safe anesthetic. Therefore, a DNR order that is applicable in the OR essentially would have to consist of no chest compressions and no cardioversion for fatal arrhythmias. Third, would resuscitation reverse the underlying cause for the arrest? Although the rate of cardiac arrest in the OR is less than 1%, when an arrest occurs because of anesthetic issues the success rate from resuscitation has been found in excess of 90% as opposed to nonanesthetic issues, when the rate is only 65%.[18] The success rate of in-the-OR resuscitations is drastically higher than other resuscitations, likely given the speed at which they are diagnosed by the anesthesia provider and the immediate access to the necessary interventions. Patients need to be aware of this advantage when considering if they want to continue their DNR order into the operative room. Fourth, is re-evaluation of the health care team's, but especially the surgeon's, views on the DNR order? One of the author's mentors used to emphatically reply, "I am not the patient's executioner," when asked if DNR orders be rescinded for the OR. Because the performance of a surgical procedure is an active process, many surgeons feel culpable if a patient does die during the procedure as opposed to when a patient dies on the ward, where the patient's death is perceived more as a result of an underlying disease process. This perceived personal failure is partly what leads some surgeons to insist on the removal of DNR orders prior to going to an OR. The other part of the equation is the surgeon's belief of "in for a penny, in for a pound." If patients consent to an invasive procedure, they also need to consent to the less-invasive procedure of CPR if they truly understand the risks of the operative process. Fifth, have all relevant parties clearly communicated what the final course of action will be? Frequently, DNR orders are created prior to a surgeon ever being involved in the care of the patient. It is essential that it discussed among the health care team what limitations are going to be placed and for what period of time, when the DNR will be rescinded, and when it will be restored. This needs to be clearly documented within a patient's medical record. It should be made easy to reference, because, by its very nature, the DNR status becomes relevant in a crisis situation. A simple DNR order or remove DNR status is not sufficient to explain the details involved in this complex decision. The decision on how long a DNR order is rescinded after a procedure frequently depends on frame of reference. Surgeons frequently think it should be rescinded for the entire hospital course[17]; anesthesiologists, for the time in OR, the postanesthesia recovery unit, and the day of surgery; and other health care providers, for only the time in the OR. Frequently patients' views vary significantly from physicians', and the distinctions that are clear to the providers are not as clear when presented to patients.

DEFINING FUTILITY

Attempts to define futility, on the surface, are as simple as, "you know it when you see it"; in practicality, however, futility is hard to define. Futility was first defined as a distinction between a treatment being effective and a treatment being beneficial.[19] Certain treatments, although effective at causing a measurable physiologic change, may not help patients achieve their goals of care, thereby remaining a futile treatment. Discussions of futility became commonplace in the medical literature with the evaluation of outcomes from attempts at resuscitation in long-term care facilities. These discussions have moved to the acute setting, with intensivists trying to define futility in patients who will not survive a costly and painful ICU course.

Brody and Halevy[20] attempted to better define futility and created 4 categories of futility. The first category is a treatment that would not cause the desired effect. This is frequently called physiologic futility. An example of this is a lung transplant to treat adult respiratory distress syndrome caused by sepsis. The proposed treatment is not an effective treatment of the condition. The second category is clinical futility or imminent demise futility. The absurdly simple example of imminent demise futility is performing CPR on a decapitated torso. No amount of CPR allows for a correction of the underlying problem. A more practical example is a trauma patient with an Injury Severity Score that predicts greater than 90% chance of mortality. The third category is lethal condition futility. An example of this is performing hemodialysis on an end-stage cancer patient. Although the dialysis corrects the patient's renal failure, it does not change the fact that the patient continues to have end-stage cancer, which will cause death. The fourth category is qualitative futility. This is when an intervention fails to restore adequate quality of life or restore a patient to functioning as a human who can interact with the environment. This is frequently seen in patients with severe brain injuries.

Resource or financial futility is increasingly suggested as a possible additional category of futility as the cost of end-of-life care continues to increase due to the addition of new, more costly therapies. It has been found that advance directives and utilization of futility policies have not resulted in a difference in the cost of end-of-life care between groups of patients in which these policies have been used and in those groups in which they have not been used.[21] Another study found similar results in the pediatric ICU population. Days on which patients met one of the futility criteria were no costlier than on other days when futility criteria were not met.[22]

Because it is difficult to clearly define futility, even using the previous parameters, a more nuanced definition of futility was developed. This definition stated that futility is an intractable disagreement between doctors and patients (or surrogates) about the appropriateness of providing marginally beneficial treatment. There are, therefore, 2 components to determining futility using this definition. First, the patient or surrogate has to determine the goals of therapy. Second, the doctor has to determine the probability of success.[23] Conflict, and thereby futility, arises when a patient's goals are deemed unreasonable by the treatment team or when a patient or surrogate disagrees with a physician's determination that a treatment has a low probability of success. If both parties are in agreement, the concept of futility is not applied. Therefore, futility is functionally an interpersonal disagreement and not an objective matter of fact. Because futility involves disagreement between parties, procedural processes have been proposed to help resolve the conflict.[24,25]

Pellegrino added a third dimension to the definition of futility.[26,27] In this definition, futility is defined as weighing the effectiveness, benefits, and burdens of a treatment. Effectiveness is determined by physicians by their evaluation of the medical literature. Benefit is subjective and determined by patients through the evaluation of how treatment helps patients achieve medical goals. Burdens are determined by both physician and patient and have to consider the cost of a treatment in physical, psychological, scarcity, and monetary aspects. Futility remains, however, a negotiation between physician and the patient (or surrogate).

Examples of Futility in Surgical Context

Fortunately, the incidence of futility seems to be low. In a study in the ICU setting, patients with imminent demise futility had a frequency of 0.3% of patient bed-days; lethal condition, futility 16.4% of bed-days; qualitative futility, 3.6% of bed-days; and no patients with physiologic futility.[28] In another ICU study, 80% of patients were judged to have never received futile care during their ICU admission; 9% probably received some futile care; and 11% were judged as receiving some futile care.[29] This study also attempted to show the accuracy of the determination of futile care by reporting an 85% 6-month mortality rate, with the remaining 15% of patients in severely compromised health in those patients deemed receiving futile care.[29]

There are a few surgical clinical circumstances where it is easier to identify poor prognosis and outcomes that are also substantiated by data. Using these conditions as examples, it can begin to be elucidated what futility looks like. Trauma and acute care surgery may provide the best examples of futility for several reasons: the disease entities are easily defined; the interventions are often extreme; and there are good clinical data for the outcomes of these interventions.

Severe Traumatic Brain Injury

The interventions for patients with selected presentations of severe traumatic brain injury (TBI) provide examples of futility. The management of severe TBI can be defined by Glasgow Coma Scale (GCS) and imaging findings. Patients who have fixed and dilated pupils with a GCS score of less than 7 have been shown to have no meaningful long-term neurologic function. Honeybul and colleagues[30] define futility in neurosurgery as a greater than 90% chance of an unacceptably poor outcome. A pitfall to using severe TBI as a model of futility is the societal benefit of organ recovery. Many patients with severe TBI may be candidates for organ donation, and these decisions not to treat are further complicated by the need for donated organs.

Interventions for penetrating severe TBI, particularly from gunshot wounds, demonstrate qualitative futility. Patients presenting with a GCS score of 3, 4, or 5 have been demonstrated to have very poor outcomes in a pooled analysis: more than 90% persisting in a vegetative state after intervention, more than 95% having a disability requiring institutionalization, and a small percentage having a good outcome.

The DECRA (Decompressive Craniectomy) trial demonstrates physiologic futility in regard to the intervention of nonpenetrating severe TBI.[31] It has provided level 1 data in which the study randomized 155 patients to groups who would receive either standardized medical management with early craniectomy at 72 hours or medical management alone. The intervention succeeded in decreasing intracranial pressures, but outcomes did not differ or favored foregoing surgical intervention. There was no difference in mortality between the 2 groups whereas there was a significant difference with an improved functional status in the group who received only medical interventions.

Pulseless Trauma Patient

In both blunt and penetrating trauma patients, if a patient arrests in the trauma bay, an emergency department thoracotomy (EDT) is indicated if there are the resources to perform the procedure. The decision to perform EDT is well defined by data and part of the decision on who receives EDT is an example of imminent demise futility. The survival for blunt trauma patients who receive ED thoracotomy is almost universally reported as less than 2%, with a large meta-analysis reporting 1.4%. Survival after thoracotomy for penetrating injury has been reported from 4% to 38%, with meta-analysis reporting 8.8%. Some traumatologists have advocated broadening the criteria for EDT. The American College of Surgeons published a retrospective series that showed no neurologically intact survivors among extended criteria EDT for penetrating trauma compared with 8.5% surviving in the group who received standard criteria EDT.[32] Although the effectiveness and societal burdens of EDT are definable, due to the nature of EDT patients, there is almost never a discussion between surgeon and patient about the patient's goals of treatment.

Mesenteric Ischemia and Massive Enterectomy

Unlike the previous 2 examples, mesenteric ischemia cases are seen infrequently and there are no guidelines or extensive literature to guide management. There are no level 1 data for patients with this disease process and the authors rely on case series to determine the outcome and in turn futility. Mortality in adults who present requiring total or near-total enterectomy has even been defined in large series by the judgment of the surgeon not to attempt resection of necrotic bowel.[33] With a substantial intestinal remnant, the survival is higher, drawing an important distinction between elderly patients with a significant remnant of 120 cm having a much higher survival.[34] Some practitioners believe that intestinal transplant is changing the treatment of these diseases, but in individuals with significant comorbidities, there is no practical application. Mesenteric ischemia, therefore, frequently goes back to the "you know it when you see it" definition of futility, combining aspects of physiologic, qualitative, and imminent death and lethal condition futility. In those patients with presumed mesenteric ischemia, it is important to discuss with the patients, if possible with their surrogate present, what the postoperative goals are of the patients prior to going to surgery, because interoperative decisions may have to be made based on those patient-defined benefits and burdens.

SUMMARY

Although obtaining an informed consent is a commonly taught and role-modeled portion of surgical education, preoperative discussions regarding patients' advance directives frequently are not. This may be partly because surgeons want to portray confidence in front of patients and are concerned that discussions about what patients want if things do not go well undermine that confidence. If done in the context of a well-established doctor-patient relationship, however, patients should be reassured that their surgeons are looking out for their entire well-being. Although preoperative advance directive discussions can be difficult, and at times uncomfortable, it is much more difficult to deal with surrogates and vague prewritten advance directives in a crisis situation that requires a decision in a matter of seconds.

REFERENCES

1. American College of Surgeons. Statement on advance directives by patients: "do not resuscitate" in the operating room. Bull Am Coll Surg 2014;99(1):42–3.
2. Yang AD, Bentrem DJ, Pappas SG, et al. Advance directive use among patients undergoing high-risk operations. Am J Surg 2004;188(1):98–101.
3. Schwarze ML, Bradley CT, Brasel KJ. Surgical "buy-in": the contractual relationship between surgeons and patients that influences decisions regarding life-supporting therapy. Crit Care Med 2010;38(3):843–8.
4. Pecanac KE, Kehler JM, Brasel KJ, et al. It's big surgery: preoperative expressions of risk, responsibility, and commitment to treatment after high-risk operations. Ann Surg 2014;259(3):458–63.
5. Barnet CS, Arriaga AF, Hepner DL, et al. Surgery at the end of life: a pilot study comparing decedents and survivors at a tertiary care center. Anesthesiology 2013;119(4):796–801.
6. Schwarze ML, Redmann AJ, Alexander GC, et al. Surgeons expect patients to buy-in to postoperative life support preoperatively: results of a national survey. Crit Care Med 2013;41(1):1–8.
7. Bradley CT, Brasel KJ, Schwarze ML. Physician attitudes regarding advance directives for high-risk surgical patients: a qualitative analysis. Surgery 2010; 148(2):209–16.
8. Swetz KM, Mueller PS, Ottenberg AL, et al. The use of advance directives among patients with left ventricular assist devices. Hosp Pract (1995) 2011;39(1):78–84.
9. United States Catholic Conference. Advance directives: a guide to help you express your health care wishes. Washington, DC: U.S. Catholic Conference, n.d. 2007.
10. Mirarchi FL, Costello E, Puller J, et al. TRIAD III: nationwide assessment of living wills and do not resuscitate orders. J Emerg Med 2012;42(5):511–20. http://dx.doi.org/10.1016/j.jemermed.2011.07.015.
11. Martin ND, Stefanelli A, Methvin L, et al. Contrasting patient, family, provider, and societal goals at the end of life complicate decision making and induce variability of care after trauma. J Trauma Acute Care Surg 2014;77(2):262–7.
12. Tomlinson T, Brody H. Futility and the ethics of resuscitation. JAMA 1990;264(10): 1276–80.
13. Diem SJ, Lantos JD, Tulsky JA. Cardiopulmonary resuscitation on television. Miracles and misinformation. N Engl J Med 1996;334(24):1578–82.
14. President's Commission for the Study of Ethical Problems in Medicine and Biomedical and Behavioral Research. Deciding to forego life-sustaining treatment: a report on the ethical, medical, and legal issues in treatment decisions. Washington, DC: Government Printing Office; 1983.

15. Ethical guidelines for the anesthesia care of patients with do-not-resuscitate orders or other directives that limit treatment. Park Ridge (IL): American Society of Anesthesiologists; 2008. p. 1–2. Available at: https://www.asahq.org/.../Standards%20Guidelines%20Stmts/Ethical%20.
16. Nurok M, Green DS, Chisholm MF, et al. Anesthesiologists' familiarity with the ASA and ACS guidelines on Advance Directives in the perioperative setting. J Clin Anesth 2014;26(3):174–6.
17. Cohen CB, Cohen PJ. Do-not-resuscitate orders in the operating room. N Engl J Med 1991;325(26):1879–82.
18. Olsson GL, Hallén B. Cardiac arrest during anaesthesia: a computer-aided study in 250,543 anaesthetics. Acta Anaesthesiol Scand 1988;32:653–64.
19. Schneiderman LJ, Jecker NS, Jonsen AR. Medical futility: its meaning and ethical implications. Ann Intern Med 1990;112(12):949–54.
20. Brody BA, Halevy A. Is futility a futile concept? J Med Philos 1995;20(2):123–44.
21. Emanuel EJ, Emanuel LL. The economics of dying. The illusion of cost savings at the end of life. N Engl J Med 1994;330(8):540–4.
22. Sachdeva RC, Jefferson LS, Coss-Bu J, et al. Resource consumption and the extent of futile care among patients in a pediatric intensive care unit setting. J Pediatr 1996;128(6):742–7.
23. Lantos JD, Singer PA, Walker RM, et al. The illusion of futility in clinical practice. Am J Med 1989;87(1):81–4.
24. Medical futility in end-of-life care: report of the Council on Ethical and Judicial Affairs. JAMA 1999;281(10):937–41.
25. Texas Advance Directives Act. Texas Health and Safety Code. Chapter 166, Sections 166.ool-166.166. Vernon.
26. Pellegrino E. Futility in medical decisions: the word and the concept. HEC forum 2005;17:308–18.
27. Grant SB, Modi PK, Singer EA. Futility and the care of surgical patients: ethical dilemmas. World J Surg 2014;38(7):1631–7.
28. Halevy A, Neal RC, Brody BA. The low frequency of futility in an adult intensive care unit setting. Arch Intern Med 1996;156(1):100–4.
29. Huynh TN, Kleerup EC, Wiley JF, et al. The frequency and cost of treatment perceived to be futile in critical care. JAMA Intern Med 2013;173(20):1887–94.
30. Honeybul S, Gillett GR, Ho K. Futility in neurosurgery: a patient-centered approach. Neurosurgery 2013;73(6):917–22.
31. Cooper DJ, Rosenfeld JV, Murray L, et al, DECRA Trial Investigators, Australian and New Zealand Intensive Care Society Clinical Trials Group. Decompressive craniectomy in diffuse traumatic brain injury. N Engl J Med 2011;364(16):1493–502.
32. Working Group, Ad Hoc Subcommittee on Outcomes, American College of Surgeons, Committee on Trauma. Practice management guidelines for emergency department thoracotomy. Working Group, Ad Hoc Subcommittee on Outcomes, American College of Surgeons-Committee on Trauma. J Am Coll Surg 2001;193(3):303–9.
33. Sitges-Serra A, Mas X, Roqueta F, et al. Mesenteric infarction: an analysis of 83 patients with prognostic studies in 44 cases undergoing a massive small-bowel resection. Br J Surg 1988;75(6):544–8.
34. Thompson JS. Short bowel syndrome in the elderly. Nutr Clin Pract 2002;17(2):110–2.

Index

Note: Page numbers of article titles are in **boldface** type.

Surg Clin N Am 95 (2015) 453–466
http://dx.doi.org/10.1016/S0039-6109(15)00028-6 surgical.theclinics.com

K

L

M

R

Printed and bound by CPI Group (UK) Ltd, Croydon, CR0 4YY
03/10/2024
01040490-0009